EXAMINATION REVIEW
FOR RADIOGRAPHY

EXAMINATION REVIEW FOR RADIOGRAPHY

Shelley L. Giordano, DHSc, RT (R)(MR)(ARRT)
Chair, Diagnostic Imaging Department
Quinnipiac University
Hamden, CT

Wolters Kluwer | Lippincott Williams & Wilkins
Health

Philadelphia · Baltimore · New York · London
Buenos Aires · Hong Kong · Sydney · Tokyo

Senior Editor: Michael Noble
Product Manager: John Larkin
Marketing Manager: Shauna Kelley
Senior Designer: Stephen Druding
Compositor: Absolute Service, Inc.

First Edition
Copyright © 2014 Lippincott Williams & Wilkins, a Wolters Kluwer business

351 West Camden Street
Baltimore, MD 21201

Two Commerce Square
2001 Market Street
Philadelphia, PA 19103

Printed in China

9 8 7 6 5 4 3 2 1

Library of Congress Cataloging-in-Publication Data

Giordano, Shelley, author.
  Examination review for radiography / Shelley Giordano. — First edition.
    p. ; cm.
  Includes bibliographical references.
  ISBN 978-1-4511-1871-1
  I. Title.
  [DNLM: 1. Radiography—Examination Questions. 2. Technology, Radiologic—Examination Questions. WN 18.2]
  RC78.15
  616.07'572076—dc23

                                                                                    2013020793

DISCLAIMER

To purchase additional copies of this book, call our customer service department at **(800) 638-3030** or fax orders to **(301) 223-2320**. International customers should call **(301) 223-2300**.

Visit Lippincott Williams & Wilkins on the Internet: http://www.lww.com. Lippincott Williams & Wilkins customer service representatives are available from 8:30 am to 6:00 pm, EST.

DEDICATION

To Poppy Louie,

A grandfather fills our lives with joy and hearts with love.
Love and miss you!

PREFACE

USE OF THIS REVIEW TEXTBOOK

This review textbook is meant to be used in conjunction with other educational materials in preparation for the American Registry of Radiologic Technologists (ARRT) certification examination in radiography. Students who have completed or are near completion of a formal radiography program would benefit from this text. This textbook is not meant to be used as a primary resource in an educational program. The content of this book follows the content specifications outlined by the ARRT. The text is divided into 6 chapters; the first is the Introduction, which provides information on the examination and study habits and outlines the content specifications for the examination. Chapters 2 to 6 correlate to the content specifications and include the following: Radiation Protection, Equipment Operation and Quality Control, Image Acquisition and Evaluation, Imaging Procedures, and Patient Care and Education. The chapters are structured as both bulleted lists and short paragraphs to allow for quick review and reference of material.

The ARRT examination is a multiple-choice examination; consequently, at the end of each chapter, there are at least 15 multiple-choice questions to review the specific chapter content. A comprehensive 220-question examination covering all content specification categories is included at the end of the textbook. Answers to all questions are included at the end of the book with an explanation. In addition, the text offers access to online mock registry Examinations in Radiography. The online examinations are populated from a large test bank of questions and randomly select 220 questions for each attempt. The online examinations may be taken on a timed basis (3.5 hours) as preparation for the actual examination.

INSTRUCTOR RESOURCES

Approved adopting instructors will be given access to the following additional resources:
- **PowerPoint slides**—The PowerPoint slides are designed to assist instructors in presenting lecture material.
- **Image bank**

STUDENT RESOURCES

- **Online Exam Simulator**—The Exam Simulator provides students with the opportunity to experience what the actual AART exam will be like. Questions are based on the AART specifications and percentages. There are approximately 2,600 questions available, with 220 questions per exam.

ACKNOWLEDGMENTS

I would like to acknowledge Wolters Kluwer Health for their support of this project, specifically John Larkin for his patience, encouragement, and continual support. I would also like to thank the faculty in the Department of Diagnostic Imaging at Quinnipiac University who contributed to this review textbook despite all their commitments: Tania Blyth, Alicia Giaimo, Bernadette Mele, and Natalie Pelletier. I would also like to thank Bernard Grindel from Quinnipiac University for his assistance with the Introduction chapter and Robert Lombardo for his assistance with digital imaging.

A very special recognition goes out to my family for their support in all my professional projects, their tireless ears listening to me, and their encouragement to keep moving forward no matter the circumstances. Without each of you I would not be where I am today; thank you to my wonderful husband Pasquale, my children Julianne and Jake, and my parents Louis and Audrey Mascola—this book truly took a village to create!

REVIEWERS

CAROLYN CIANCIOSA
Empire State College
Cheektowaga, NY

KENDALL DELACERDA
Northwestern State University
Alexandria, LA

MARLENE JOHNSON
University of Utah
Salt Lake City, UT

TRICIA LEGGETT
Zane State College
Zanesville, OH

LEANNA NEUBRANDER
Adventist University of Health Sciences
Orlando, FL

GLEB SCOSYREV
Concorde Career College
Memphis, TN

CONTENTS

CHAPTER 1

Introduction

INTRODUCTION

Congratulations on completing a radiography program and starting the preparation process for the American Registry of Radiologic Technologists (ARRT) comprehensive certification examination in radiography. This review textbook is designed to work in cooperation with your formal education program to prepare you for the examination. This review textbook is not meant to function as a primary textbook but as an accompaniment to the material learned during your radiography education. As you prepare for the examination, use this review textbook, textbooks used during your formal program, and all notes taken during course work to develop a well-rounded study program. Remember, no one book can completely prepare you for the exam; this review textbook is meant to provide you with just that: a review of key terms, concepts, and ideas to support your study efforts.

This review book is divided into six chapters including this introduction. Chapters 2 to 6 focus exclusively on the content areas outlined by the ARRT. The content specifications used to develop this review book are based on the *Radiography Didactic and Clinical Competency Requirements* and the *Content Specifications for the Examination in Radiography* effective for January 2012 by the ARRT.[1] Chapters 2 to 6 are divided with the same heading titles as those listed on the content specifications provided by the ARRT. The ARRT provides all applicants a summary of the components of each content area and is extremely useful when preparing a study guide for the comprehensive examination.

Radiography Examination Specifics

The ARRT examination in radiography is a 220-question multiple-choice examination. Of the 220 questions, 20 are pilot questions that are not scored; however, these pilot questions are not identified to the examinee. Students taking the ARRT radiography examination are given 3.5 hours to complete the 220 questions. Examinees are provided a 20-minute tutorial prior to beginning the exam and a 10-minute survey at the conclusion of the exam, resulting in a total administration time of 4 hours. The test is administered by computer; the ARRT provides comprehensive information on its website regarding the computer-based test process. It is

strongly suggested you review the information available on the ARRT website regarding the examination well in advance of your test date. The best preparation for such an examination is not only to study material but also to be familiar with the test process, so go to www.ARRT.org and search; you will be amazed by the support you will find!

The 200 questions of the examination (not counting the 20 pilot questions) are divided between five content areas. The division is not equal, meaning not each content area has an equal number of questions asked. Table 1-1 below provides a breakdown of the number of questions for each content area and the percentage of the test these questions equal.

It is important for the student not to base studying strategies on the number of questions per content area. The student needs to approach the examination and each content area with equal attention and effort. Often, students will focus a greater amount of attention on the higher-percentage content areas such as Radiation Protection or Imaging Procedures and extremely limited time on the areas of Equipment Operation and Quality Control or Patient Care and Education; this is a mistake that can result in a nonpassing grade on the examination. Remember, the percentages and numbers of questions listed in Table 1-1 are not based on the importance of the content but rather the amount of specific information in each content area. All content is im-

T A B L E	**1-1**	ARRT Examination in Radiography: Content Breakdown	
Content Area		Number of Questions	Percentage of the Examination
Radiation Protection		45	22.5%
Equipment Operation and Quality Control		22	11%
Image Acquisition and Evaluation		45	22.5%
Imaging Procedures		58	29%
Patient Care and Education		30	15%

SOURCE: American Registry of Radiologic Technologists (2010).*Radiography didactic and clinical competency requirements and the content specifications for the examination in radiography.* http://www.arrt.org/pdfs/Disciplines/Content-Specification/RAD-content-specification.pdf. Accessed May 14, 2013.

portant and thus each question, regardless of content area, is weighed the same. So remember: You are studying for a comprehensive examination and each area is equally important.

The ARRT content specifications are listed on the ARRT website and also in the front of the application packet. The content specifications include guidelines on the material that will be tested. These guidelines are just that—a guide—and should be used as such; they are not meant to be the primary source of information for curriculum development nor do they provide you with specific information that will be presented on the examination. The content specifications, however, are beneficial when mapping your study strategy. The following is the URL for the content specifications on the ARRT website: www.arrt.org/pdfs/Disciplines/Content-Specification/RAD-Content-Specification.pdf. In addition, the content specifications are included in the application packet that every student receives.

Application Process

Each student who would like to be considered for the ARRT certification examination in radiography must complete an application process. The application process is the responsibility of the student to complete and is not submitted by the program. The ARRT outlines in the application handbook the specific requirements for the application. It is important that the student read the directions extremely carefully; the applicant needs to use his or her legal name (i.e., if legal name is William, it must be submitted as such, not as Bill) and the name on the application must match the photo identification (ID) presented at the time of the examination. Any variation from this procedure will result in ineligibility to take the examination and forfeiting of the application

fee. In addition, applicants must attach a photo that is no older than 6 months to the application form. All photos must be of high quality. Photos may be black and white or in color but must not include any hats, visors, sunglasses, or other attire that alters a person's appearance. The ARRT has final determination if a photo is acceptable. A passport-quality photo is required and must be taped to the application.

An application for the radiography examination can be submitted not earlier than 3 months before the graduation date stated on the form. Once an application is received and processed, the applicant will receive a Candidate Status Report (CSR). This may take 4 weeks or longer depending on date of receipt of the application or other extenuating circumstances (Ethics Review required). Scheduling of your examination date is outlined on the CSR. You will have 90 days from the Wednesday after the application is processed to book a test date. The ARRT provides an example in the application handbook to clearly define this window. In addition, the handbook outlines procedures for cancelling an examination date, failing to book an examination date within the required 90-day window, Americans with Disabilities Act (ADA) accommodation requests, name and address changes, and requests to change the examination window.

All ARRT certification examinations are administered by an outside company. The ARRT handbook provides detailed information on scheduling an examination appointment. You are encouraged to read the information carefully regarding scheduling an appointment and be prepared to provide all necessary information to the test center when scheduling. Your failure to provide accurate information may result in the test center refusing to let you take the examination.

Day of the Examination

On the day of the examination, you are required to bring two forms of ID to the test center. The ARRT defines these two forms of ID as primary and secondary. Primary ID includes the following: government-issued driver's license, state ID card, or passport. The secondary ID may be one from the primary list or any of the following: government-issued ID (e.g., Social Security card), employee ID or work badge, school ID, ATM card, or credit card. Any ID provided MUST have your complete name and signature.

Besides the ID above, do not bring any paper, notes, pens, pencils, books, or calculators. The test center will provide you with an erasable board and pen. The computer has a built-in basic and scientific calculator for use during the examination. Upon request, the test center will provide a handheld basic calculator. If at any time during the examination you require assistance, raise your hand and wait for a test center employee to come to you. Do not leave your computer to seek assistance.

Examination Results

At the conclusion of the computer-based examination, you will see a preliminary score. This is NOT your final score but a preliminary result of the answers provided. The preliminary score is also not a notification of ARRT certification in the modality. Once the examinee's score and documentation are reviewed, a final score report will be mailed to the examinee's address on file with the ARRT. You may also check the ARRT website to verify your credentials. Passing of the ARRT certification examination in radiography requires a scaled score of 75 or higher. A scaled score takes into consideration the difficulty of specific tests in comparison to other incidences of test administration. The ARRT provides a thorough explanation of scoring on its website.

EXAMINATION PREPARATION

The Pleasures of High-Stakes Testing

You probably never intended for your education to be condensed into one 3.5-hour-long experience, but that's the state of affairs in health care education today. You will take the radiography certification exam to verify the knowledge and abilities it took years to build. X hours to ratify Y credits of classes, Z hours of lab work, and countless hours and days of reading, studying, and learning. It hardly seems fair. But there is good reason for the multiple-choice certification exam—it's the only feasible way that everyone can be evaluated using the same measure. In that way, it's the fairest means available to safeguard the integrity of the diagnostic imaging profession. Certification (i.e., passing the exam) serves as a public acknowledgment of your achievements and paves the way for a rewarding professional future.

Apart from the obvious advantages of certification, passing the certification exam brings other positive outcomes. First, this is an opportunity to review all the material you've learned in the past 2 years and put it together into a coherent body of knowledge. All the work you did for individual evaluations (midterms, quizzes, lab practicals, and final exams) can finally be assembled into one unit. The outcome of the exam should be a feeling of mastery over all that you've been learning and an assurance that you understand the "big picture" that professors and clinical practitioners talk about. Second, and less obviously, the certification exam allows you to revisit topics that eluded you the first time you encountered them. In many instances, students reviewing material that they "failed" to learn earlier find that subsequent experiences give them the perspective to understand the previously daunting topics. Investigating these topics will also give you the opportunity for a third outcome: review of your favorite topics. Some students tend to focus exclusively on troublesome material to the exclusion of topics that seemed to come easy or were intrinsically interesting. This is a mistake—in a comprehensive review of this nature, you should be prepared both to revisit past trouble spots and to remind yourself of past successes. In other words, the goal of reviewing for a comprehensive exam like the ARRT radiography certification examination is to build on your overall sense of the field, to create the big picture understanding that's required for licensure, and to do so by building on past strengths and filling in gaps in your knowledge.

Some Thoughts on the Struggle between Life and Test

If you're like most people, you're a little bit obsessed with taking and passing your certification exam, and with good reason. But ask yourself this: Is being a certified radiologic technologist the be-all and end-all of your life? Or is there more to you than just a professional certification? Hopefully your answers are "no" and "yes," respectively. A little bit of anxiety and self-doubt are probably good since they help motivate and focus a test-taker, but too much can be debilitating. Given that anxiety (targeted on a specific object) is related to stress (a general measure of tension in one's life), it makes sense to find balance in the preparation for the exam so that the day of the test itself does not turn into a made-to-order anxiety attack situation. In fact, addressing the common sources of stress can be just as important to passing the exam as reviewing course work.

The academic success you've experienced to this point has probably been due, at least in part, to the beneficial habit of scheduling. Preparation for the certification exam will require even more efficient use of time, so prepare for more scheduling. To help with this task, there are two aspects of time use that deserve particular attention: prioritization and task management. Working hand in hand, these two modes of decision making will provide you with more opportunities to pursue the activities that will lead to personal and professional satisfaction. In fact, so important are these issues that long after technology changes and many of the things you've learned to do as a radiologist have changed, you will still practice the important behaviors of prioritization and task management. But what do these terms mean? And does one employ both skills simultaneously?

If you've ever procrastinated or been caught short of time to study for a test or to complete an assignment, you've most likely committed an error in prioritization. It should be simple to prioritize activities, so why does it seem that so many of us so often do things that aren't in our best interests or don't serve our long-term goals? Prioritization means putting the most important activities first so that they are sure to be completed, and putting less important things last so that there's little loss if they are not even attempted. The diagram in Figure 1-1 below helps explain how prioritization mistakes happen.

Any activity or task can be categorized into one of the four boxes in this grid. High-importance activities are those that help you achieve long-term goals or maintain core values. Low-importance activities do not achieve those ends. High-urgency activities are those that happen in the current moment, whereas low-urgency activities are more under your control (i.e., they can be delayed with little effort). Most people have no problem identifying high-importance/high-urgency needs. How many of us would forget to study for an important exam the night before or neglect to pick up toilet paper if there's an urgent need at home? When the need is pressing and the task must be done soon, it's pretty clear how time should be spent.

Similarly, many of us make a common mistake when it comes to high-urgency and low-importance tasks. When there's not an obvious deadline to meet, we can be found pursuing high-urgency/low-importance activities. Walk around a college campus and count the number of people on Facebook, playing video games, or chatting on their phones. Are they engaged in highly important activities? Maybe, but probably not. In their homes, many others can be found watching TV or surfing the web—again, probably not highly important tasks. So why do we do it? In short, because we have short time horizons. The game is on TV now even though we don't care about either team, the sale ends soon so we have to shop now even though we have no money to spend, updates appear by the dozens even though these aren't really our friends. We tend to answer the call when it comes rather than thinking critically about our priorities.

So, how do we combat this tendency? Ask simple questions: Will the next hour of (fill in the blank) allow me to pursue my personal or career goals? Will it help me maintain my sense of self? If the answer is no, then start asking whether there are highly important activities that lie in the future; if so, what can you do now? If you've been following along to this point, you're probably thinking that your licensure exam is clearly the highly important but not quite urgent thing that you should attend to. And that's the point of this exercise, to remind you that the high-importance tasks are the ones that you are committed to, the ones that should give you the best return on your investment of time. Remind yourself of the prioritization grid and you'll find that you make better time-use choices on a more consistent basis.

But what if prioritization isn't your problem? What if your challenge is simply finding the time to do those tasks that you know you need to accomplish? Figure 1-2 is another visual guide that can help you maintain sanity and do the studying that you know you need.

In this chart, you can plot all your time used over the course of a week. The best practice is to use a weekend day to look back over the week and assess

	HIGH IMPORTANCE	LOW IMPORTANCE
HIGH URGENCY		
LOW URGENCY		

FIGURE 1-1

	Monday	Tuesday	Wednesday	Thursday	Friday	Saturday	Sunday	Key code
								ACTIVITY
6:00 AM								Required
6:30 AM								Scheduled
7:00 AM								Discretionary
7:30 AM								
8:00 AM								
8:30 AM								
9:00 AM								
9:30 AM								
10:00 AM								
10:30 AM								
11:00 AM								
11:30 AM								
12:00 PM								
12:30 PM								
1:00 PM								
1:30 PM								
2:00 PM								
2:30 PM								
3:00 PM								
3:30 PM								
4:00 PM								
4:30 PM								
5:00 PM								
5:30 PM								
6:00 PM								

FIGURE 1-2

your time use. The activity code in the upper right-hand corner names the three types of time use that you can assign to any given task. Simply write your tasks into each hour or half-hour block of time and designate the task required, scheduled, or discretionary. Required tasks are those that must be done but over which you exercise some control of when to do them (e.g., sleeping or eating). Scheduled tasks are those that are done at a planned time (e.g., work, class, or bowling league). Discretionary activities are those that you don't have to do or can put off indefinitely, and over which you have complete control of when to do them (e.g., Facebook, watching TV, spontaneous bowling games). There is a high degree of subjectivity in assigning tasks to a category. One person's "required" is another's "discretionary," but in the end the results are the same. Wherever you find discretionary tasks that should be planned, there you have the opportunity to increase the effectiveness of your time use.

At this juncture, an important term needs to be introduced: chunking. A chunk of time is 15, 20, or maybe 30 minutes. In fact, you can define your own chunk of time just so long as it's not more than 30 or 45 minutes, the time that you can sit down and pay exclusive attention to one task. Any long task, like reviewing an entire textbook or answering hundreds of practice questions, can be chunked into a number of smaller tasks. Having a realistic appraisal of how much you can accomplish in a chunk of time is vital. If you tell yourself that you can read 30 textbook pages (and remember the material!) in 30 minutes when it really takes you 90 minutes, then you will not do well with chunking. But if you realize that in 30 minutes you can carefully read 10 textbook pages, then you can start planning accurately. Determine how many chunks of time it will take to complete a task, then distribute those chunks across the days and hours that you have available to you. Do the same with all your other important tasks and you have the beginnings of a schedule. In other words, rather than treating your study tasks as discretionary, you now are able to consider planning for them.

Using the prioritization grid, the 24/7 time use assessment tables, and chunking, you should be able to overcome procrastination, poor prioritization, and other time-wasting tendencies. Remember that you don't have to stick to a specific time management system or plan every single moment of your life—the point is to think about how you value your time and to make sure that you use your time in ways that correspond to those values.

Reading and Study Tips that Work

There are a myriad of techniques for reading and studying and there's some truth in each of them. The fact of the matter is that most any system can work for you, but only if you make it right for you. Therefore, this section does not advocate any particular reading or study system; rather, it will provide some specific pointers to help you think about how you read and study, suggest some resources if you want to find a particular system to follow, and put you on the road to creating your own personalized and effective reading and study regimen.

First, you should think about where, when, and how you study best. Students typically say that their bedrooms, whether at home or at school, are the default places for study, but is a bedroom really the best study environment? If you have to share space, if there will be distractions or people competing for your attention, then the answer is probably no. There are certain study tasks that require sustained concentration and focus. For activities related to reading text or reviewing notes for understanding, it's best to have a quiet place where you can be left alone. We've already looked at time and task management above, but in relation to having a place to study, the issue of time becomes important again. Be sure to have an explicit agreement with your living companions about when and where you can have alone/quiet time. The corollary to the time management idea of a chunk of time is the space idea of a proper place to study. Thinking about time and space together will help you plan where to study exactly what. In other words, you'll want to determine which tasks you'll accomplish and where you will take them on.

Once you have your time and place issues sorted, the next task is to consider how you study. For many students, there is a strong disconnect between the manner in which information is typically presented in the classroom (lecture, textbooks) and the manner in which they like to learn (hands-on, practice). This disconnect

is particularly visible in the health sciences. In the experience of this writer, most health science students cannot get enough of clinical experience, a reflection of their hands-on or kinesthetic preference in learning (by contrast, the vast majority of history majors probably want nothing more than time alone to read). For an easy-to-use learning styles assessment, visit the VARK site (www.vark-learn.com/english/index.asp). So it is vitally important to plan a study strategy that accounts for your preferred method of learning. This shouldn't be a Herculean undertaking either. You've succeeded to this point because your study skills have been good. Think of the following suggestions as improvements and refinements rather than a total revamping of your approach to studying.*

Textbook reading can be the bane of even the most enthusiastic learners because textbook authors rightly prioritize completeness and coherence over entertainment value. But that leaves you with the burden of finding interest and engagement. One suggestion that works, even though it's counterintuitive, is to commit to going over the text multiple times. Many students put textbook reading into a special category of drudgery; they set aside hours and hours to do nothing but read, with the result that the task of reading seems like it can only be accomplished all at once. Instead, try an approach to reading and studying that allows you to dip into the text over and over again, each time with a specific purpose and focus.

One suggestion, based in part on the SQ3R method (Survey, Question, Read, Recite, Review), is to skim a chapter before reading it. Skimming is looking over the introductory paragraphs to sections, the first sentence in each paragraph, and the bolded/highlighted terms in the text. If there are charts and graphs, you should also look over these while skimming. The purpose of skimming is to familiarize yourself with key terms and ideas, not to understand them in their entirety. As a prereading exercise before a class, skimming is the most time-efficient manner of using the textbook. Skimming over old class notes can revive memories and assist in building comprehensive knowledge. If nothing else, skimming

---

*A complete approach to being a better student can be found in Dave Ellis, *Becoming a Master Student*, now in its 14th edition from Wadsworth (although any recent version will do fine). There's more than you need in *Becoming a Master Student*, but at the least it can serve as a good reference. A popular reading approach is SQ3R (for Survey, Question, Read, Recite, Review). A useful summary can be found at studygs.net/texred2.htm along with a host of other study tips.

through an entire textbook or semester's collection of notes will give you a sense of how the various chapters and topics fit together. Skimming through all your textbooks and class notes as a first step in a comprehensive review will allow you to establish the outlines of the big picture, the often-mentioned but seldom-defined sense of knowing a discipline inside and out.

The term *big picture* is something of a mystery to many students, so a few words to clarify the image are appropriate. Big picture thinking means being able to grasp the relations between the various parts of a field of knowledge, for example, the relationship between the arrangement of bones in the wrist (anatomy) and the various methods for taking an image of a patient's wrist. And that's a fairly obvious example. Big picture thinking implies an ability to work both with details as well as general principles, all in the same situation. Therefore, to have big picture knowledge, you must have exposure to many different sources of information, you must have strong memory for seemingly countless details, and you must be able to understand how the many details fit together to make up general principles. Another way to look at the big picture: Having this kind of understanding allows you to fit new information into the frame, to understand something different and unfamiliar in a way that relates the new item to the material you've already mastered. Big picture thinking does not mean ignoring details nor does it mean that understanding starts at the level of detail. The big picture is an integrated whole, and when you achieve big picture thinking and knowledge, you should be ready to ace your certification exam.

If you've used skimming to help start your big picture, it's time for more detail-oriented work. For this level of review, a good start is to use your class lecture notes as the skeleton on which to build a comprehensive review guide. It might be necessary to recopy or reformat your notes in order to have enough room to add in necessary information from different sources. Luckily, this process does not have to be done all at once and many students find that there's more than enough space in their class notes. When creating a review guide, the first order of business is determining what you know and what you don't know. "Know" in this case means to have an understanding of the material that allows you to explain it to another diagnostic imaging student while using your notes. Absolute memorization of details is not yet necessary. "Don't know" means that in a perfect world, you would like to have the professor or a clinical instructor explain or demonstrate to you alone in terms that you are guaranteed to

understand. Simply marking "know" and "don't know" in the margin of your newly created review guide will save you hours of time if you prioritize the "don't knows" for the next round of textbook reading.

With the fundamental understanding of material accomplished, it's now time to tack down all the details. For this task, there are as many valid processes as there are students, so if you have something that works, then don't feel you need to change it. On the other hand, if you find that tests are taxing because you often aren't sure about detailed information, then try one of the following approaches, test your knowledge with some practice tests, and use the approach that works best by allowing you to be the most confident.

First option: rote memorization (the classic). Rote memorization means going through the information repeatedly until it's all committed to memory. Some of the more popular methods are rewriting the study guide over and over, reading the notes aloud over and over, covering up notes and progressively revealing them line after line over and over, and quizzing from notes with other students. All of these methods can result in a recall memory that works—you know you've succeeded when you anticipate the next line in your review guide even before you see it or are prompted to think about it. Rote memorization can be a very powerful means of learning, but for most students it takes a lot of time and it doesn't promote critical thinking and problem solving, both of which are skills you will be tested on.

Second option: problem-based learning. Problem-based learning works well for health-care learning because it allows learning to reflect the complexity of real-life experience rather than separating topics that are really inextricable. You can use problem-based learning alone or in a group or alternate between the two; the key thing is to pose problems that require answers from more than one slide in a lecture or one section in a textbook. An appropriate problem would typically be based on a clinical situation or scenario and may not have one and only one solution. To solve this problem would take, ideally, the resources from radiographic procedures. To study using problem-based learning, it would be wise to work with fellow students and, more importantly, faculty to be sure that the problems cover all the material that might be covered on the comprehensive exam. Problem-based learning will not completely replace other modes of study because it may be necessary to use those traditional techniques to lock down the details of complex subjects, but it does allow you to create more memorable mental landmarks. For students who chafe under the burden of rote memorization, problem-based learning allows a more real-life study experience that can add interest and sustain effort.

Third option: two-column notes (Cornell method). This method of studying is something of a middle ground between rote memorization and problem-based learning. The traditional Cornell or two-column note-taking method is a means of controlling the overload of information in a lecture, but experience shows that the approach also works well as a means of studying. To create a two-column study guide, simply leave the left one-third of the page blank while writing your review guide in the right two-thirds. Once the guide is finished, start using the left-side area. The first time through the notes, you should use the left-hand column to mark "knows" and "don't knows" as well as key words that you should know the definitions of. The second time through, work through the "don't knows" and try to recall as much as you can about each key word. At this time, you can also start posing questions in the margins. Useful questions can be like the clinical or scenario questions for problem-based learning or they can be more direct, possibly predictions of the sorts of questions you might be asked about the material. The left column can also be a place to sketch out diagrams, tables, or charts that help you visualize important information. As you read through the guide multiple times, your focus should be more and more on the left-hand column. Ideally, by the time of the exam, you would be able to read through the key words, questions, and notes in the left column and recall all the relevant descriptions, details, and definitions in the review guide to the right. This approach emphasizes recall learning, forcing yourself to produce answers from memory rather than simply reciting by memory. The difference is slight but significant: Practicing recall based on memory landmarks that relate to the application of knowledge rather than the order of notes gives you more options for using the information and practicing the kind of thinking that you'll have to perform when taking the test.

At this point, you should be asking, when will I know that I'm ready for the exam? If you've followed some of the advice above, you will be studying effectively. You're ready for the test when you find that your study sessions no longer involve trying to understand fundamental theories or concepts, when study does involve much review of details, and when you find the majority of the review repetitive and predictable. One last study tip: Use practice questions as much as you can. Forcing yourself to recall information as if

taking a test will raise your comfort level when faced with the real thing. As you get closer to your test date, make a practice of sequestering yourself in a quiet room for an hour or more to practice nothing but answering practice questions. Especially valuable are questions that have rationales for their answers, as you can check the rationales against your own knowledge and review guide.

Pointers on Effective Test Taking

High-stakes testing can be nerve wracking, but there's no reason for multiple-choice phobia to detract from your performance. In the following pages, you will find some time-tested tips to help you navigate through the difficulties of taking a test. Remember, nothing replaces adequate knowledge of the material, but these techniques should help you attain a score that more closely matches your knowledge.

Anatomy of a Multiple-Choice Question

In the following example, the bolded print is the question stem.

Which of the following do patients have under the Patient's Bill of Rights?

a. Access to their medical records
b. Information regarding hospital policies
c. Advance directives
d. All of the above

The question stem helps you identify the topic of the question (in this case, the Patient's Bill of Rights) and determine which specific information you should consider (in this case, the rights that patients are granted under this law). The answer choices are listed under the question stem and should be considered a separate entity, related to the question by a shared topic but not part of a grammatical unit.

Tip 1: Glance at, but don't read through, the answer choices before you read the question stem thoroughly. The question stem is the basis of a productive reading of a question. If you were answering the above question, you would read the stem, glance at the answers to find they are individual terms rather than long descriptions, and then recall the salient points about the Patient's Bill of Rights.

Tip 2: If you can, preanswer the question before reading through the answer choices.

In the following example, the question stem is a "regular" question that could appear on a short-answer exam. In other words, you don't need the answer choices to provide a correct answer.

Assault is defined as:

a. Threatening to restrain a patient if they do not cooperate
b. Applying a tourniquet to a patient without obtaining consent for an intravenous injection
c Using positioning aides during the exam
d. Physically harming a patient

In this case, you should recall the definition of assault, say it to yourself (silently when you're taking the real exam), and then find the example that most closely fits your definition.

Tip 3: If there are multiple correct answers to a question stem, don't try to predict all of them. Instead, you should think about the general outlines of a correct answer and then find the answer choice that most closely relates to your general guidelines. In the example below, a "which of the following" phrase alerts you to the fact that there are multiple possible correct answers.

A consent form must contain which of the following?

a. Name of the facility
b. Name of the physician
c. Name of the procedure
d. All answers must be present on a consent form

Tip 4: When in doubt, treat each of the answer choices as a true/false statement with regard to the topic raised in the question stem. In the above example, you would find that answers a, b, and c are all true, so d would be the right answer. This technique is particularly useful when choosing between two answers. It is also helpful in the following example, when you are looking for the false answer.

Which of the following is NOT included in the HIPAA legislation?

a. Patients must submit payment for medical services electronically.
b. Health providers must notify patients of their privacy practices.
c. Patients have the right to access their medical records.
d. Violations of HIPAA may include civil and criminal penalties.

In this case, the capitalized "not" lets you know to look for the false answer. In fact, you can ignore the "not" once you employ the true/false technique as you simply look for the answer that's not like the others (Yes, this means you learned how to analyze this sort of question when you sang "Which one of these is not like the others? Which one of these is not the same?" as a preschooler watching Sesame Street).

Tip 5: When you get lost, reread the question stem. Too many students blitz through the question stem and spend all their test time comparing answer choices to each other. Remember that the majority of the answer choices are wrong! Don't waste time considering information that's intentionally misleading, incorrect, or incomplete. Rereading the question stem can clarify the issues that confuse you when choosing in a 50/50 situation.

Tip 6: Simplify complex questions. The following example is typical of a scenario question that presents multiple points of information that must be analyzed to find the correct answer:

A patient presents to the emergency department post-MVA by ambulance; she is conscious but has multiple injuries. The patient seems disoriented and confused regarding her whereabouts. She cannot tell the ER staff her name or DOB. The patient requires medical treatment to stabilize her injuries. What type of consent would this situation require?

Confronted with such an array of clues, many students will quickly skim through the question to find the main point (type of consent) and then spend most of their time trying to choose an answer. Then they will narrow things down to two answers and then not be able to choose the correct one. Instead of comparing the two answers to each other, a student would do better to draw slashes in the question to separate the different clues:

A patient presents to the emergency department/ post-MVA by ambulance;/ she is conscious /but has multiple injuries./ The patient seems disoriented and confused regarding her whereabouts./ She cannot tell the ER staff her name or DOB./ The patient requires medical treatment to stabilize her injuries./ What type of consent would this situation require?

With the question marked in this way, it's easier to reread it, comparing each clue to the remaining two questions in order to find the clue that rules out one of the remaining answer choices. But if you're taking a computerized test, you can't mark up the question. In that case, practice first with printed questions and when you're comfortable with the technique, start practicing with computer questions, mentally slashing them into component clues.

Tip 7: Never spend more than twice the average time for a question on any particular question. If you let even a handful of questions take up too much time, you lose the chance to spend sufficient time on other questions. Alternately, you might put so much time pressure on yourself at the end of the test that you find yourself simply guessing at answers.

Tip 8: If you want to change an answer to a question or if you're stuck between two equally good answers, write down why you are choosing the answer that you finally mark down. Writing forces you to articulate your thinking about the relation between your chosen answer and the topic of the question stem. Writing also allows you to see if your reasons for being undecided about an answer are relevant. Sometimes a student will think that an answer is "too obvious" or will mistrust the fourth "c" in a row. Writing down such doubts allows you to ignore them, as you should.

Last Thoughts about Test Preparation and Test Taking

The task of preparing yourself for a comprehensive licensure exam will seem daunting, but it's also a terrific opportunity. This is when all the hard work that you've done to date will pay off. The notes and hints in this chapter should put you on the right path to organizing and reviewing the vast amount of knowledge you've already mastered. Just remember to have a plan for organizing your time, reviewing information, and analyzing test questions. And don't hesitate to ask for help if you need it—your faculty, academic support personnel, and fellow students may be your most important assets.

REFERENCE

1. American Registry of Radiologic Technologists. Content specifications for the examination in radiography. http://www.arrt.org/pdfs/Disciplines/ Content-Specification/RAD-content-specification.pdf. Published 2010. Accessed May 14, 2013.

CHAPTER 2

Radiation Protection

The Radiation Protection portion of the ARRT Examination in Radiography comprises 22.5% of the examination, corresponding to 45 total questions on the examination. The content specifications for this examination category include four sections:

1. Biological Aspects of Radiation
2. Minimizing Patient Exposure
3. Personnel Protection
4. Radiation Exposure and Monitoring

BIOLOGICAL ASPECTS OF RADIATION

Cells are the basic functional unit in plants and animals and fundamentally the basic building blocks of life. The human cell consists of the following:

Nucleus—major structure that contains the target molecule, DNA, some RNA, protein, and water

Cytoplasm—major structure that contains all molecular components except DNA

Endoplasmic reticulum—acts as a channel or series of channels that allows for communication between the nucleus and the cytoplasm

Nucleolus—rounded structure attached to the nuclear membrane that contains most of the RNA

Mitochondria—large bean-shaped structures that digest macromolecules in order to produce energy for the cell

Ribosomes—small speck-like structures located throughout the cytoplasm or the endoplasmic reticulum; the site where protein synthesis occurs

Lysosomes—small pealike sacs that contain enzymes which help control contamination within the cell by digesting cellular fragments and the lysosome itself

There are two types of cells in the human body:

1. Genetic or germ:
   • Sexually reproducing cells
   • Function is to reproduce the species
   • Distinguished as female gametes that are referred to as oocytes and male gametes referred to as spermatozoa
   • Contain unpaired chromosomes or one-half the normal number (i.e., 23, haploid, or n number) of chromosomes
2. Somatic:
   • Refer to all other cells in the body
   • Contain identical, paired chromosomes or the normal number (i.e., 46, diploid, or 2n) of chromosomes
     Human beings contain 46 chromosomes in the nucleus of somatic cells.
     Of these 46 chromosomes, 44 are autosomes and 2 are sex chromosomes.
     Cell growth and division differ based on the type of cell: somatic or genetic.

Cell growth and division may occur in two ways:

1. Mitosis—All somatic cells of the body replicate in this manner. A diploid cell divides into two identical diploid cells, which is necessary for growth and tissue repair by way of the cell cycle. The cell cycle is made up of two phases: interphase and mitosis.
   a. Interphase is subdivided into G_1, S, and G_2:
      • G_1—gap or growth phase; pre-DNA synthesis and cell maintenance occurs
      • S—DNA replication occurs
      • G_2—gap or growth phase; post-DNA synthesis and cell preparation for mitosis occurs
   b. The mitosis phase of cell division has four stages:
      • Prophase—First stage of mitosis, during which the chromosomes condense and spindle fibers that are formed between centrioles move toward opposite poles of the cell. Disappearance of the nuclear membrane occurs and there is no visible nucleolus.
      • Metaphase—Second stage of mitosis, during which spindle fibers from each centriole attach

to the centromeres of the chromosomes and paired chromosomes line up at the cell's equator. The nuclear membrane completely disappears and centromeres divide.

- Anaphase—Third stage of mitosis, during which centromeres divide and sister chromatids detach and are pulled to opposite poles. Resulting chromatids are now separate chromosomes and form two complete and distinct sets.
- Telophase—Final stage of mitosis, during which the chromosome sets elongate, becoming thinner and indistinct as they reach the cell poles. DNA unravels to form chromatin and formation of new nuclear membranes occurs along with the reappearance of the nucleolus. Cell division is almost complete. The final steps include division of the cytoplasm with a new cell membrane and two daughter cells are formed.

2. Meiosis—All genetic cells of the body undergo this process to reproduce the species.
   - Occurs in sexually mature people. Ova and sperm have n or 23 chromosomes.
   - In females, meiotic process is referred to as oogenesis.
   - In males, meiotic process is referred to as spermatogenesis.
   - Referred to as reduction division; this means that the cells divide twice but chromosomes are only duplicated once.
   - At the end of mitotic phase one in meiosis, resulting daughter cells reenter a second stage, causing a second division of cellular material but without DNA replication.
   - Results in the production of four gametes, each containing haploid number or 23 chromosomes.

Cell division and proliferation is not perfect and requires proofreading and repair. Enzymes do the work of an editor by evaluating DNA replication and correcting any errors that may occur during synthesis.

- Enzymes that proofread DNA ensure that the errors are corrected prior to mitosis.
- Errors that are missed by proofreading enzymes may alter cell function and may result in cell death.

Cell theory states that radiation interaction at the atomic level may result in molecular changes leading to abnormal cell growth and/or metabolism.

- Sequence of events resulting from radiation exposure provides opportunity for damage repair and recovery.
- Radiation exposure, whether by direct effect through ionization or excitation through interaction with water,

may lead to alterations in molecular structure within the human body.

- The radiation response of humans is the result of x-ray interaction at the atomic level resulting in ionization or excitation of orbital electrons, which ultimately leads to the deposit of energy in body tissue.
- The energy deposited may cause measurable changes in critical molecules.

Critical molecules consist of five major groups:

1. Water
2. Protein
3. Lipids
4. Carbohydrates
5. Nucleic acid

Water is the most abundant molecule in the human body, yet is not considered to be a macromolecule like others in the group.

- The body is composed mainly of water.
- Water is composed of two hydrogen (H) atoms and one oxygen (O) atom and makes up approximately 80% of the body's structure.
- Water exists in free and bound states and aids in maintaining body temperature and homeostasis. It is involved in reactions within the human body.
- Water is also one of two end products in catabolism, a result of metabolism.

Metabolism is essential to bodily processes and results in not only catabolism but also anabolism.

- Catabolism refers to the breaking down of macromolecules into smaller parts.
- Anabolism refers to the production of large molecules from small parts.
- Metabolism and its by-products may result in harmful adverse effects.

Proteins:

- Make up about 15% of the body's molecular composition
- Consist of amino acids, which are essential to protein synthesis
- Are required for structure and support in the human body
- Are needed for function in enzymes, hormones, and antibodies
- Are represented by the formula $C_nH_nO_nN_nT_n$

Additional macromolecules include the following:

- Enzymes are molecules that allow biochemical reactions to progress within the body.

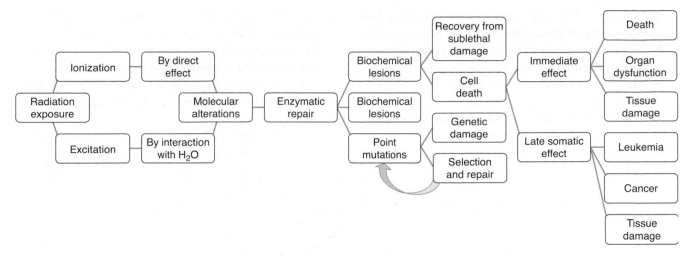

FIGURE 2-1   Biological Effect of Ionizing Radiation

- Hormones are molecules that provide regulatory control over body functions and are secreted by glands within the human body.
- Antibodies possess a molecular structure that provides a defensive front to infection and disease that may attack a person.

Lipids:

- Are inherent to the body and are composed of carbon (C), H, and O
- Are represented by the formula $C_nH_nO_n$
- Contain both one molecule of glycerol and three molecules of fatty acid
- Provide structure to cell membranes
- Insulate the body from the environment
- Provide energy to the body by storing it until it is needed (however, it is more difficult to access energy in this manner)

Carbohydrates:

- Also contain C, H, and O but have a different structure than that of lipids
- Ratio of H to O atoms is 2:1 in carbohydrates
- Referred to as saccharides or sugars
- Serve to provide the main source of energy within the body for cell metabolism

Nucleic acids that are essential to cell metabolism:

- DNA is located within the cell's nucleus and contains genetic information.
- RNA is located within the cell's cytoplasm and is further distinguished as messenger RNA (mRNA) and transfer RNA (tRNA).

DNA is considered to be the radiation-sensitive target molecule.

- Consists of deoxyribose
- Four different nitrogenous bases:
  Adenine
  Guanine
  Thymine
  Cytosine
- Adenine binds with thymine, while guanine binds with cytosine in sugar-phosphate bases
- Double helix alternating configuration
- Disruption of this configuration may result in abnormal protein synthesis and other harmful effects

RNA contains:

- Ribose as its sugar component
- Single spiral configuration
- Four different nitrogenous bases:
  Adenine
  Guanine
  Uracil
  Cytosine

RELATIVE TISSUE RADIOSENSITIVITIES

1. Linear energy transfer (LET)
   - Measure of the rate at which energy is transferred from ionizing radiation to soft tissue
   - Another method of expressing radiation quality and determining the value of radiation weighting factor (W_R)
   - May be expressed in kiloelectron volt per micrometer (keV/μm); LET of diagnostic x-rays is 3 keV/μm

- As LET increases, the ability of biologic response to ionizing radiation increases
- High LET results in more ionizations and increased risk to target molecule

2. Relative biologic effectiveness (RBE)
   - Directly proportionate to LET
   - As LET increases, the ability of biologic response to ionizing radiation increases
   - RBE of diagnostic x-rays is 1

Radiation dose delivered over a long period of time may result in a lower dose effect. Higher dose is required to produce the same effect and may be accomplished in two ways:

1. Protraction—indicates a dose of radiation that is delivered continuously but at a lower dose rate
2. Fractionation—indicates a dose of radiation that is delivered at the same dose rate but in equal fractions of dose over a 24-hour period; will reduce effect as a result of cell repair and recovery between doses; basis for radiation oncology

Cells and tissues are distinguished by the rate at which they divide and their stage of development. The Bergonié-Tribondeau law discusses the radiosensitivity of cells based on the following four concepts:

1. Cells that are considered highly radiosensitive include:
   - Lymphocytes
   - Spermatogonia
   - Erythroblasts
   - Intestinal crypt cells
2. Cells that have an intermediate radiosensitivity include:
   - Endothelial cells
   - Osteoblasts
   - Spermatids
   - Fibroblasts
3. Cells that have low radiosensitivity include:
   - Muscle cells
   - Nerve cells
   - Chondrocytes
4. Cell radiosensitivity depends on where the cell is in the cell cycle.
   - Most radiosensitive: mitosis and passage from late G_1 into early S
   - Most radioresistant: mid-to-late S

Factors that are associated with affecting radiosensitivity in individuals vary and include age, metabolism, recovery, O effect, chemical agents, and hormesis.

Age—most sensitive before birth and in old age
Metabolic rate—rapidly dividing cells at increased risk

Recovery—human cells have the ability to recover from damage caused by exposure to radiation; however, survival depends on the dose:

1. Intracellular response states:
   - Cells that are radiated and survive will have the opportunity to recover and may proceed to replicate.
   - Cells that are radiated and destroyed before interphase are beyond repair.
2. Organ or tissue response states:
   - If sufficient radiation dose is experienced, shrinking or atrophy will occur as a result of cell death and disintegration.
   - If sublethal radiation damage occurs, proliferation and repopulation of tissue or organ may occur.
3. Whole-body response states:
   - Repopulation of the surviving cells must occur during recovery as a result of sublethal radiation damage.

Oxygen effect—states the following:
   - Tissues are more radiosensitive when they are oxygenated.
   - Radio-resistant behavior occurs as a result of conditions that are anoxic or hypoxic.
   - Diagnostic x-ray is performed under fully oxygenated conditions.

Oxygen enhancement ratio (OER)—ratio of radiation dose required to cause a particular biologic response in cells or organisms in an environment deprived of O to radiation dose required to cause the exact same response in an environment with natural oxygenation

Chemical agents—must be present at the time of irradiation and have the ability to change the radiation response of cells, tissues, and organs
   - Radiosensitizers—enhance the effect of radiation and have an effectiveness ratio of approximately 2; only half the radiation dose will be needed to produce the same effect in the presence of a sensitizing agent
   - Radioprotectors—include molecules that contain sulfur and H bound together and have an effectiveness ratio of approximately 2; twice the amount of radiation dose would be required to produce the same effect in the presence of a radioprotective agent

Hormesis—the idea that small amounts of radiation are beneficial due to their ability to stimulate hormones and immune responses to other toxic environmental agents.

   - At very low doses, irradiated subjects experience less response.
   - Observation of radiation response in humans after receiving doses less than 10 rad (100 milligray [mGy]) has not been performed.

Dose-Response Relationships

Dose-response relationships are mathematical relationships between varying levels of radiation dose and the magnitude of the observed response. These relationships have two important applications in radiology:

1. To design therapeutic treatment routines for cancer patients
2. To determine the effects of low-dose irradiation to provide the basis for radiation control activities

Human response falls into two categories as a result of these dose-response relationships:

1. Deterministic—radiation responses that usually follow a high-dose exposure and result in an early response such as a radiation-induced skin burn
2. Stochastic—radiation responses that usually follow a low-dose exposure and result in a late radiation response such as cancer, leukemia, or genetic effects

Every radiation dose-response relationship has two characteristics:

1. Linear versus nonlinear
2. Threshold versus nonthreshold

Linear dose-response relationships indicate a response that is directly proportionate to the dose.

Linear, nonthreshold types:

- Dose-response relationships intersect the dose axis at or below zero.
- Any dose is expected to produce a response.
- At zero, the relationship will demonstrate a measurable yet natural response.
- Even without exposure to radiation, this response will be observed.
- Radiation-induced cancer, leukemia, and genetic effects follow a linear, nonthreshold dose-response relationship.

Linear, threshold types:

- Dose-response relationships demonstrate an interception of the dose axis greater than zero.
- Doses below these thresholds are not expected to produce a response.

All other radiation dose-response relationships are nonlinear. There are two types of nonlinear dose-response relationships:

1. Nonlinear, nonthreshold
   - Large response results from a small radiation dose.
   - Incremental doses in very low dose range produce very little response.
   - Higher doses with the same increment of dose produces a greater response.

2. Nonlinear, threshold
   - Doses below the threshold produce no measurable response.
   - Doses implemented above the threshold become increasingly more effective at each increment until inflection point of curve (the area at which the curve stops bending up and begins bending down) is reached.
   - Deterministic response that occurs will be reflected through this sigmoid-type dose-response relationship curve.
   - Doses above the inflection point become less effective.
   - High-dose fluoroscopic procedures that cause skin effects will follow the sigmoid-type dose-response relationship.

Molecular and Cellular Radiobiology

Injury that can be seen as a result of radiation exposure in humans occurs at the molecular level. Irradiation of macromolecules results in molecular lesions both in vitro and in vivo:

In vitro—the irradiation of macromolecules outside of the cell or body. Considerable dose is required to produce a measurable effect. Results in three major effects:

1. Main-chain scission
   - Breakage of the backbone of the long-chain macromolecule
   - Results in reduction of a long, single molecule into many smaller molecules
   - Main-chain scission reduces viscosity
2. Cross-linking
   - Small, spurlike side structures develop off the main chain of a macromolecule after irradiation
   - Spurs cause the main chain to become sticky
   - Spurs attach to neighboring macromolecules or another segment of the same molecule
   - Cross-linking increases viscosity
3. Point lesions
   - Result in disruption of single chemical bonds through interaction with radiation
   - Point lesions are not detectable
   - May cause small changes that will result in cell malfunction
   - Point lesions that result from low radiation doses are considered to be the cellular radiation damage that results in late effects at whole-body level

In vivo—the irradiation of macromolecules within the human body. Indicates that the macromolecules are more radiosensitive in their natural state.

DNA:

- Contains genetic information for each cell
- Can be damaged without visible detection
- Damage may result in abnormal metabolic activity including rapid and uncontrolled proliferation
- Observable damage a result of considerable radiation exposure
- Damage that is not detectable may produce responses at the cellular or whole-body level
- Point or genetic mutations are common with low LET radiations and may be transferred incorrectly to daughter cells

Radiation effects on DNA may cause chromosome aberrations or cytogenic damage. The response of DNA to radiation exposure may include the following:

- Main-chain scission with only one side rail severed
- Main-chain scission with both side rails severed
- Main-chain scission and subsequent cross-linking
- Rung breakage causing a separation of bases
- Change in or loss of a base

The principal observable effects that may result from irradiation of cells are:

1. Cell death
2. Malignant disease
3. Genetic damage

Malignant disease and genetic damage at the molecular level conform to the linear, nonthreshold dose-response relationship.

Radiolysis of water is the dissociation of water into other molecular products:

- The human body is made up of approximately 80% water molecules.
- Irradiation of water is the principle radiation interaction in the body.

Cell Survival and Recovery

In order to determine lethal effects of radiation, observations surrounding cell survival must be assessed. Cell survival is evaluated using two methods:

1. Single-target, single-hit—applies to biologic targets including enzymes, viruses, and bacteria
   - May occur in G_1 or G_2 phases of cell cycle
   - Irradiation to chromosomes may be direct or indirect hit
   - Chromosome hits cause a visible chromosome change
   - Numerous molecular bonds may have interference
   - Interference may cause severing of DNA
   - Represent critical DNA damage

- Breakage of a chromatid results in a chromatid deletion
- May result in a missing chromosome fragment and missing genetic material
- May occur at doses given in diagnostic radiology

2. Multitarget, single-hit—applies to more complicated biologic systems including human cells
   - May occur in G_1 or G_2 phases of cell cycle
   - In G_1 phase, two hits that may occur on one chromosome produce ring chromosomes
   - Also in G_1 phase, one hit to two neighboring chromosomes that recombine produces dicentric fragments: a chromosome with two centers or two centromeres
   - In G_2 phase, chromosomal abnormalities similar to those mentioned above may also occur but are rare
   - Represent major cell damage
   - In mitosis, may result in daughter cells missing important genetic information
   - Reciprocal translocations are types of multitarget, single-hit methods and involve a rearranging of the genetic material and improper code sequencing

The effects to the chromosomes have been discussed extensively and may result in not only structural direct or indirect changes but also indirect ionization resulting in breakage of the chromosome. Damage to chromosomes may occur from both low and high radiation doses; the effects on chromosomes are nonspecific and never desirable.

Somatic Effects

The amount of biologic damage sustained by an individual or individuals as a result of radiation exposure is dependent on several factors:

The amount of ionizing radiation that is delivered to the individual or individuals

The ability of the ionizing radiation to produce ionization in the tissue of the affected person or persons

The length of time that the body or body area is exposed to ionizing radiation

The body parts that are exposed to ionizing radiation

Short-term versus Long-term Effects

Short-term somatic effects may also be referred to as acute or early effects. Characteristics include:

Appearance within minutes, hours, days, or weeks after radiation exposure

Nausea

Fatigue

Skin erythema

Hair loss

Intestinal disorders

Fever

Blood disorders

Shedding of the outer layer of skin

Acute Radiation Syndromes

Acute radiation syndromes are inferred from the relationship of the signs and symptoms to an organism's exposure to whole-body radiation. Three conditions must be present in order for total-body radiation syndrome to be considered:

1. Acute radiation exposure must have occurred within seconds or minutes.
2. The entire body must have been exposed to the irradiation.
3. The source that caused the exposure must have come from an external source of x-radiation or gamma radiation.

   Acute radiation exposure:

- Shortens the life span of the organism (dependent on the dose)
- Decreases life span from moderate to high dose of total-body radiation and may be instantly fatal
- Requires no medical intervention

   Survival times of people or organisms affected by the same dose of whole-body radiation vary. They are related through the survival of the people under the same circumstances within the same population within a specific time period.

- $LD_{50/30}$—refers to the lethal dose required to kill 50% of a population in a 30-day time period and requires no medical intervention
- $LD_{50/60}$—refers to the lethal dose required to kill 50% of a population past the 30-day time period but within 60 days; 250 to 300 rad (2.5 to 3 Gy)

   Even though many organs and systems within the human body may be altered by exposure to radiation, there are three body systems that may be greatly affected. Responses to radiation exposure are represented in four stages:

1. Prodromal stage
   - Consists of nausea, vomiting, and diarrhea
   - Can occur with a dose as low as 50 rad (500 mGy)
   - Lasts from a few minutes to a few days
   - Dose dependent
2. Latent stage
   - Affected individual appears symptom-free
   - Internal changes lead to recovery or death
   - Lasts from weeks in doses below 500 roentgens (R) to hours or less at doses greater than 10,000 R

3. Manifest illness stage
   - Noticeable illness in specific syndrome of organ system damaged
   - Lasts from minutes to weeks
   - Dose dependent
   - Recovery or death occurs as a result of damage from radiation exposure
4. Recovery or death
   - Recovery will be complete for a time period of a week to years with the possibility of stochastic effects
   - Death may occur within 1 to a few months

   Failure of a system or death of an organism may result in the following systems:

1. Hemopoietic system
2. Gastrointestinal system (GI)
3. Central nervous system (CNS)

Hemopoietic

- The hemopoietic system will be affected at doses between 100 and 1,000 R
- Results in bone marrow syndrome, hematologic syndrome, or hematopoietic syndrome
- Death occurs within 6 to 8 weeks at 200 R
- Exposure range between 100 and 300 R may result in sufficient bone marrow repopulation to sustain life, with a large number of survivors fully recovering during the 3rd week to 6 months postexposure
- Doses from 400 to 600 R result in fewer survivors
- Survival at doses of 1,000 R not evident and will cause death within 2 weeks
- $LD_{50/60}$ for humans is approximately 450 R or 250 to 300 rad (2.5 to 3 Gy)
- Destruction of bone marrow occurs
- Mechanism of death caused by reduction of red blood cells (RBCs), white blood cells (WBCs), and platelets
- Death results from anemia and infection
- Without medical intervention, death will occur in approximately 4 to 6 weeks in the 300 to 500 R range but in 2 weeks in the 500 to 1,000 R range

   The stages of the bone marrow, hematologic, or hematopoietic syndrome include:

1. Prodromal stage
   - Occurs a few hours after exposure
   - Involves nausea and vomiting
2. Latent stage
   - Extends from a few days up to 3 weeks postexposure
   - Circulating blood cells are not severely depressed
   - Bone marrow stem cell death occurring
   - Fewer mature cells produced
   - Lower numbers of cells in circulating blood

3. Manifest illness stage
   - Occurs 3 to 5 weeks postexposure
   - Reduction of blood cell count
   - Depression of blood cell counts (cytopenia)
   - Resulting anemia and infections

Gastrointestinal System

- Symptoms appear in all animals at doses between 1,000 and 10,000 R
- In humans, symptoms may appear at threshold dose of 600 R, and full syndrome manifests at 1,000 R
- Results in GI syndrome as a result of damage to the GI tract and bone marrow
- GI tract lining, especially the small intestine, is damaged by doses
- Causes depletion of the crypts of Lieberkühn—radiosensitive precursor cells in villi cell populations
- Decreased absorption results in depletion of these cells
- Dehydration results from leaking GI fluids
- Systemic bacterial infection
- Depletion of WBCs
- Irreversible damage to bone marrow will cause death
- Death occurs regardless of dose and results from infection, dehydration, and electrolyte damage
- Death in humans occurs within 3 to 10 days without medical intervention and within approximately 2 weeks with medical intervention

The stages for the GI syndrome occur more rapidly than the stages for the hematologic syndrome and include:

1. Prodromal stage
   - Occurs within hours postexposure
   - Involves nausea, vomiting, cramps, and diarrhea
2. Latent stage occurs through the 5th day
3. Manifest illness stage
   - Reoccurrence of nausea, vomiting, and diarrhea with fever
   - Perseveres from the 5th through the 10th days

Central Nervous System

- The CNS will be affected at doses greater than 5,000 R in humans
- Results in CNS syndrome
- Damage may result from:
  Damage to the blood vessels that support the CNS, causing edema in the cranial vault
  Vasculitis
  Meningitis
- Death may occur within hours or up to 3 days postexposure
- Exposed individual does not live long enough to exhibit many of the symptoms from CNS syndrome

The stages for the CNS syndrome include:

1. Prodromal stage
   - Dependent on dose
   - May last from a few minutes to a few hours
   - Results in nervousness, confusion, nausea, vomiting, loss of consciousness, and burning skin sensations
2. Latent stage may last several hours.
3. Manifest illness stage
   - Occurs 5 to 6 hours after exposure
   - Results in diarrhea, convulsions, coma, and death

Organ and Tissue Response

- Partial body irradiation may also occur as a result of exposure to radiation
- Organs and tissues may be affected, with death to some of the cells in these areas resulting in atrophy
- Atrophy may lead to a nonfunctioning organ or tissue
- Organ or tissue may recover as a result of atrophy
- Tissue or organ response depends on three things:
  1. Radiosensitivity
  2. Reproduction rate
  3. Maturation rate

To discuss the issue of local tissue damage, three main areas that may demonstrate tissue or organ response to irradiation include the skin, eyes, and gonads.

Effects to skin include:

- Inflammation—swelling
- Erythema—redness that may be induced by x-radiation or sun exposure
- Desquamation—peeling

Skin is composed of:

- Epidermis—outer layer; consists of mature nondividing cells on the surface and immature dividing cells in the basal layer
- Dermis—middle layer of connective tissue
- Subcutaneous layer—fat and connective tissue
- Follicles—accessory hair structures that originate out of the dermis and are actively growing
- Sebaceous glands—secrete oil
- Sweat glands—secrete water
- Sensory receptors—allow for touch

The characteristics of the epidermis basal cells and the hair follicles make the skin radiosensitive, while the sebaceous and sweat glands are relatively radioresistant.

- Skin redness or mild erythema may be seen within 1 to 2 days after a single dose of 100 to 1,000 rad (1 to 10 Gy)
- Followed by a more severe erythema in about 2 weeks
- Follows a nonlinear, threshold dose-response relationship

- Despite the radiosensitivity of the epidermis, exposure to moderate doses does not deter regeneration of cells or healing; however, exposure to high doses results in late changes consistent with:
  Atrophy
  Fibrosis
  Pigmentation changes
  Ulcers
  Necrosis
  Cancer
- Despite the radiosensitivity of the hair follicles, exposure to moderate doses may result in merely temporary epilation or alopecia; however, exposure to high doses results in permanent epilation
- Despite the radioresistance of the sebaceous and sweat glands, exposure to high doses causes atrophy to the glands and fibrosis that lead to minimal or nonexistent function

Effects to the eyes as a result of irradiation are:

- Dependent on the dose received
- Likely to cause radiation cataractogenesis

The lens of the eye contains radiosensitive cells that are likely to be damaged or destroyed by exposure to radiation.

- The body is not able to remove damaged cells from the eyes.
- Damaged cells accumulate and form cataracts.
- This damage is described as a threshold, nonlinear dose-response relationship.
- Threshold dose is approximately 200 rad (2 Gy).
- Doses greater than 700 rad (7 Gy) result in cataract development in all people.
- Average latent period is 15 years for formation of cataracts.
- High LET has a high RBE for cataractogenesis by a factor of two or more.
- Protective eyewear for radiation personnel and patients undergoing radiologic procedures will reduce the risk of forming radiation-induced cataracts.

The human reproductive system is extremely radiosensitive.

- Doses as low as 10 rad (100 mGy) have caused observable responses.
- Male testes and female ovaries react differently to radiation exposure.
- Differences are attributed to the rates and times for the ova and sperm to develop from stem to mature cells.
- Female germ cells multiply only during fetal development and may reach numbers up to 7 million and decline throughout life.

- Male germ cells multiply throughout the life of the human male.

Males

- Majority of male tissue is radioresistant.
- Testes contain mature and immature spermatogonia.
- Mature spermatogonia are radioresistant.
- Immature spermatogonia are radiosensitive.

The main effect of irradiation in males is damage to and reduction in the number of spermatogonia, which leads to maturation depletion.

1. Following testicular irradiation, fertility may be altered despite the radioresistance of the mature sperm.
2. The dose delivered may result in temporary or permanent sterility.
3. The cause of sterility is the loss of immature spermatogonia that results from irradiation; immature spermatogonia are unable to replace the mature sperm lost from the testes.
4. A dose of 200 to 250 rad (2 to 2.5 Gy) produces temporary sterility.
5. An acute dose of 500 to 600 rad (5 to 6 Gy) produces permanent sterility.

Additional effects of irradiation in males may result in:

- The production of chromosomal abnormalities that may be passed on to offspring
- Damage to the chromosomes in functioning spermatogonia as a result of temporary sterility
- Damage to the chromosomes in immature spermatogonia

Females

- Ova are classified as small, intermediate, and large within the follicles.
- Intermediate follicles contain ova that are the most sensitive.
- Small follicles contain ova that are most resistant.
- Mature follicles contain ova that are moderately sensitive.

The effect of irradiation in females depends on the phase of menstruation, fertilization, or ovulation that may be occurring.

1. Moderate dose of radiation to the ovaries results in an initial period of fertility.
2. This is caused by presence of moderately resistant mature follicles that may release an ovum.
3. Fertile period is followed by either temporary or permanent sterility.
4. Sterility is caused by ova damaged in the radiosensitive intermediate follicles that are restricting their maturation and release.

5. A dose of 10 rad (100 mGy) may restrain and slow menstruation.
6. Sterility occurs with age; the fetus and child, especially, are more radiosensitive.
7. Sensitivity decreases until the age of 30 years but increases with age thereafter.
8. Doses of 200 rad (2 Gy) produce temporary sterility.
9. Acute dose of approximately 500 to 600 rad (5 to 6 Gy) will cause permanent sterility.

Additional concerns in females resulting from exposure to radiation include:

• Anxiety over genetic changes in functional ova
• Potential chromosomal damage to ova postexposure
• Genetic abnormalities may be produced in offspring
• Nonvisible mutations may be manifested in future generations

The hemopoietic system is composed of the bone marrow, circulating blood, lymph nodes, spleen, and thymus. In response to radiation, the hemopoietic system may suffer:

• Low radiation dose will result in a slight decrease of stem cells with a rapid recovery a few weeks postexposure.
• Moderate to high radiation dose will result in a more intense depletion of stem cells and a longer, slower, or incomplete recovery of stem cells.
• Most sensitive stem cells are the erythroblasts, the precursors for RBCs.
• Moderately sensitive stem cells are the myelocytes, the precursors for WBCs.
• Least sensitive stem cells are the megakaryocytes, the precursors for platelets.

Long-term somatic effects may also be referred to as chronic or late effects.
Characteristics include:

Appearance within months or years after radiation exposure
Cancer
Birth defects
Cataract formation

Late somatic effects may be further distinguished as late nonstochastic and late stochastic somatic effects.
Characteristics that define late nonstochastic somatic effects include:

Cataract formation
Fibrosis
Organ atrophy
Loss of parenchymal cells

Reduced fertility
Sterility

Characteristics that define late stochastic somatic effects include:

Cancer
Birth defects

Acute versus Chronic Effects
Acute effects may be preventable when exposure to radiation is limited:

Below the threshold for adverse biologic effects
Daily threshold of 0.2 R was recommended by the International X-Ray and Radium Protection Commission (now known as the National Council on Radiation Protection and Measurements [NCRP]) in 1934[1]
In 1936, the daily threshold was reduced to 0.1 R after assessment of late effects of radiation exposure were evaluated

Chronic effects are evaluated when exposure to radiation occurs and are the basis for the focus on minimizing exposure to radiation.

Carcinogenesis
Cancer is the important late stochastic somatic effect resulting from exposure to ionizing radiation. Two risk models are used in predicting the incidence of cancer:

1. Absolute risk—predicts that a set number or excess cancers will occur from exposure to radiation
2. Relative risk—predicts that the number of excess cancers will increase as the natural incidence of cancer increases within an aging population

To further understand the process by which carcinogenesis occurs, discussion surrounding cancer-inducing events is presented.

Radiation-induced cancer may occur 5 years or more after exposure to ionizing radiation.
Painters of watch dials in the 1920s and 1930s used paint containing radium to apply fine lines on the dials, often placing the tip of the brush to their lips to draw the bristles into a fine point. Ingestion of radium led to accumulation of this toxic substance and eventual radium poisoning.
Uranium miners in Arizona and New Mexico inhaled dust and drank water tainted by the radioactive substance, leading to deaths caused by cancer and respiratory illnesses. Families of uranium miners were also affected by the contaminated clothing worn by workers and became at risk for developing radiation-induced cancers.

Early medical radiation workers including radiologists, dentists, and technologists were exposed to large amounts of ionizing radiation, putting them at risk for increased incidence of aplastic anemia and leukemia because protective measures and devices were not available.

From 1925 to 1945, patients undergoing diagnostic angiography were injected with the contrast agent Thorotrast, which emitted radioactive particles into the livers and spleens of these patients, leading to late somatic effects 15 to 20 years postexposure. Cancers of the liver and spleen as well as angiosarcomas and biliary duct carcinomas were seen at this time.

Infants with enlarged thymus glands in the late 1940s and early 1950s were administered therapeutic doses of x-radiation to reduce the size of the glands. Incidence of thyroid nodule and carcinoma development in patients treated during infancy occurred approximately 20 years postexposure.

Incidence of breast cancer in radiation treatment of benign postpartum mastitis is still a concern and raises awareness of the need for mammography in screening and diagnostic purposes.

Children of Marshall Islanders developed thyroid cancer after being inadvertently subjected to high levels of radiation fallout during an atomic bomb test in March of 1954.

Japanese atomic bomb survivors suffered from radiation injuries including leukemia and breast cancer.

Evacuees from the Chernobyl nuclear disaster are still being evaluated for radiation-induced leukemias, thyroid cancers, and other malignancies as a result of the disaster.

Embryonic and Fetal Risks

The growth of a human being results in rapid proliferation of cells to develop cells, tissues, organs, organ systems, and the eventual organism. Based on the Bergonié-Tribondeau law, it can be determined that the embryo is very radiosensitive.

The embryo's response to radiation is based on these factors:

- The total dose delivered
- The rate of the dose delivered
- The quality of the radiation
- The embryonic stage of development

The fetus develops through three stages:

1. Preimplantation
   - Joining of the sperm and the egg into a zygote until day 9
   - Zygote attaches to intrauterine wall
   - Rapid proliferation into highly undifferentiated cells
   - Irradiation at this time can result in prenatal death, low incidences of congenital abnormalities, and all-or-nothing survival of embryo
   - Critical times of radiation exposure are 12 hours postconception and at 30 to 60 hours when the first two divisions begin
2. Major organogenesis
   - Occurs at 10 days to 6 weeks after conception
   - Developing fetus is most at risk for radiation-induced congenital abnormalities
   - Undifferentiated cells start to differentiate into organs with the exception of the CNS
   - CNS develops during 12th year of life
   - Irradiation effects include mental retardation, growth inhibition, microcephaly, genital deformities, and damage to sense organs
   - Late-stage organogenesis with fatal abnormalities will cause neonatal death
   - High doses of radiation will also cause death
3. Fetal or growth stage
   - Skeletal damage from exposure to radiation occurs during week 3 to week 20
   - Irradiation during this stage may present as cancer or other functional childhood disorders after birth

The effects of irradiation of the fetus include the following:

- Prenatal or neonatal death
- Congenital abnormalities
- Growth impairment
- Reduced intelligence
- Genetic abnormalities
- Cancer induction

Genetic Impact

Genetic impact, or effects on future generations as a result of exposure to ionizing radiation, varies and is based on the impact to DNA in the mature sperm or ova. Genetic information may be faulty or inconsistent, which may lead to diseases or malformation in resulting offspring.

There are natural spontaneous mutations that may occur without a known cause and result in permanent alterations to the genetic material, which may be passed on to future generations. These spontaneous mutations do not occur as a result of exposure to ionizing radiation.

Mutagens responsible for genetic mutations are another way in which genetic information may be altered because of changes in the environment relating to temperature, viruses, and chemicals; ionizing radiation is also considered a mutagen that may cause a change.

Genetic alterations or impacts may result from exposure to the mutagen ionizing radiation and from any of the following methods:

- Radiation interaction with DNA macromolecules—The structure of a macromolecule may be modified from breaks in the DNA, resulting in a deletion or alteration which changes the genetic information in the cell. This type of mutation may be passed down to future generations without correction.
- Cellular damage repair by enzymes—The repair of damage caused to the chromosomes hit by ionizing radiation may or may not be successful. A successful repair results in normal cell function, while a repair that is not successful may result in apoptosis or cell death.
- Incapacities of mutant genes—Improper control or chemical balance within a cell due to the presence of a mutant gene may result in a variety of genetic diseases. Improper sequencing during synthesis results in defects in proteins, which are necessary for proper cell function.
- Dominant or recessive point mutations—Dominant point mutations will most likely be demonstrated in resulting offspring, while recessive mutations are less common. However, recessive point mutations may be expressed in offspring as the following:
  Allergies
  Slight alteration in metabolism
  Decreased intelligence
  Predisposition to certain diseases

Genetically Significant Dose

Genetically significant dose (GSD) assesses the impact of gonadal dose and is based on the genetic influence of low doses of radiation to the entire population.

- Gonadal dose differs in males and females; therefore, the importance of protecting the reproductive organs is a concern in diagnostic radiology.
- Exposure to females is higher because of the location of the reproductive organs. The ovaries are located within the pelvis, which places them in the primary beam for radiographs of the abdomen and pelvis; exposure to the female reproductive organs is three times more than that of male reproductive organs in this area.

GSD considers the following:

There are people who are at risk of irradiation to their reproductive organs on an annual basis.

There are people who are not at risk of irradiation to their reproductive organs on an annual basis.

Individuals who are no longer in childbearing years are not genetically impacted.

The average annual gonadal equivalent dose (EqD) to childbearing people in a population includes children who are expected to be conceived in an exposed population in a given year.

Sherer states, "According to the U.S. Public Health Service, the estimated GSD for the population of the United States is about 0.20 millisieverts (mSv) (20 millirem [mrem; rem = roentgen equivalents human])."[2]

Goals of Gonadal Shielding

Gonadal shielding is performed to minimize the effects of ionizing radiation in patients during radiographic procedures.

- Proper collimation should be incorporated to include only the area of clinical interest
- Gonadal shielding must be used in the primary beam or within 5 centimeters (cm) (2″) of it
- Gonadal shielding must contain 1 millimeter (mm) of lead or lead equivalent
- Popular theory states that gonadal shielding should be used only for anyone of reproductive age
- Should not be used when it interferes with necessary diagnostic information on a radiographic image
- Used as a secondary protective measure to the collimation of the beam
- Contact shields used on female reproductive organs reduce exposure by 50%
- Contact shields used on male reproductive organs reduce exposure by 90% to 95%

Types of gonadal shielding include the following:

1. Flat contact shields—made of rubberized lead strips that are laid directly over the patient's gonads and may be secured with tape; excellent for recumbent studies
2. Shadow shields—made of a radiopaque material; suspended from the x-ray tube housing, casting a shadow over the patient's gonadal region; useful in operating rooms or in sterile fields during special procedures
3. Shaped contact shields—made of lead and worn by male patients and held in place by a supporter; useful for performing oblique, lateral, and erect studies; rare to find these in current use
4. Clear lead shields—transparent lead-plastic material impregnated with 30% lead by weight; for gonadal and breast regions

Photon Interactions with Matter

Photons may interact with matter in five different ways:

1. Coherent scattering
   - Also known as classic, elastic, or unmodified scattering

- Results in no loss of energy as x-rays scatter
- Low-energy photon (less than 10 keV) interacts with atom, causing vibration and change in direction; results in Rayleigh scattering
- May result in radiographic fog (unwanted density) in diagnostic radiology
- In addition to Rayleigh scattering, Thomson scattering may occur when low-energy photon interacts with one or more free electrons
- Does not affect radiography but affects visible light

2. Compton scattering
   - Also known as incoherent, inelastic, or modified scattering
   - Responsible for most of the scattered radiation produced during radiologic procedures
   - Scatter may occur in any direction and is the reason for providing protection for personnel and patients
   - Incoming x-ray photon interacts with a loosely bound electron of an atom of the irradiated object
   - Incoming x-ray surrenders a portion of its kinetic energy to dislodge the electron from its orbit, causing ionization
   - The freed electron is referred to as the Compton scattered electron, secondary, or recoil electron
   - The Compton scattered electron loses its kinetic energy through collisions with nearby atoms and recombines with an atom that needs another electron within a few micrometers of the initial Compton interaction
   - The Compton scattered electron or photon may interact with other atoms through photoelectric absorption or subsequent Compton scattering
   - It may also emerge from the patient and degrade the radiographic image by causing additional fog or expose others present in the room

3. Photoelectric absorption
   - Most important interaction between x-ray photons and atoms of the patient's body to produce useful radiographic images in mammography and radiographic procedures
   - Interaction between an x-ray photon and an inner-shell electron (K or L shells) that is tightly bound
   - Dislodgement depends on the kinetic energy of the incoming x-ray photon, which must be as great as or greater than the amount of energy that is binding the electron in its orbit
   - Upon interaction in the orbit, the incoming x-ray photon surrenders all of its kinetic energy to the orbital electron and ceases to exist
   - Electron that is hit is ejected from its inner shell, causing a vacancy

- Ejected orbital electron is called a photoelectron (may interact with other atoms, causing excitation or ionization) until all kinetic energy has been spent
- Increased patient dose contributes to biologic damage to tissues
- The original ionized atom is unstable from this interaction and attempts to restabilize; an electron from a higher shell drops down to fill the vacancy by releasing energy as a characteristic photon
- Cascade effect of dropping electrons continues until the original atom regains its stability

4. Pair production
   - Does not occur unless the energy of the incident x-ray photon is at least 1.022 megaelectron volts (MeV)
   - Incoming x-ray photon strongly interacts with the nucleus of an atom of the irradiated biologic tissue and disappears
   - The energy of the photon is transformed into two new particles: a negatron (electron) and a positron (positively charged electron)
   - Electron loses its kinetic energy by exciting and ionizing atoms in its path
   - Positron and electron annihilate each other, resulting in two 0.511 MeV photons moving in opposite directions
   - Probability for occurrence from at least 1.022 MeV, but becomes significant at 10 MeV x-ray energies and above
   - Annihilation radiation used in positron emission tomography (PET)
   - Useful in therapeutic radiology

5. Photodisintegration
   - Interaction that occurs above 10 MeV in high-energy radiation therapy treatment machines
   - Energy range is far above useful diagnostic range
   - High-energy photon collides with the atom's nucleus, which absorbs all of the photon's energy
   - Energy excess in the nucleus creates an instability that is alleviated by the emission of a neutron by the nucleus
   - May also result in emission of a proton or proton–neutron combination (deuteron) or alpha particle
   - Results in a radioactive nucleus

Attenuation by Various Tissues

Attenuation is the reduction in the number of primary photons in the x-ray beam through absorption (loss of radiation energy) and scatter (change in direction of travel resulting in loss of radiation energy).

Thickness of Body Part

The density of different body structures affects and influences attenuation.

The denser a body part is, the more photon absorption occurs.

Density and atomic number (Z) of body structures play a role in determining attenuation.

Bone is twice as dense as soft tissue and will absorb approximately nine times as many photons in the diagnostic range as soft tissue.

The thickness factor of a body part is a linear relationship.

A thicker structure will absorb twice as many photons.

Type of Tissue

Based on the type of tissue involved in the procedure, the following are true:

Z increases as the energy of the photon decreases

Compact bone has a Z of 13.8

Calcium has a Z of 20

Soft tissue has a Z of 7.4

Air has a Z of 7.6

MINIMIZING PATIENT EXPOSURE

Exposure Factors

Technical exposure considerations should be taken into account when reducing exposure to patients. The radiographer is primarily responsible for the chosen technical factors used during a radiographic examination.

Kilovoltage Peak

Kilovoltage peak (kVp) determines the energy level of the photons in the x-ray beam. The quality of the x-ray beam and its penetrating power is controlled by this factor.

- Increase in kVp without compensation for other factors results in increased patient dose.
- Decrease in kVp is desirable to reduce patient dose.
- Increase in kVp with compensation results in a significant reduction in patient dose.
- kVp is dependent on generator phase.

Milliamperes per Second

Milliamperes per second (mA/s) is the product of the electron tube current and the amount of time in seconds that the x-ray tube is activated. It is also the main determinant of how much radiation is directed toward the patient.

- Decrease in mA/s results in less patient dose
- Increase in mA/s with compensation by a decrease in kVp results in an increase in patient dose

- Inverse relationship between mA/s and kVp in maintaining radiographic density

Selection of appropriate technical factors to ensure sufficient penetration, adequate density, and a balanced amount of radiographic contrast between adjacent tissue densities is based on:

Mass of the clinical area of interest

Densities of the tissues

Film-screen combination or other type of image receptor

Source-to-image distance (SID)

Type and quantity of filtration used

Type of x-ray generator used

Balance of radiographic density and contrast

Use of standardized technique charts when automatic exposure control (AEC) is not available:

Uniform selection of exposure factors

Efficient imaging on each unit

Minimal patient dose with diagnostic radiographic image produces:
- Higher-quality images
- Fewer repeated images

Use of high kVp and low mA/s will reduce patient dose but will produce a poor-quality image.

Increase in kVp with a decrease in mA/s reduces radiographic contrast.

Diagnostic information may be reduced as a result.

Choose the highest practical kVp and the lowest possible mA/s to yield sufficient information on the image.

Shielding

In order to minimize exposure to the patient, proper protective apparel must be available in lead or lead-equivalent material.

Beam Restriction

In addition to shielding, other types of protective devices and equipment must be incorporated into the radiographic examination room.

X-ray beam limitation devices may be employed to ensure automatic collimation of the primary beam, which in modern equipment is provided through light-localizing variable-aperture rectangular collimators. Types include:

- Light-localizing variable-aperture rectangular collimator—consists of two sets of adjustable lead shutters which help to reduce off-focus or stem radiation and further confine the radiographic beam to the area of interest

- Positive beam limitation (PBL)—consists of electronic sensors in the cassette holder that, when activated, automatically adjust the collimators so the field matches the size of the image receptor; state regulations state that PBL must be within 2% to 3% of the SID
- Aperture diaphragms—the most simple beam limitation device; consists of a flat piece of lead with a hole of designated size and shape cut in its center; used in trauma imaging, chest radiography, and dental radiographic procedures
- Cones—may be used for areas such as the head or projections of the paranasal sinuses; circular metal tubes that attach to the x-ray tube housing to limit the x-ray beam to a predetermined size and shape; used in dental radiography
- Cylinders—similar to cones

Purpose of Primary Beam Restriction

Primary beam restriction is employed in radiography to decrease the area of the x-ray beam, helping reduce the amount of radiation absorbed and scattered by the patient.

Filtration

In order to minimize patient exposure, conventional x-ray tubes possess additional filters made of aluminum to aid in reducing low-energy photons so that the resulting x-ray beam is of higher quality and energy.

This hardening of the beam may be accomplished in two ways:

1. Inherent filtration
   - The glass envelope encasing the x-ray tube, the insulating oil surrounding the tube, and the glass window in the tube housing amount to 0.5 mm aluminum equivalent.
   - Light-localizing variable-aperture rectangular collimator provides an additional 1 mm aluminum equivalent through the reflective surface of the collimator mirror.
2. Added filtration
   - Usually consists of sheets of aluminum (or equivalent) of appropriate thickness
   - Located outside the glass window of the tube housing above the collimator's shutters
   - Readily accessible to service personnel and may be changes as the tube ages

Effect on Skin and Organ Exposure

- Use of filtration on the skin and organs assists in reducing exposure to the patient.
- Absorption of low-energy photons results in a decrease of the intensity of the radiation.

- The photons that are not absorbed by the filtration are more penetrating.
- Patient-absorbed dose is decreased.

Effect on Average Beam Energy

- Use of filtration on average beam energy results in less low-energy photons that are absorbed.
- The quality of the beam is improved.
- Average beam energy is hardened.

NCRP Recommendations for Minimum Filtration in a Useful Beam

Minimum standards for filtration are as follows[1]:

- Total filtration of 2.5 mm aluminum equivalent for fixed x-ray units operating above 70 kVp
- Total filtration of 1.5 mm aluminum equivalent for fixed x-ray units operating at 50 to 70 kVp
- Total filtration of 0.5 mm aluminum equivalent for fixed x-ray units operating below 50 kVp
- Total filtration of 2.5 mm aluminum equivalent for mobile diagnostic units and fluoroscopic units

Exposure Reduction

Radiographic imaging equipment is designed for optimal reduction in exposure to the patient, radiologic technologist, and all personnel in the department. In order to properly ensure safety in the radiographic room, the following must be present:

1. Radiographic equipment, devices, and accessories
   - Protective tube housing
     Composed of lead-lined metal
     Leakage radiation measured at a distance of 1 meter (m) (3¼ feet) from the x-ray source does not exceed 100 milliroentgens per hour (mR/h) (2.58×10^{-5} coulombs per kilogram per hour [C/kg/h])
   - Correctly functioning control panel
     Technical factors including mA and kVp are seen indicators on panel
     Located behind a protective barrier that allows for patient observation during procedure
     Electrically connected to the x-ray equipment
     Indicates the exposure conditions and when the x-ray tube is energized through both visible (light) and audible (tone) signals
   - Radiographic examination table
     Strong enough to sustain the weight of a patient
     May have a floating tabletop or magnetic controls
     Uniform thickness and as radiolucent as possible
     Minimal absorption of radiation to aid in reducing patient dose
     Composed of C fiber

- SID indicator

  Measures the distance from anode focal spot to image receptor

  Manual measurement of distance via attached tape measure

  Lasers may be used to aid in deciphering distance

  Accuracy must be within 2% of the indicated SID

2. X-ray beam limitation devices

   - Ensures that the collimation does not exceed the size of the image receptor
   - Accomplished by providing the x-ray unit with a mechanism to adjust size and shape of beam automatically or manually:

     Light-localizing variable-aperture rectangular collimator—most commonly seen in modern equipment.

     Aperture diaphragm—simplest of all beam limitation devices

     Cones—may be flared metal tubes or straight cylinders, as well as beam-defining cones that are attached directly to the x-ray tube housing or variable rectangular collimator

3. Filtration

   - Reduces exposure to the patient's skin and superficial tissue by absorbing most of the lower-energy photons
   - Increases the quality of the x-ray beam by hardening the beam
   - Two types:

     a. Inherent filtration

        Includes the glass envelope encasing the x-ray tube, the insulating oil surrounding the tube, and the glass window in the housing

        Amounts to approximately 0.5 mm aluminum equivalent

        Light-localizing variable-aperture collimator mirror provides additional 1 mm aluminum equivalent

     b. Added filtration

        Consists of aluminum sheets of appropriate thickness located outside the glass window of the tube housing above the collimator shutters

        Readily accessible to service personnel and may be changed as needed

   - Total filtration is determined by kVp of x-ray unit.

     For fixed units operating below 50 kVp: 0.5 mm aluminum equivalent

     For fixed units operating between 50 and 70 kVp: 1.5 mm aluminum equivalent

For fixed units operating above 70 kVp: 2.5 mm aluminum equivalent

Mobile and fluoroscopic units require total permanent filtration of 2.5 mm aluminum equivalent

- Mammographic equipment filtration

  Mammographic equipment produces photons with energy ranging from 17 to 20 keV

  Molybdenum (Z = 42) and rhodium (Z = 45) used in filters

  Molybdenum filters require filtration of 0.03 mm

  Rhodium filters require filtration of 0.024 mm

- General radiographic equipment filtration

  Aluminum (Z = 13) is the metal used most frequently in filters because of its ability to effectively remove low-energy x-rays without decreasing the intensity of the beam

  Half-value layer (HVL) must be able to decrease the intensity of the x-ray beam by 50% of its initial value

- Compensating filters

  Composed of aluminum, lead-acrylic, or other materials

  May be used when partially attenuating x-rays are striking anatomy of varying thickness

  Wedge filter—provides uniform density by attaching to the lower rim of the collimator and is positioned so that the thicker part of the filter is directed toward the thinnest anatomy and the thinner part is towards the thickest anatomy

  Trough or bilateral wedge filter—compensating filter used in dedicated chest radiographic units to allow for adequate x-ray penetration and uniform density

4. Grids

   - Devices used to remove scattered x-ray photons that emerge from the patient before reaching the film or other image receptor
   - Made up of parallel radiopaque strips that alternate with low-attenuation strips of aluminum, plastic, or wood
   - Improves radiographic contrast and visibility of detail
   - Used when the thickness of the part is greater than 10 cm
   - Increases patient dose, but compromises by improving the quality of the recorded image and allowing for a greater quantity of diagnostic information to be presented
   - Higher-ratio grids lead to increases in patient dose but a better-quality image

- Different types of grids may be used during exams:
  Stationary
  Oscillating
5. Fluoroscopic equipment, devices, and accessories
   - Patient radiation exposure rate
   - Fluoroscopic imaging systems
   - Image intensification fluoroscopy
   - Intermittent, or pulsed, fluoroscopy
   - Limiting fluoroscopic field size
   - Technical exposure factors
   - Filtration
   - Source-skin distance (SSD)
   - Cumulative timing device
   - Exposure rate limitation
   - Primary protective barrier
   - Fluoroscopic exposure control switch
   - Mobile C-arm fluoroscopy
     C-shaped portable x-ray unit with an x-ray tube at one end of the arm and an image intensifier attached to the other end
     Used in operating room, cardiac imaging, and interventional procedures
     Potential for large radiation doses to patients and operators
     Minimal source-to-end-of-collimator-assembly distance of 12″ (30 cm)
     Minimal patient–image intensifier distance to reduce entrance dose
     X-ray tube position should be under patient to lessen scatter radiation to patient and surrounding personnel
   - Cinefluorography
     Film size
     High-dose-rate procedures
     Filming frame rate
     Inference of patient dose from tabletop exposure levels
     Collimation
     Dose-reduction techniques
     Patient dose determined by procedure
   - Digital fluoroscopic equipment, devices, and accessories
     Pulsed progressive systems for dose reduction
     Last-image-hold feature for dose reduction
   - High-level-control interventional procedures
     Justification for use of high-level-control fluoroscopy (HLCF)
     Public health advisory regarding dangers of overexposure of patients and exposure rate limits
     Use of fluoroscopic equipment for nonradiologist physicians

Patient Communication

- Effective communication through an exchange of information to alleviate patient's uneasiness during examination
- Verbal messages and body language play an important role in establishing rapport with a patient
- Clear and concise instructions will result in increased cooperation with the patient
- Reduce the incidence of repeat examinations through good and honest communication

Digital Imaging

The use of the computer in imaging has transformed how radiography is evolving. Technologists now have the ability to access images at several workstations.

Pediatric Dose Reduction

Children are most vulnerable to biologic damage caused by exposure to ionizing radiation. Late somatic and genetic effects are greater for children who undergo diagnostic x-ray studies. Appropriate radiation protection methods should be employed to reduce pediatric dose.

- Smaller radiation doses: entrance exposure below 5 mR
- Patient motion and motion reduction methods: use of short exposure times and effective immobilization techniques
- Cooperation methods: rooms that are pediatric friendly with entertainment devices, restraint devices, cartoons, posters, and puppets
- Gonadal shielding: varies based on the age and size of the child, especially girls
- Gonadal dose: dose caused by internal scatter
- Collimation: extremely important in pediatric procedures
- Patient protection for children: particularly in CT scanning protocols; adult routines are not appropriate for children and must be adjusted accordingly

As Low as Reasonably Achievable (ALARA) Concept

Set in motion by the National Committee on Radiation Protection (now known as the National Council on Radiation Protection and Measurements or NCRP) in 1954, the ALARA concept states the following:

- Occupational exposure of the radiographer and other occupationally exposed individuals should be kept ALARA with consideration of economic and social factors

- Actual effective and EqD values should be kept far below allowable maximum limits
- Linear, nonthreshold relationship stating that biologic effect and radiation dose are directly proportional
- Requires the use of radiation control procedures

Sources of Radiation Exposure

Radiation sources are generated in an x-ray room and are classified as primary, scatter, and leakage radiation. Scatter and leakage radiation are categorized as secondary radiation.

Primary X-ray Beam

- The primary radiation that is emitted from the x-ray tube is known as direct radiation.
- Energy from direct radiation has not been degraded from scatter.
- Energy from direct radiation has not been attenuated.
- A wall that is in the direct path of the primary x-ray beam must be properly shielded to be safe for the workers and the general public.

Secondary Radiation

Secondary radiation includes the categories of scatter and leakage radiation.

- Scatter radiation: results whenever a diagnostic x-ray beam passes through matter; is the occupational hazard in diagnostic radiology; Compton interactions result from this type of radiation; the patient is the main source of scatter radiation; use of beam limitation devices, collimation or PBL, and variable apertures decrease the incidence of Compton scatter
- Leakage radiation: results from the radiation generated in the x-ray beam that is not emitted through the collimator opening but from the housing; permissible exposure rate of 100 mR/h at 1 m
- Patient as source: scattered radiation as a result of Compton interaction may be minimized at a 90-degree angle to the primary x-ray beam at a distance of 1 m; scattered x-ray intensity is approximately 1/1,000 of the intensity of the primary x-ray beam in this location

Basic Methods of Protection

The basic methods of protection are demonstrated in the triad of time, distance, and shielding.

Time

Minimize the amount of time that a radiation worker is exposed to ionizing radiation. Risk of exposure is directly proportional.

Distance

The most effective means of protection from ionizing radiation is based on the inverse square law (ISL). The ISL states, "the intensity of radiation is inversely proportional to the square of the distance from the source."[3]

Shielding

Shielding is used when it is not possible to use time and distance to minimize occupational radiation exposure. Common materials used in structural protective barriers include:

Lead
Concrete

Common protective apparel is made of lead-impregnated vinyl and includes:

Aprons and gloves—must be at least 0.25 mm thickness of lead; 0.5 or 1 mm lead equivalent offers greater protection; 0.5 mm lead equivalent is recommended as the minimum for occupationally exposed individuals

Neck and thyroid shields—should possess a minimum of 0.5 mm lead equivalent

Protective eyeglasses—should possess a minimal lead equivalent of 0.35 mm; wraparound frames are available in 0.5 mm lead equivalent

The protective apparel provides protection from ionizing radiation when structural protective barriers including stationary (fixed) or mobile barriers are not available. Effectiveness of the shielding materials depends on the Z, density, and thickness used.

Protective Devices

Within facilities that house radiation-emitting equipment used for diagnostic purposes, protective structures must be established to ensure the safety of the workers and the general public.

Types

Lead sheets and lead-equivalent or concrete barriers of appropriate thickness are used in shielding in primary and secondary protective barriers.

Primary protective barriers prevent direct or unscattered radiation from reaching others on the opposite side of the barrier.

- X-ray photons in the primary beam follow straight-line paths.
- Primary protective barriers are located perpendicular to the path of the beam.

Secondary protective barriers protect against secondary radiation leakage and scatter radiation that has been deflected from the primary beam.

- Leakage from the tube housing a concern

Control-booth barriers protect the radiographer during an examination.

- Must extend 7 feet upward from floor and must be secured to it
- Diagnostic x-rays must scatter at least two times before reaching any area behind the barrier
- Intercepts only leakage and scatter radiation
- Personnel must remain completely behind booth for maximal protection
- Exposure of the radiographer will not exceed a maximum of 1 mSv (100 mrem) per week
- Exposure cord must be short enough that the exposure switch can only be operated from behind the control-booth barrier

Clear lead-plastic secondary barrier is another option for a facility.

- Contains approximately 30% lead by weight
- Provides a modern appearance to a facility
- Allows a complete view of the examination room
- Modular x-ray barriers are shatter resistant

Clear lead-plastic overhead protective barrier may be used in addition to a special procedures or interventional radiology suite.

Attenuation Properties
The attenuation properties of the protective devices used

Minimum Lead Equivalent
- Primary barriers consists of $\frac{1}{16}''$ lead and extends 7 feet from the floor with the x-ray tube 5 to 7 feet from the primary wall.
- Secondary barrier should overlap primary protective barrier by about $\frac{1}{2}''$ and consists of $\frac{1}{32}''$ lead.
- Lead glass in booth contains 1.5 mm lead equivalent.
- Clear lead-plastic secondary barriers extend 7 feet upward from floor and are available in lead equivalency from 0.3 to 2 mm.
- Clear lead-plastic overhead shielding available at 0.5 mm lead equivalent.[1]

Fluoroscopy
Personnel protection during fluoroscopic procedures ensures protection from scattered radiation coming from the patient.

- Radiographer should stand as far away from the patient as possible yet close enough to assist when needed.

- Protective apron of 0.5 mm lead equivalent must be worn with protective lead gloves of 0.25 mm lead equivalent.
- Thyroid shields of 0.5 mm lead equivalent should also be worn.
- Stand behind the radiologist or behind the control booth barrier until needed.
- If assistance is required during exam, personnel should wear wraparound protective aprons.
- Protective drapes or spot film device protective curtain contains a minimum of 0.25 mm lead equivalent and are positioned between the fluoroscopist and the patient to intercept scatter above the tabletop.
- Protective Bucky slot cover contains a minimum of 0.25 mm lead equivalent and automatically covers the Bucky slot opening during standard fluoroscopic procedures. Cover provides protection at the gonadal region of the radiologist and radiographer. Exposure rate without device would exceed 100 mR/h at a distance of 2 feet from the side of table.
- Rotating schedules mean radiographers spend less time in higher-radiation tasks to decrease exposure and employ time as a means of radiation protection.
- Cumulative timer must be provided and used with each fluoroscopic unit. The timer is resettable and sounds an alarm after 5 minutes of use. Total fluoroscopic beam time is indicated and documented for each procedure.

Guidelines for Fluoroscopy and Portable Units
- NCRP mandates that the SSD be no less than 15″ for stationary fluoroscopes
- NCRP mandates that the SSD be no less than 12″ for mobile fluoroscopes
- Exposure rate limitation indicates that current federal standards limit entrance skin exposure rates to a maximum of 10 R per minute (/min)
- High-level control units permit 20 R/min
- Primary protective barrier of 2 mm lead equivalent for the image intensifier unit
- Fluoroscope must not be activated when in parked position
- Fluoroscopic exposure control switch must be of deadman type[1,4]

RADIATION EXPOSURE AND MONITORING

Despite NCRP-recommended dose limits of 50 mSv per year (/y) (5,000 mrem/y) for radiologic technologists, it is more beneficial to keep occupational radiation exposure for technologists at or below 1 mSv/y (100 mrem/y).[6] Generally speaking, radiologists will receive higher exposures than technologists due to radiologists' participation in fluoroscopic procedures and their relation to the patient as the radiation source.

Units of Measurement: Conventional and SI Units

- Absorbed dose (rad)
- Dose equivalent (rem)
- Exposure (R)

NCRP Recommendations for Personnel Monitoring

- The NCRP provides the most recent guidance on radiation protection: "to prevent the occurrence of serious radiation-induced conditions (acute and chronic deterministic effects) in exposed persons and to reduce stochastic effects in exposed persons to a degree that is acceptable."[5]
  Occupational exposure
  Public exposure
  Fetus exposure
  ALARA and EqD limits
  Evaluation and maintenance of personnel dosimetry records

MEDICAL EXPOSURE OF PATIENTS

- Detailed in NCRP Report No. 160[6]
- Typical effective dose per exam
- Comparison of typical doses by modality

REVIEW QUESTIONS

1. The principle effect of radiation on humans is:

   a. Direct effect
   b. Indirect effect
   c. Target theory
   d. None of the above

2. Damage to vital biologic macromolecules occurs as a result of which types of interactions?

   a. Characteristic and coherent
   b. Compton and k-edge
   c. Photodisintegration and characteristic
   d. Photoelectric and Compton

3. Radiolysis results in production of damaging _____.

   a. Hydrogen radical (H*) and hydroxyl ion (OH−)
   b. Hydroxyl ion (OH+) and hydrogen ion (H−)
   c. H* and hydroxyl radical (OH*)
   d. O_2H_2

4. During direct-hit interactions, x-ray photons "hit" the target molecule and the damage becomes apparent during which phase of the cell cycle?

   a. G_1
   b. Metaphase
   c. S
   d. Telophase

5. Irradiation of macromolecules within the human body is referred to as:

   a. In vivo
   b. In vitro
   c. Ex vivo
   d. Ex vitro

6. Identify the three observed effects that occur after a population has been exposed to an acute radiation exposure.

   a. Cell mutation, genetic anomalies, human death
   b. Cell death, point lesions, sterility
   c. Mutations, cancer, infertility
   d. Malignancies, apoptosis, genetic deviations

7. Tissues that are _____ with a _____ metabolic rate are more radiosensitive.

   a. Immature, low
   b. Immature, high
   c. Mature, low
   d. Mature, high

8. _____ is a measure of the rate of energy that is transferred from ionizing radiation to soft tissue.

   a. LET
   b. RBE
   c. MeV
   d. OER

9. A protracted dose of radiation is given:

   a. Over a long period of time
   b. All at one short exposure
   c. In a series of separate doses
   d. In two large doses

10. The tissue in the _____ is more radiosensitive than _____ tissue.

    a. Bone marrow, skin
    b. Brain, cornea
    c. Muscle, gonadal
    d. Brain, lymphoid

11. Tissue is _____ radiosensitive under high O conditions and _____ radiosensitive under hypoxic conditions.

    a. Less, equally
    b. Less, more
    c. More, less
    d. More, equally

12. Radiation-induced cancer, leukemia, and genetic effects follow which type of dose-response relationship?

    a. Linear, nonthreshold dose-response
    b. Nonlinear, threshold dose-response
    c. Linear, threshold dose-response
    d. Nonlinear, nonthreshold dose-response

13. The dose of radiation that causes 50% of irradiated subjects to die within 60 days is referred to as:

    a. $LD_{60/50}$
    b. $LD_{50/50}$
    c. $LD_{30/50}$
    d. $LD_{50/60}$

14. The human application of radioprotective agents would _____.

    a. Double radiation damage
    b. Be fatally toxic
    c. Reduce radiation effects by half
    d. Reduce radiation effects by one-fourth

15. The amount of radiation that is permitted to escape from the x-ray tube is less than _____ at 1 m from the tube housing.

    a. 5 mR/h
    b. 50 mR/h
    c. 10 mR/h
    d. 100 mR/h

REFERENCES

1. National Council on Radiation Protection and Measurements. Report no. 102: medical x-ray, electron beam and gamma-ray protection for energies up to 50 MeV (equipment design, performance and use). http://www.ncrppublications.org/Reports/102. Published June 1989. Accessed April 4, 2013.

2. Sherer M, Visconti P, Ritenour ER. *Radiation Protection in Medical Radiography*. 6th ed. Maryland Heights, MO: Mosby Elsevier; 2011: 259.

3. Sherer M, Visconti P, Ritenour ER. *Radiation Protection in Medical Radiography*. 6th ed. Maryland Heights, MO: Mosby Elsevier; 2011: 287.

4. US Food and Drug Administration. *Food and drugs.* 21 CFR. http://www.accessdata.fda.gov/scripts/cdrh/cfdocs/cfCFR/CFRSearch.cfm. Updated April 1, 2012. Accessed April 4, 2013.

5. National Council on Radiation Protection and Measurements. Report no. 116: limitation of exposure to ionizing radiation. http://www.ncrppublications.org/Reports/116. Published March 1993. Accessed April 4, 2013.

6. National Council on Radiation Protection and Measurements. Report no. 160: ionizing radiation exposure of the population of the United States. http://www.ncrppublications.org/Reports/160. Published March 2009. Accessed April 4, 2013.

SUGGESTED READINGS

Bushong S. *Radiologic Science for Technologists: Physics, Biology and Protection*. 9th ed. St. Louis, MO: Mosby; 2008.

Forshier S. *Essentials of Radiation Biology and Protection*. 2nd ed. Clifton Park, NY: Delmar Cengage Learning; 2009.

Shapiro J. *Radiation Protection: A Guide for Scientists, Regulators, and Physicians*. 4th ed. Cambridge, MA: Harvard University Press; 2002.

Stabin M. *Radiation Protection and Dosimetry: An Introduction to Health Physics*. New York, NY: Springer Science+Business Media, LLC; 2010.

CHAPTER 3

Equipment Operation and Quality Control

The Equipment Operation and Quality Control portion of the ARRT Examination in Radiography comprises 11% of the examination, corresponding to 22 total questions on the examination. The content specifications for this examination category include three sections:

1. Principles of Radiation Physics
2. Imaging Equipment
3. Quality Control of Imaging Equipment and Accessories

PRINCIPLES OF RADIATION PHYSICS

X-ray Production

The production of x-radiation is the result of the interaction of rapidly moving electrons from the cathode end of the x-ray tube with the atoms within the target. There are three requirements associated with x-ray production:

1. Source
2. Force
3. Target

Source of Free Electrons

- The phenomenon of thermionic emission occurs at the cathode within the filament, which is located in the focusing cup of the tube.
- Thermionic emission results in electrons being released from a heated filament within the tube.
- The higher the temperature of the filament, the greater the number of electrons released through thermionic emission; with a high filament temperature, outer shell electrons of the filament atoms are "boiled off" and ejected from the filament, making them available for the production of x-rays.
- These free electrons, when emitted from the filament, are then held near the vicinity of the filament in the negatively charged focusing cup within an electron cloud called the *space charge*.

- The space cloud prevents additional electrons from being released from the heated filament because of electrostatic repulsion referred to as the *space charge effect*.
- This cloud of electrons is now available for the production of x-radiation.

Focusing of Electrons

- The negatively charged focusing cup that contains the electron cloud or space charge aids in the centering of the x-ray beam as kilovoltage (kV) is applied.
- With the acceleration of negatively charged electrons from the cathode to the anode's target, the electron beam will have the tendency to spread beyond the target without a focusing cup.
- The focusing cup size, shape, and negative charge help it to electrostatically confine the projectile electrons to a small area of the anode's target.
- This allows for a greater number of projectile electrons to be directed toward the target atoms, allowing for the production of x-radiation.

Acceleration of Electrons

- Kinetic energy in the form of kV is applied to the free electrons located at the cathode.
- This applied kV determines the wavelength of the resulting radiation as well as the efficiency of the production of the x-ray.
- The purpose of this energy is to promote the movement of the electrons from the cathode to the anode. As the kinetic energy of the electrons increases, the efficiency of x-radiation produced also increases. In addition to this, the intensity (quantity) and the energy (quality) of the x-ray beam increases.
- These electrons in motion are referred to as *projectile electrons*; projectile electrons travel the distance between the filament and the x-ray target. The distance travelled is approximately 1 centimeter (cm).

- Electrons in motion also make up the current within the x-ray tube; this current, through the application of kV, comes into direct contact with the heavy metal atoms of the x-ray tube target located in the anode.
- Energy transfers from the projectile electrons to the target atoms through these initial interactions.

Deceleration of Electrons

Electron interactions occur through a shallow depth into the target; however, they result in the deceleration and eventual stoppage of these projectile electrons.[1] As a consequence of these interactions, the projectile electrons may do either of the following:

- Slow down as they come into close proximity to the nuclear field
- Interact with the electrons located in the target atom's orbital shells

Target Interactions

As the projectile electrons interact with the target atoms:

- The interactions that occur with the outer shell electrons do not transfer enough energy to knock them out of orbit or to ionize them; yet, the excitation of these outer shell electrons is enough to raise their energy level.
- Through the leveling off of this raised energy level, outer shell electrons emit a large amount of infrared radiation.
- This infrared radiation or heat makes up approximately 99% of the kinetic energy of the projectile electrons.
- The remainder, less than 1% of the kinetic energy, is available for the production of x-radiation. This remaining less than 1% may result in two types of radiation:
  1. Bremsstrahlung radiation
  2. Characteristic radiation

Bremsstrahlung Radiation

Radiation that refers to the interaction of the projectile electron that is influenced by the nuclear field of the target atom is called *bremsstrahlung*.[2] With bremsstrahlung (brems) or braking radiation, the following occurs:

- The projectile electron loses its kinetic energy as it interacts with the nuclear field of the target atom and is also converted into electromagnetic (EM) radiation.
- Owing to the positive charge of the target atom's nucleus and the negative charge of the projectile electron, an electrostatic force draws these participants closer, causing a varying degree of kinetic energy loss.
- This varying degree of kinetic energy loss results from the slowing down or braking of the projectile electrons as they pass the nucleus of the target atom; this force causes a change in direction, a loss of kinetic energy that comes off as an x-ray photon.
- The amount of energy that comes from bremsstrahlung radiation is dependent on what kV is used for the exposure; brems can be produced at any projectile electron energy. Therefore, the range of energies is wide when associated with brems interactions and depends on:
  Electron speed
  Proximity to nucleus
- Low-energy brems x-rays result in the projectile electron being poorly influenced by the strength of the nuclear field.
- In contrast, maximum-energy brems x-rays result in the projectile electron losing all kinetic energy and drifting away from the nucleus.
- The majority of radiation that is produced at the target atom is classified as bremsstrahlung and occurs between the low- to maximum-energy extremes listed above.
- At 100 kilovoltage peak (kVp), 85% of radiation produced is bremsstrahlung; the remaining 15% of radiation can be classified as characteristic radiation.

Characteristic Radiation

Radiation that refers to the interaction of the projectile electron with a k-orbit electron in the target may result in ionization and eventual production of characteristic radiation.[2] With characteristic radiation, the following occurs:

- Projectile electron interacts with a tightly bound k-orbit electron in the target of the anode.
- This k-shell electron experiences enough energy to knock it out of its place in the orbit; the projectile electron is successful in totally removing the electron from its orbit, therefore making it an ion.
- This opening in the k-orbit is then replaced by an outer shell electron through a process referred to as *transition*.
- This transition is accompanied by the release of characteristic radiation and energy resulting from the difference between the binding energies of the orbital shells involved in this replacement process.
- The effective energy of characteristic x-rays increases with target elements of higher atomic number. The x-ray energies associated with characteristic

radiation have precisely fixed energies and form discrete spectrums.

- Characteristic x-rays may occur in orbital shells other than k-orbits, but only the k-characteristic x-rays of tungsten are useful for imaging; characteristic x-rays other than k x-rays have very low energy.

X-ray Beam

The x-ray beam occurs in the x-ray tube and originates via the space charge effect and thermionic emission at the filament within the focusing cup of the cathode. Through the application of kV, the electron cloud is accelerated in the form of projectile electrons in this x-ray beam to interact with the target at the anode.

Frequency and Wavelength

EM radiation in the form of x-rays possesses wavelength and frequency. The relationship between these properties is inverse; as wavelength increases, frequency decreases and vice versa.

- Frequency
  May be expressed as hertz (Hz).
  Can be described as the number of wavelengths that pass the point of observation per second.
- Wavelength
  May be expressed as meters (m).
  Can be described as the distance from one crest or point on a sine wave to another on the next.

Beam Characteristics

The quality (kV) and quantity (in milliamperes or mA) of the x-rays produced in the tube may be affected by changes in other factors as well; these factors include voltage ripple, target atomic number, and added filtration. While the majority of the characteristics of the heterogeneous x-ray beam depend mainly on two exposure factors, these additional factors must be taken into consideration when evaluating x-ray emissions through graphical representation.

1. Quality (voltage)
   The higher the kVp, the higher the effective energy of the x-ray beam, which translates to greater quality of the x-ray production. On the x-ray emission spectrum, this would be demonstrated by the average energy shifting to the right, indicating a hardening of the x-ray beam.
2. Quantity (current)
   The larger the area under the emission spectrum, the greater the amount of radiation energy produced or the higher the x-ray intensity. On the x-ray emission

spectrum, this would be demonstrated by the average energy increasing in height and quantity.
3. Filtration
   The use of added filtration externally in the x-ray tube aids in the selective removal of low-energy x-rays from the beam. While this reduces the intensity of the x-ray produced, filtration increases effective energy of the x-ray beam.
4. Target material
   The composition of the target material affects both the amplitude (quantity) and the energy (quality) of the x-rays produced.
   - The higher the atomic number, the greater the efficiency of brems radiation produced.
   - In addition to this, the high-energy x-rays increase in number over the low-energy x-rays.
5. Voltage waveform and generator
   The type of voltage waveform and generator used in the production of x-rays has an effect on quantity and quality of the resulting beam.
   - The less efficient the generator, the greater the voltage ripple.
   - The greater the voltage ripple, the lesser the intensity and energy of the x-ray beam produced.
   - The greater the efficiency of the generator, the less voltage ripple will occur.
   - The lesser the voltage ripple, the greater the intensity and energy of the x-ray beam produced.

Primary versus Remnant (Exit) Radiation

1. Primary radiation
   - Radiation that is produced in the x-ray tube
   - Emerges from the x-ray tube target
   - Consists of x-ray photons with heterogeneous energies
   - Produced when the target is bombarded with the electrons streaming at a high speed from the cathode end of the tube and these projectile electrons interact with the target atoms
2. Primary beam
   - Radiation that passes through the tube window.
   - X-ray photons in this beam can interact with atoms of the patient's body.
   - This energy transfer to the tissue is called *absorption*.
3. *Leakage radiation* refers to any x-rays present other than the primary beam.
4. Remnant radiation
   - Refers to the primary beam that exits the patient
   - May also be referred to as *exit radiation*
   - Is the radiation responsible for the formation of an image

Inverse Square Law

- The *inverse square law* refers to the way intensity of radiation decreases rapidly as the distance increases from the source.
- EM radiation is inversely related to the square of the distance from the source.
- This law may be applied to distances greater than seven times the longest dimension of the source.
- Should the distance from the source of radiation be doubled, the intensity of the radiation is reduced by 25% or one-fourth.
- Should the distance from the source of radiation be reduced by 50% or one-half its original distance, the intensity of the radiation is increased by a factor of four.

Fundamental Properties

- EM radiation such as x-rays depends on different factors.
- Photons are the measurement of EM energy, whether that radiation refers to x-rays or gamma rays.
- Energy of x-rays ranges from about 1 kiloelectron volt (keV) to 50 megaelectron volts (MeV) to gamma. Radiowaves give off the least amount of energy. Microwaves give off slightly more energy.
  Visible light gives off more energy than microwaves or radiowaves.
  X-rays and gamma are capable of giving off the most amount of energy.
- Frequency of the photons may be expressed as 10^{18} to 10^{23} Hz.
- Wavelength of the x-ray can be expressed as 10^{-9} to 10^{-12} m.
- Photons move at the speed of light, have no mass, and possess both electric and magnetic fields that constantly change in sine waves.
- EM energy may be described by three wave parameters:
  1. Velocity (constant)
  2. Frequency
  3. Wavelength
- Should frequency or wavelength of EM energy change, the value of the other will change accordingly. Velocity does not change and remains a constant (speed of light).
- Ionizing EM radiation is characterized by the energy contained in a photon.
- X-ray photons possess a higher frequency and shorter wavelength as compared to other types of EM energy.
- X-rays are produced outside of the nucleus in the electron shells of the excited atom for use in diagnostic imaging systems.

IMAGING EQUIPMENT

Components of a Radiographic Unit

Operating Console

The console of an x-ray system is where the technologist controls the energy that will produce an x-ray. There are normally four controls that are used:

1. The power switch to turn the system's power supply on or off
2. The kilovoltage control (kVp) to vary the amount of x-ray energy for proper penetration of an anatomical part
3. The mA control to vary the amount of current, which controls the density of the x-ray
4. The timer to control the amount of time the x-ray is on to make the correct exposure, measured in mA per second or mA/s

The X-ray Tube

The x-ray tube's major components are all housed in a leaded-glass casing and operate in a vacuum. The *anode* is a disk connected to a motor that spins at high speeds during an exposure. The outer edge of the disk is cut to an angle approximately 12 to 15 degrees. This angle is called the *target* and is made up of tungsten. The anode is positively charged.

On the other side of the x-ray tube is a component called the *cathode*. The cathode is negatively charged and emits electrons. During an x-ray exposure, electrons are accelerated toward the anode at an extremely high speed from the cathode. This high-speed flow of electrons directly hits the rotating anode disk (target). The resulting high-speed impact of electrons hitting the target on the rotating anode causes a large amount of heat along with a small percentage of x-rays, which deflect off the angled target and exit the x-ray tube to create an exposure.

- The anode is a rotating disk that is positively charged.
- The target is an angle cut on the outside edge of the rotating anode.
- The cathode emits electrons and the electrons are accelerated toward the target, creating heat and x-rays.

Electron Source

Electrons in an x-ray tube come directly from the cathode end of the tube, which contains a spiral wire made of tungsten. The tungsten wire is the source of the electrons. Most x-ray tubes have two wires of different sizes set in a small recessed area of the cathode. This recessed area is called a *focusing cup*. An electrical current is applied to one of the tungsten wires, resulting in heating. The filament glows just like the filament in a light bulb. The filament emits a small cloud of electrons through the glowing process. When the anode and cathode are energized, the electrons from the glowing filament are propelled and accelerated at a very high speed, striking the anode and creating the x-ray. The majority of the energy is dissipated as heat.

- Most x-ray tubes have two different-sized spiral wires to emit electrons (a dual-focus tube).
- Spiral wires glow like a light bulb, emitting a cloud of electrons.
- An x-ray is produced when the electrons are propelled to strike the anode target.

Target Materials

The anode side of the x-ray tube is a positively charged disk that rotates at high speed during the x-ray process. The outer edge of the anode is cut at an angle to deflect the x-ray energy out of the x-ray tube. This outer angled edge is called the *target* and is constructed of tungsten. During the x-ray process, high amounts of heat are generated in the x-ray tube when the electrons are striking the target. Tungsten is a very hard material that has a high melting point and is able to withstand the high heat generated during the exposure process. The production of x-rays creates high heat that needs to be dissipated. X-ray tubes have a cooling system that circulates oil in the insulation to carry off the heat.

- The target of a rotating anode is made of tungsten.
- High amounts of heat are generated at the target during the x-ray exposure.
- The x-ray tube uses oil to dissipate the heat.
- Tungsten is an extremely hard material with a high melting point.

Induction Motor

The induction motor of a rotating anode in an x-ray tube needs to be made of a material resistant to high heat. The motor is made up of two parts, the *stator* and the *rotor*.

The stator is made up of a series of magnets around the tube near the neck designed to operate together to create a current to spin the rotor. The rotor is made up of copper bars and soft iron. When the rotor spins at a high rate, the heat that is generated at the target is dissipated over a large area for better cooling of the x-ray tube and more load capacity.[1]

- An induction motor of an x-ray tube needs to be made of a material resistant to high heat.
- There are two parts of an induction motor: the stator and the rotor.

- The rotor spins at a high rate during the x-ray process to dissipate heat.

Automatic Exposure Control

Automatic exposure control (AEC) is a device incorporated into the x-ray system that measures the correct amount of radiation reaching image detectors. These detectors use *ionization chambers* that respond to the x-ray beam. During the x-ray exposure, when a predetermined density is reached, the x-ray exposure is terminated automatically. Sensors are normally located in x-ray tables and chest units. There are usually three sensors, and depending on specific anatomical interest, the radiologic technologist (RT) will position the patient over the appropriate sensor and choose one of the three to obtain the proper image density. Proper positioning is very important when using AEC. AEC can be adjusted in small increments above or below set exposure values. The settings usually average from a −2 up to a +2 density. These small adjustments may be necessary depending on patient size and/or pathology. In AEC systems, a backup timer is used to override the x-ray exposure system. It is a safety feature built into the x-ray system to shut down if it reaches the maximum exposure level or if the x-ray is on for an extended period of time, limiting excessive radiation to the patient. Backup timers are also needed in the event of an equipment malfunction or operator error to safely shut down the x-ray exposure.

- AEC measures the correct amount of radiation during an exposure.
- Using AEC, the radiologist needs to properly position the patient over the exposure detectors.
- Small adjustments using plus or minus settings can be made using AEC depending on patient size and/or pathology.
- Backup timers are used to limit exposure when maximum radiation levels are reached or when there is a possible equipment malfunction or operator error.

Manual Exposure Controls

Manual exposure control allows the RT to control a kVp value, which determines how much energy is required to penetrate the part of interest. Excessive amounts of kVp can produce an image that may have loss of detail and less than desirable contrast. Insufficient kVp values may underpenetrate the patient, resulting in lighter, undiagnostic areas.

Another manual x-ray control is the mA control. This is used in conjunction with the time control to make an x-ray exposure. mA is used to set the proper density of an x-ray image; it controls the quantity of radiation. The timer is used to deliver the mA in milliseconds. Proper kVp, mA, and time will produce an image with good penetration along with good contrast and detail.

- Manual exposure control allows the imaging specialist the ability to manipulate kV, mA, and time to properly make an x-ray exposure while reducing radiation dose to the patient.
- kV values control penetrating radiation; too much or too little will affect the image quality.
- mA controls the quantity of radiation and is used along with the exposure time to deliver the amount of radiation in a given time.
- mA used with a given amount of time is calculated in mA/s.

Beam Restriction Devices

Beam-restricting devices control the size and shape of the x-ray beam to help reduce patient exposure and improve image quality. There are three different types of beam restriction devices:

1. Adjustable collimator on an x-ray tube.
2. Aperture diaphragm
3. Cones and cylinders

The collimator has a set of movable rectangular shutters that open and close and is located just below the x-ray tube. The collimator helps reduce dose to the patient and also eliminates areas that do not pertain to the part that is being x-rayed.

The aperture diaphragm consists of a flat piece of lead with a hole that is cut out of the center. The aperture can be cut to any size desired or bought in various sizes. The aperture diaphragm's function is the same as a collimator's, but the diaphragm is not manually adjustable. The diaphragms are attached just below the x-ray tube. The aperture diaphragm may cause a loss of resolution at the peripheral edges of the primary beam.

Other types of beam-restricting devices are cones and cylinders. These devices are similar to an aperture diaphragm; they have a specific opening but have an extended flange attached to the aperture. These are attached just below the x ray tube, like the aperture diaphragm. Cones and cylinders perform better than an aperture diaphragm at limiting unsharpness.

- Beam-restricting devices control the size and shape of the x-ray beam.
- A collimator is the most popular device used and has adjustable shutters to limit the area upon which the x-ray beam is projected.

- An aperture diaphragm is a cut hole in a piece of flat lead that is not adjustable and may cause some outer area unsharpness.
- Cones and cylinders are similar to an aperture diaphragm but will help limit unsharpness.

X-ray Generator, Transformers, and Rectification System: Basic Principles

Most x-ray systems have three main components:

1. High-voltage power supply to provide the energy to create the x-ray
2. Control unit to manipulate the power for the x-ray
3. X-ray tube to generate the x-ray

The high-voltage power supply consists of a transformer that takes incoming voltage and steps it up to a higher voltage required for x-ray production. There are two other types of x-ray transformers: The second type is a step-down transformer where the incoming voltage is stepped down to supply voltage to the filament of the x-ray tube. The third type of transformer is the autotransformer, which allows the operator to select the voltage needed to make an x-ray exposure.

In order for an x-ray tube to generate an x-ray, the voltage needs to be converted from alternating current (AC) to direct current (DC). DC is required because the anode needs to have a positive charge and the cathode needs to have a negative charge. In an AC circuit, the current would alternate from positive to negative on both anode and cathode and radiation could not be produced.

Once the step-up transformer provides the necessary power, it needs to be *rectified*, or changed from AC to DC. Changing from AC to DC will allow a difference in potential between the anode and cathode to produce an x-ray. When an exposure is made, electrons will accelerate to the anode side, striking the target and producing an x-ray.

Main components of an x-ray system:

- Transformer to step up the power
- Rectifier to change AC to DC
- X-ray tube to generate the x-ray

Phase Pulse and Frequency

The incoming power to supply an x-ray system is classified in phases. A system that uses one source of power is classified as *single phase*. A single-phase system uses one power line to supply energy to an x-ray system. The one power source would be displayed as a single sine wave showing a positive and negative peak. Each positive and negative peak is called a *pulse*; therefore, each wave contains 2 pulses. The power sources used in the United States alternate at a frequency of 60 Hz or 60 times per second or 120 pulses. X-ray systems operate using DC to make an exposure in the x-ray tube; therefore, the power has to be rectified.

When rectification occurs, a single-phase (single) sine wave is changed by taking the negative peak (or pulse) of the waveform and flipping it to the positive side of the sine wave. The waveform would look like two humps instead of a typical S pattern. Portable x-ray units use a single-phase system.

Three-phase x-ray systems are designed to use more power and are used in stationary x-ray equipment, as in a hospital. As a single-phase system uses only one sine wave, a three-phase system would take three power sources or three sine waves and stagger each 120 degrees out of phase, then rectify all three power sources. The resultant sine wave would take all the negative waveforms and flip them to the positive side, creating many multiple humps or peaks. Each sine wave operating at a frequency of 60 Hz or cycles per second would have 120 pulses. Since there are three power sources, there would be 360 pulses. Using three-phase power increases the efficiency of the x-ray unit.

- Single-phase power operates at 60 cycles per second or 60 Hz and consists of a positive and a negative pulse.
- Three-phase power combines three single-phase power sources and staggers or places them 120 degrees out of phase.
- Single-phase and three-phase power need to be rectified to create a difference of potential on the anode and cathode.

Components of Fluoroscopic Units (Fixed or Mobile)

A fluoroscopic unit is a real-time x-ray system that displays live images. A system consists of the following:

- Operator
- X-ray tube
- Image intensifier
- Display screen

The x-ray tube is normally positioned under the patient with the image intensifier above the patient. As the radiation passes through the patient, it strikes the large surface of the image intensifier called the *input phosphor*. The input phosphor converts the x-ray energy to light, and the image is projected and focused to a small area called the *output phosphor* at the top of the image intensifier. This process is called *minification*. Since the output phosphor is smaller than the input phosphor, the image gains brightness. At the top of the image intensifier is a small TV camera that displays the image on a screen for real-time viewing. The TV system is connected to a recorder where live digital images can be recorded for playback.

There are two types of fluoroscopy systems: conventional and digital. Conventional units use an image intensifier to create an image to display on a TV monitor. Digital fluoroscopy uses flat-panel detectors that replace image intensifiers. Digital fluoroscopy is more sensitive and operates at a lower dose than conventional fluoroscopic systems. Both systems incorporate automatic brightness control or ABC. As the position of the fluoroscopic unit changes over different body thicknesses, the ABC will adjust kVp or mA to give the operator consistent viewing of the displayed image.

The recording of fluoroscopic images can be done by a spot film device, which uses a film or digital cassette to record an image. Newer systems can acquire images digitally for immediate review.

- Fluoroscopic x-ray systems are used when real-time (live) images are needed.
- There are two types of fluoroscopic systems: conventional, where x-rays pass through an image intensifier and the image is projected on a TV monitor, and digital fluoroscopic x-ray systems, where flat-panel detectors are used.
- ABC automatically changes the kV or mA to provide a consistent viewing image as the thickness of a body part changes.

Components of Digital Imaging (Computed and Digital Radiography)

Digital imaging is a technology that is filmless and employs a reusable image receptor or imaging plate (IP). In computed radiography (CR), the image receptor uses a photostimulable phosphor (PSP) to capture an x-ray image. This latent image is stored in the image phosphor. In the processing sequence, the image phosphor is excited by a laser, which makes the stored image phosphoresce, and the image is captured through a series of optics and converted to a digital image. Even after the digital image is extracted from the IP, the latent image is still stored in the plate, which needs to be erased in order for the IP to be reused. The erasure process is the last step in the processing sequence. Once the image is converted to a digital image, the IP is exposed to a series of fluorescent lights, which removes the image and returns the IP back to a nonexcited state. The normal erasure process can take 60 seconds or more depending on how much energy was used in making an exposure. The more x-ray energy used to make an image, the longer the erasure process.

Flat-panel detectors are used in another type of digital imaging system called *digital radiography* (DR), where the image receptor (DR panel) has an array of electronic detectors that receives an x-ray image, converts the image electronically, and then converts it to a digital signal sent to a computer for viewing. There are two types of DR systems: direct and indirect. Indirect detectors use a scintillator, which is a device that detects and measures radiation, converts the x-ray energy to light, and then converts the light into an electronic charge from which the image is digitized and sent to a computer for viewing. A direct DR panel uses amorphous selenium, which is a material that directly converts an x-ray image to an electrical charge. The electrical charges from the image are then converted to a digital image and are sent to a computer for viewing.

The start-up and shut-down procedure in a CR or a DR system is a simple process. Both types of systems use computers, mostly PC-based programs. Depending on the manufacturer, there may be a procedure where the system reader needs to be shut down or started prior to viewing the system. In the shut-down sequence, depending on the manufacturer, there may be a procedure to turn off the IP reader or detector first, then a simple shut-down as in a standard PC. Improper start-up and shut-down may cause conflicts with the imaging program.

- Digital imaging employs a reusable IP or panel.
- There are two types of digital imaging systems: CR and DR.
- CR uses a PSP that retains an image where it is excited by a laser and optically extracted and converted to a digital image.
- A DR panel has two types of systems: indirect and direct.
- Indirect panels convert an image to light and then converts the light to an electronic signal and sends it to the computer.
- Direct panels convert an image directly to an electronic signal and send it to the computer.
- CR IPs are erased by using a bank of fluorescent lights to return them to their preexposed normal state.

Types of Units (Chest and Tomography)

Dedicated chest systems may incorporate automatic collimation, vertical tracking, AEC, and a Bucky. Older systems may have film stored in a magazine; once an image is taken, the film would be automatically fed into a film processor and developed.

Tomography uses an x-ray tube and image receptor that are directly connected and move in opposite directions during an exposure. During an exposure, the x-ray tube and image receptor move in an arc. The movement of the x-ray tube and image receptor creates a central axis or pivot point called the *fulcrum*. The patient is placed on the table and the fulcrum is placed at the area or plane of interest. During the exposure sequence, as the x-ray tube and image receptor move in an arc, the area of the fulcrum remains in focus while the areas above and below the fulcrum level remain out of focus and will be seen in the resulting image as a blur. The area where the fulcrum is set will be the only area of the image that is focused.

- Dedicated chest unit is a freestanding system designed for upright radiography.
- Dedicated systems can be digital or film-type systems.
- Digital chest units can use CR image detectors or DR panels.
- Tomography system can be an x-ray device where an x-ray tube and image receptor are connected and move in opposite directions. The center point is called the *fulcrum*.

Accessories

Grids are devices that filter out scatter or secondary radiation that may reduce image quality and detract from diagnostic interpretation. They are made up of lead strips that are minutely spaced in one direction corresponding to the direction of the x-ray beam. There are two types of grids commonly used in medical radiography: stationary and reciprocating.

Stationary grids can be incorporated into a standard film or digital image receptor or can be a separate plate placed on top of an image receptor. Since the grid is stationary, grid lines are usually detected on the resultant image, but not enough to deter image quality. A reciprocating grid is commonly called a *Bucky*. A Bucky grid is a system that moves the grid during an x-ray exposure. This movement of the grid blurs out the grid lines that would normally be seen with the use of a stationary grid and produces a clearer, uniform image. The Bucky system consists of an assembly that fits under an exam table or behind a freestanding chest unit. It contains a film tray to accommodate an image receptor and the grid, which is attached to a motor device that will move the grid during an exposure. Bucky systems can be moved along the table length to allow proper positioning under the anatomical area of interest.

- Grids filter out scatter radiation that may interfere with image quality.
- Stationary grids can be incorporated into image receptors, such as film, CR cassettes, or portable DR panels.

- Reciprocating grids are used in Bucky systems, in which the grid is motorized and moves during an x-ray exposure, blurring out the grid lines for a clearer image.
- All stationary grids can be used with all size image receptors and are used where it is not possible to use a Bucky, such as in cross-table laterals or portable examinations.

QUALITY CONTROL OF IMAGING EQUIPMENT AND ACCESSORIES

Beam Restriction

Beam restriction testing compares the light field produced by collimation to the radiation field. A simple method to compare the light field to the corresponding radiation field is to use radiopaque markers on the edges of the collimated area. In the United States, the x-ray field and light field need to be aligned to within 2% of the source-to-image distance (SID).

Another type of an alignment test uses a fluorescent plate that has a measured scale printed on the surface alignment, which allows checks to be performed without an image detector. When the plate is exposed, it produces a green fluorescence, which is visualized and lasts for a few minutes after the radiation ceases. The image can then be compared to the scaled lines on the plate.

Central ray alignment testing is done to ensure the x-ray beam is perpendicular to the image receptor. A tube is placed in the center of the image receptor or a fluorescent screen with the x-ray tube perpendicular to the plane of the x-ray tube. The tube is approximately 6″ high and approximately 1″ in diameter and can be plastic or aluminum. A low kVp and mA/s is used to make an exposure. The resultant test will show a concentric circle on the image if the beam is aligned properly. If the circle is not concentric, it will indicate a central ray adjustment is required.

- Occasional testing should be performed on beam restriction in collimators.
- Using an image receptor and radiopaque markers placed on coned edges of an x-ray light field is a simple test to check both the light field and the actual x-ray field.
- A commercially manufactured fluorescent plate can also be used; it will produce a green fluorescence after exposure to compare the light field with the radiation field.
- Central ray alignment can be tested using a 1″ diameter plastic or aluminum tube placed perpendicular to the x-ray beam on an image receptor to see if there is a concentric circle, indicating proper beam alignment.

Digital Imaging Receptor Systems
Artifacts

Digital imaging receptors are subject to artifacts. Artifacts can be debris shown on an image receptor, scratches, or even electronic problems from the software or hardware transport operations of the digital system.

Debris artifacts are usually seen as a light density where the image phosphor or panel behind the debris did not absorb the transmitted energy to produce the latent image. This debris can also deposit on the light guide in the CR optics, causing a light artifact as well.

Scratches can occur in CR and DR systems. Scratches are more common in CR where the IP can be subject to mechanical movement during the processing or erasure sequence, causing scratches on the imaging phosphor.

System erasure may also contribute to an imaging artifact by not uniformly erasing the image plate or panel. If a digital system does not apply adequate erasure time or there is a problem with the erasure system, a ghost image artifact will appear on the next image. In DR systems, the charge from a previous exposure can be trapped. If the DR panel is used again and erased, a ghost image appears on the next image.

Image detectors are subject to fogging. If they are not used for a period of time, an accumulation of fog will result. In CR, the image detector can absorb the inherent radiation that is in the environment. Over time, this inherent radiation will collect to a point that it would be seen on an exposure. It is recommended that before a detector is used at the beginning of each work day, it be placed in the erase cycle to clear up any fog on the detector.

Display monitors in a digital imaging system are subject to artifacts, which have a direct effect on digital image quality. The digital viewing monitor should be checked daily, monthly, and quarterly. An SMPTE (Society of Motion Picture and Television Engineers) pattern is an image commonly used to check the viewing monitor. The pattern consists of various line pairs that are computer generated to monitor sharpness, distortion, and luminescence and can be checked to assure the digital image is viewed properly.[3]

- Imaging artifacts can result from debris, scratches, software, or mechanical issues with digital imaging equipment.
- Improper erasure can contribute to imaging artifacts by producing a ghost image.
- Regular maintenance of digital equipment is required to ensure the safety of the patient and operator.
- Image detectors are subject to fog over a period of time if not used regularly. All digital imaging detectors

should go through an erase cycle at the beginning of the day to remove any accumulation of fog.

- Viewing monitors are subject to artifacts. Monitors should be checked daily, monthly, and quarterly.
- An SMPTE pattern is commonly used to check image quality and performance of viewing monitors.

Shielding Accessories

Periodic testing of lead aprons, gloves, and gonadal shields is important for patient and operator safety. Periodic tests of any shielding accessories should be performed regularly. Cracks and holes in shielding equipment can occur because of the frequent handling and use of these items. Shielding should be checked visually for any tears or possible cracks. The most commonly used test to check shielding is to "look-view"

it under fluoroscopy. Using fluoroscopy, any holes or cracks would be seen on the monitor. This is usually done on the manual setting. Automatic setting may cause excessive radiation when viewing shielding. Any holes in the shielding would show as a lighter density while the shielding would show as a darker density. Any defective shielding should be removed from service and properly disposed of to an environmentally secure organization or facility.

- Periodic testing of shielding is an important factor for patient and operator safety.
- Shielding should be visually checked for any tears or cracking.
- The most common way to test shielding is by using fluoroscopy.
- Any defective shielding should be properly disposed of.

REVIEW QUESTIONS

1. The component that controls the quantity of radiation is called a _____.

   a. kV controller
   b. mA controller
   c. Timer
   d. kV controller and timer

2. The charge of the anode is:

   a. Positive
   b. Negative
   c. Neutral
   d. Both positive and negative

3. The device in the x-ray tube that produces electrons is called:

   a. The filament
   b. The focusing cup
   c. The target
   d. The anode

4. The outer edge of an anode is constructed of which material?

   a. Copper
   b. Steel
   c. Tungsten
   d. Nickel

5. This device measures the amount of radiation reaching the image detector.

   a. Image intensifier
   b. Backup timer
   c. kVp selector
   d. AEC

6. Which of the following factors are important to consider specifically when using AEC?

   a. Proper patient positioning
   b. Voltage
   c. Image receptor size
   d. All of the answers are correct

7. The most commonly used beam restriction device used by the RT is:

   a. Collimator
   b. Aperture diaphragm
   c. Cone
   d. Cylinder

8. In order for x-radiation to occur, it is necessary for rapidly moving electrons to travel from the cathode end of the x-ray tube to the target of the anode. Three requirements associated with the production of x-ray are:

   a. Source
   b. Force
   c. Target
   d. All of the answers are correct

9. Interactions that occur in the tube result in:

   a. 99% of kinetic energy available for x-ray production
   b. 99% of kinetic energy available for infrared radiation production
   c. 1% of kinetic energy available for x-ray production
   d. 1% of kinetic energy available for infrared radiation production

10. These interactions within the x-ray tube may result in two types of radiation:

    a. Bremsstrahlung and Compton
    b. Bremsstrahlung and characteristic
    c. Coherent and Compton
    d. Coherent and characteristic

11. The radiation caused by the interaction of the projectile electron with a tightly bound k-orbit electron in the target of the anode is referred to as:

    a. Characteristic
    b. Compton
    c. Bremsstrahlung
    d. Coherent

12. EM radiation that results from the loss of kinetic energy in the projectile electron as it interacts with the nuclear field of the target atom is referred to as:

    a. Characteristic
    b. Compton
    c. Transition
    d. Bremsstrahlung

13. The amount of energy that comes from bremsstrahlung radiation is dependent on the kilovoltage applied in the exposure; therefore, it can be determined that brems radiation _____.

    a. Has a wide range of energies
    b. Has a discrete peak of energies
    c. Is only produced at low energy levels
    d. May or may not be produced with high mA/s

14. Low-energy brems x-rays may be the result of the projectile electron being:

    a. Greatly influenced by the nuclear field strength
    b. Poorly influenced by the nuclear field strength
    c. Uninfluenced by the nuclear field strength
    d. None of the above

15. At 100 kVp, the radiation produced is:

    a. 15% bremsstrahlung and 85% characteristic
    b. 15% characteristic and 85% bremsstrahlung
    c. 50% characteristic and 50% bremsstrahlung
    d. 30% bremsstrahlung and 70% characteristic

REFERENCES

1. Bushong S. *Radiologic Science for Technologists: Physics, Biology and Protection*. 9th ed. St. Louis, MO: Mosby; 2008.

2. Sherer M, Visconti P, Ritenour ER. *Radiation Protection in Medical Radiography*. 6th ed. Maryland Heights, MO: Mosby Elsevier; 2011.

3. Peck D. Quality assessment procedures for digital radiography. http://www.aapm.org/meetings/amos2/pdf/26-5959-83142-414.pdf. Accessed March 8, 2013.

CHAPTER 4

Image Acquisition and Evaluation

The Image Acquisition and Evaluation portion of the ARRT Examination in Radiography comprises 22.5% or 45 total questions on the examination. The content specifications for this examination category include three sections:

1. Selection of Technical Factors
2. Image Processing and Quality Assurance
3. Criteria for Image Evaluation

SELECTION OF TECHNICAL FACTORS

This section of the Image Acquisition and Evaluation portion of the ARRT examination consists of 20 total questions.

Factors Affecting Radiographic Quality

Factors affecting radiographic quality are divided into four main categories: density (brightness), contrast (gray scale), recorded detail (spatial resolution), and distortion (size or shape). Factors which influence each are listed below.

Density/Brightness

The ARRT describes density as the "degree of blackening or opacity of an area in a radiograph due to the accumulation of black metallic silver following exposure and processing of a film." Brightness is described as "the measurement of the luminance of a monitor calibrated in units of candela (cd) per square meter on a monitor or soft copy."[1] Factors affecting radiographic density or brightness are listed below.

Milliamperes and Time

The main factors controlling density are milliamperes (mA) and time (measured in seconds or s). mA controls the tube current at the filament, while the time (s) controls the length of time that the filament is charged.

The combination of mA and time is referred to as mA/s and affects the quantity of radiation and the amount of thermionic emission. mA/s and density are directly proportional: As mA/s increases, density increases; as mA/s decreases, density decreases.

Three laws describe the relationship between mA/s and density. These laws are called the laws of linearity, reciprocity, and reproducibility. The *law of linearity* states that doubling the mA/s doubles the amount of density of the resulting image, while halving the mA/s halves the density. The *law of reciprocity* states that different combinations of mA and time that produce the same mA/s will produce the same density. The *law of reproducibility* states that every time the same combination of mA and time is set on the same x-ray unit, the resulting images will demonstrate the same density.

- As mA/s increases, density increases.
- As mA/s decreases, density decreases.

Kilovoltage Peak

Kilovoltage peak (kVp) affects the quality (penetrating power) of the x-ray photons and affects density by influencing the penetration, transmission, absorption, and attenuation of x-rays. In order to ensure proper diagnosis, the anatomy of interest must be adequately penetrated. Anatomy that is underpenetrated or overpenetrated may result in poor visualization of the anatomy and possibly a missed diagnosis. As kVp increases, more penetrating x-ray photons readily pass through the anatomy, resulting in increased density. As kVp decreases, less penetrating x-ray photons are likely to be absorbed by the anatomy, decreasing the density. According to the *15% rule*, in order to double the density of an image, a 15% increase in kVp is required. To halve the radiographic density, kVp must be decreased 15%.

- As kVp increases, density increases.
- As kVp decreases, density decreases.

Source-to-Image Distance

Source-to-image distance (SID) refers to the distance from the x-ray source to the image receptor (IR). Because the x-ray beam diverges from the source, the number of x-ray photons reaching the IR will change at varying SIDs. SID and density are inversely proportional: As SID increases, density will decrease; as SID decreases, density will decrease. SID also affects radiation intensity: As SID increases, radiation intensity decreases; as SID decreases, radiation intensity increases. This is known as the *inverse square law*. The inverse square law states that the intensity of radiation is inversely proportional to the square of the distance from the x-ray source, or

$$\frac{I_1}{I_2} = \frac{(D_2)^2}{(D_1)^2}$$

In order to compensate for the change in distance, and as a result, the change in density and intensity, the *direct square law* is applied. The direct square law formula is:

$$\frac{mA/s_1}{mA/s_2} = \frac{(D_1)^2}{(D_2)^2}$$

- As SID increases, density decreases.
- As SID decreases, density increases.

Object-to-Image Distance

Object-to-image distance (OID) refers to the distance from the object being imaged to the IR. An OID of 6″ or greater (air gap) is required in order to affect density. The OID air gap causes much of the scatter radiation exiting the anatomy to miss the IR, thereby decreasing density. When the OID exceeds 6″, density will decrease. As OID continues to increase, density will further decrease.[2]

- As OID increases greater than 6″, density will decrease.

Grids

A grid is a device that contains lead strips, which are separated by an interspaced material (commonly aluminum [Al]). Grids are placed between the patient and IR and can be either reciprocating or stationary. The function of a grid is to increase contrast by absorbing scatter radiation that exits the patient, but by doing so, density will decrease. Grids are used in circumstances when large amounts of scatter will be exiting the patient; their use will degrade the image. It is suggested that grids be used when the part thickness is greater than 10 centimeters (cm) and the kVp exceeds 60.

The lead lines within a grid have a specific height, thickness, and distance between them, determining the grid ratio. The grid ratio is the ratio between the height of the lead lines and the distance between them. As the grid ratio increases, the grid will absorb more scatter. The formula for grid ratio is:

$$\frac{h}{D}$$

Grid frequency is defined as the number of lead lines per inch or cm with the usual ranges between 25 and 45 lines/cm (60 to 110 lines/inch). Grids can also be described by their pattern. Two grid patterns that are available include linear and crossed (crosshatched). Linear pattern grids contain lines that run in only one direction, whereas crossed grids contain lines that are perpendicular to each other. Crossed grids are more effective at reducing scatter, but are more difficult to use since the tube cannot be angled in any direction.

When grids are used, a portion of the primary beam is absorbed by the grid along with the scattered radiation; therefore, the use of a grid will result in a decrease in radiographic density. As the grid ratio increases, the grid will be more effective at absorbing scatter. In order to maintain density, exposure factors must be changed to compensate for the addition or removal of a grid or when changing between grid ratios.

Each grid ratio has a corresponding grid conversion factor (GCF) which is applied to a formula in order to determine the mA/s needed when a grid is used. The GCFs for common grid ratios are listed in Table 4-1.

The use of a grid results in a decrease in density; therefore, mA/s must be changed when a grid is added or removed or the grid ratio is changed. The following formula is used to compensate for the addition or removal of a grid:

$$\frac{mA/s_1}{mA/s_2} = \frac{GCF_1}{GCF_2}$$

- Because grids absorb both scatter radiation and a portion of the primary beam, the use of a grid results in a decrease in density.

TABLE 4-1 GCFs	
Grid Ratio	**GCF**
5:1	2
6:1	3
8:1	4
10:1	5
12:1	5
16:1	6
No grid	1

- As grid ratio increases, density decreases.
- As grid ratio decreases, density increases.

Filtration

The polyenergenic (heterogeneous) x-ray beam contains radiation of varying energies. The low-energy x-ray photons do not contain enough energy to penetrate the anatomy and only serve to contribute to patient dose. In an effort to minimize dose to the patient, filtration is used to absorb low-energy x-ray photons. Filtration affects density by decreasing the number of low-energy x-ray photons exiting the x-ray tube.

Two types of filtration exist: inherent and added. Inherent filtration is a permanent part of the x-ray tube construction and cannot be changed. Inherent filtration includes the glass envelope, the oil surrounding the x-ray tube, and the x-ray tube window, which result in a total filtration of 0.5 millimeters of aluminum (mm Al) or equivalent. The collimator adds an additional 1 mm Al equivalent to the filtration. Added filtration (usually a thin sheet of Al) is located between the x-ray tube housing and the collimator and adds an additional 1 mm Al. Total filtration (inherent and added) is equivalent to a minimum of 2.5 mm Al.

- As filtration increases, density decreases.
- As filtration decreases, density increases.

Film-Screen Speed

The combination of the x-ray film and the speed of the intensifying screen, or IR, used will affect the density of the resulting image. The purpose of an intensifying screen is to emit light in response to x-ray exposure, thereby decreasing patient dose. Faster-speed screens will emit more light in response to radiation exposure than slower-speed screens and will result in a higher-density image with less patient dose. IR speed (screen speed) is also referred to as *relative speed index* (RSI). Table 4-2 lists available RSIs for use in general radiography.

TABLE 4-2 Available RSIs for Use in General Radiography	
RSI	**Application**
50	Occasionally used for extremities
100	Extremities
200	Occasionally used for chest
400	Most examinations (except extremities)
800	Seldom used

The relationship between film-screen speed and density is directly proportional: As IR speed increases, density also increases; as IR speed decreases, density decreases. With changes in screen speed, in order to maintain density, the following formula is used:

$$\frac{mA/s_1}{mA/s_2} = \frac{RSI_2}{RSI_1}$$

- As RSI increases, density increases.
- As RSI decreases, density decreases.

Beam Restriction (Collimation)

Beam restriction, or collimation, changes the size of the x-ray field and, therefore, the volume of tissue being exposed to radiation. As collimation increases, the size of the light field and the volume of tissue irradiated are decreased. Increasing collimation results in a decrease in scatter production and, as a result, decreased density.

- Increasing collimation decreases density.
- Decreasing collimation increases density.

Anode Heel Effect

The anode is angled to project the x-ray photons downward through the x-ray tube window and toward the patient; however, this causes the radiation intensity exiting the x-ray tube to be nonuniform. This phenomenon is called the *anode heel effect*. The anode heel effect results in a decrease in density at the anode end of the x-ray field compared to that at the cathode end. The anode heel effect is more evident with short SIDs and decreased collimation in the cathode–anode axis.[3] In order to achieve a more uniform density throughout the image, the thicker part of the anatomy should be placed under the cathode end of the x-ray tube when imaging anatomy that requires the collimation to be open in the cathode–anode axis.

- The anode heel effect results in a decrease in density at the anode end of the x-ray field.
- The anode heel effect is more evident at short SIDs and decreased collimation in the cathode–anode axis.

Patient Size or Pathology

Patient size and radiographic density are inversely proportional: As the size of the anatomy of interest increases, density decreases; as anatomy size decreases, density will increase. To compensate for changes in patient size, for every 4 cm change in tissue thickness, mA/s will change by a factor of two. For example, a 4-cm increase in part thickness requires the mA/s to be doubled to produce an image with comparable density. Conversely, a 4-cm decrease in part thickness requires

TABLE 4-3 Additive and Destructive Pathologies

Additive Pathologies	Destructive Pathologies
Ascites	Bowel obstruction
Cirrhosis	Emphysema
Congestive heart failure (CHF)	Gout
Edema	Osteoporosis
Hemothorax	Pneumothorax
Hydrocephalus	
Pneumonia	
Pulmonary edema	

the mA/s to be halved in order to produce a radiograph of similar density.

The presence of pathology also has an effect on the radiographic density. Additive pathologies, which are more difficult for x-ray photons to penetrate, will result in a decrease in density. Destructive pathologies, which allow x-ray photons to more readily penetrate tissue, will result in an increase in density. Table 4-3 lists some additive and destructive pathologies.

Contrast / Gray Scale

The ARRT defines contrast (analog systems) as "the visible differences between any two selected areas of density levels within the radiographic image."[1] Scale of contrast refers to the number of shades of gray within the image and can be described as *long-scale contrast* or *short-scale contrast*. Long-scale contrast describes an image with many shades of gray that have slight differences between them, whereas an image with short-scale contrast contains few shades of gray that have drastic differences between them. With digital systems, scale of contrast is referred to as *gray scale*, which is controlled by the bit depth. Factors affecting contrast or gray scale are listed below.

Kilovoltage Peak

kVp is the most influential factor affecting radiographic contrast and is sometimes referred to as the *primary controlling factor*.[4] Because kVp affects the penetration of the x-ray beam, it also affects the amount of radiation being absorbed and attenuated. As kVp increases, the penetrating power of the x-ray beam increases, resulting in more x-ray photons being transmitted through the anatomy and interacting with the IR. As more photons are able to pass through the anatomy, each representing a shade of gray corresponding to the tissue density that it passed through, more shades of gray will be demonstrated. This will result in a long scale of contrast (low contrast). Likewise, as kVp decreases, x-ray beam penetration will also decrease. When fewer x-ray photons pass through the anatomy and interact with the IR, fewer shades of gray will be represented. This is referred to as a short scale of contrast (high contrast).

- As kVp increases, contrast decreases (low contrast, long scale).
- As kVp decreases, contrast increases (high contrast, short scale).

Object-to-Image Distance

With an OID greater than 6″ (air gap), much of the scatter exiting the anatomy will miss the IR, resulting in an increase in contrast.

- As OID increases over 6″, contrast increases.

Grids

As mentioned previously, grids reduce the amount of scattered radiation that reaches the IR, thereby increasing contrast. As the grid ratio increases, the grid is more effective at scatter reduction, and contrast will be further increased.

- The use of a grid increases image contrast.
- As grid ratio increases, contrast increases.
- As grid ratio decreases, contrast decreases.

Filtration

If the amount of filtration increases, more of the lower-energy x-ray photons are absorbed, increasing the average photon energy. With an increased average energy, more scatter will reach the IR, resulting in a slight decrease in contrast. It is important to note that filtration does not vary by much and the resulting change in contrast would be minimal.[5]

- Small variations in filtration can occur and would have a minimal effect on contrast.
- As filtration increases, contrast decreases (very slightly).
- As filtration decreases, contrast increases (very slightly).

Beam Restriction (Collimation)

Beam restriction (collimation) affects contrast by changing the volume of tissue that is exposed to radiation, and therefore affects the amount of scatter being produced, and as a result, the image contrast.

- As beam restriction (collimation) increases, contrast increases.
- As beam restriction (collimation) decreases, contrast decreases.

Patient Size or Pathology

The size of the patient or the thickness of the anatomy being exposed affects the total volume of tissue irradiated. As the volume of tissue irradiated increases, the amount of scatter being produced also increases, and, as a result, contrast decreases. Presence of pathology may also affect contrast.

- As patient size increases, contrast decreases.
- As patient size decreases, contrast increases.

Recorded Detail / Spatial Resolution

Recorded detail (analog systems) describes the sharpness of the structural lines that are demonstrated in the radiographic image. Spatial resolution (digital systems) refers to the sharpness of the structural edges that are demonstrated in the radiographic image. Factors that affect recorded detail are listed below.

Source-to-Image Distance

The SID affects the amount of recorded detail that exists on the image. As a result of the angle of the anode and the divergence of the x-ray beam, as SID is increased, the amount of geometric unsharpness that is visualized on the image decreases. As the SID decreases, geometric unsharpness increases.

- As SID increases, recorded detail increases.
- As SID decreases, recorded detail decreases.

Object-to-Image Distance

Like SID, OID also plays a role in the amount of recorded detail that exists on an image. As the distance between the object being radiographed and the IR increases, the structural lines within the image become blurred and the recorded detail decreases. Unless the air-gap technique is being used, it is important to place the anatomy of interest as close to the IR as possible.

- As OID increases, recorded detail decreases.
- As OID decreases, recorded detail increases.

Focal Spot Size

The focal spot size plays a role in the amount of geometric unsharpness and recorded detail that exist on the image. When selecting the focal spot, the technologist selects the size of the filament being energized for the exposure. Modern x-ray units are considered "dual focus," meaning that there are two filaments (small and large). Most radiographic units have filament sizes ranging from 0.5 to 1.2 mm, with small filaments falling in the 0.5- to 0.6-mm range and large filaments ranging from 1 to 1.2 mm.[6] The *actual focal spot* refers to the size of that area on the anode that is struck by electrons. The *effective focal spot* refers to the size of the focal spot area beneath the anode and is influenced by the anode target angle.

- As the focal spot size increases, geometric unsharpness increases and recorded detail decreases.
- As the focal spot size decreases, geometric unsharpness decreases and recorded detail increases.

Film-Screen Speed

Film-screen speed (RSI) plays a significant role in geometric unsharpness and recorded detail. In conventional radiography, common screen speeds are 50, 100, 200, 400, and 800. Computed radiography (CR) imaging plates (IPs) have a screen speed of approximately 200.[7]

In order to increase the speed of an intensifying screen, the size of the phosphor crystal or the thickness of the phosphor layer must be increased. A reflective layer can also be added to increase the speed of an intensifying screen. When x-ray photons interact with the phosphor crystals, light is produced by the phosphor crystals and is also reflected by the reflective layer of the screen. Because the phosphor crystal size is larger than that of the x-ray photon, the area of the film exposed to light from the crystal will also be larger than that affected by the original x-ray photon. This enlargement of the information on the film will result in more geometric unsharpness and decreased recorded detail.

- As screen speed increases, geometric unsharpness increases and recorded detail decreases.
- As screen speed decreases, geometric unsharpness decreases and recorded detail increases.

Motion

Motion is also referred to as motion unsharpness and results in the most significant negative effect on the recorded detail of an image. Factors that cause motion on an image are movement of the patient, x-ray tube, or IR. Short exposure times, immobilization devices, and clear instructions can help to reduce the chance of patient motion.

- Motion of the patient, x-ray tube, or IR increases geometric unsharpness and decreases recorded detail.

Patient Size/Pathology

Patient size plays a role in the recorded detail of an image. In order to maximize recorded detail and reduce geometric unsharpness, it is important to position the patient with the anatomy of interest as close to the IR as possible. With large patients, even while positioned appropriately, an increased OID may exist between the anatomy of interest and the IR, resulting in increased geometric unsharpness and decreased recorded detail.

Patient factors—such as the inability to attain the appropriate projection because of injury, illness, or physical limitations—may also affect recorded detail. When positioning such patients, the technologist should place the anatomy as close to the IR as possible and increase the SID as necessary to reduce the magnification and increase recorded detail.

Angle of the Tube / Part / Image Receptor
The angling of the x-ray tube, anatomy, or IR will decrease the amount of recorded detail that exists on the image.

Distortion
A misrepresentation of either the size or the shape of an object is referred to as distortion. Factors affecting distortion are listed below.

Source-to-Image Distance
SID is inversely related to the amount of size distortion (magnification) that exists on an image. According to the magnification factor (MF) formula, the amount of magnification that exists on the image is determined by the SID divided by the source-to-object distance (SOD). The SOD is calculated by subtracting the OID from the SID:

$$MF = \frac{SID}{SOD}$$
$$SOD = SID - OID$$

If the SID is 40″ and the OID is 1″, the MF will be calculated thus:

$$SOD = SID - OID$$
$$SOD = 40 - 1$$
$$SOD = 39$$
$$MF = \frac{SID}{SOD}$$
$$MF = \frac{40}{39}$$

MF = 1.025 (the object is magnified 2.5%)

If the SID is increased to 72″ and the OID remains 1″, the new MF will be calculated thus:

$$SOD = SID - OID$$
$$SOD = 72 - 1$$
$$SOD = 71$$
$$MF = \frac{SID}{SOD}$$
$$MF = \frac{72}{71}$$

MF = 1.014 (the object is magnified 1.4%)

- As SID increases, magnification decreases.
- AS SID decreases, magnification increases.

Object-to-Image Distance
Like SID, OID plays a role in the size distortion (magnification) of the image. Using the MF formula, magnification can be calculated as the OID changes. For example:

$$MF = \frac{SID}{SOD}$$
$$SOD = SID - OID$$

If two radiographs were taken at 40″ and the OID was increased from 1″ to 6″, we can compare the MFs of the two images:

$$MF = \frac{SID}{SOD}$$
$$SOD = SID - OID$$

Image 1:

$$SOD = 40 - 1$$
$$SOD = 39$$
$$MF = \frac{SID}{SOD}$$
$$MF = \frac{40}{39}$$

MF = 1.025 (the object is magnified 2.5%)

Image 2:

$$SOD = 40 - 6$$
$$SOD = 34$$
$$MF = \frac{SID}{SOD}$$
$$MF = \frac{40}{34}$$

MF = 1.176 (the object is magnified 17.6%)

- As OID increases, magnification increases.
- AS OID decreases, magnification decreases.

Patient Size
The size of the patient will affect the amount of size distortion on a radiograph. As the size of the patient increases, the anatomy farthest from the IR will be more magnified compared to that anatomy closer to the IR.

Angle of the Tube / Part / Image Receptor
Any angling of the x-ray tube, anatomy of interest, or IR will result in distortion of the natural shape of the anatomy, which will be visualized on the resulting image. As with lordotic views of the chest and many other projections, angling of the x-ray tube or the anatomy of interest is purposely performed to better demonstrate specific anatomical areas, to elongate anatomy, or to minimize superimposition. In trauma situations

(as with traumatic cervical spine variations to demonstrate the intervertebral foramen), or when the patient is unable to attain the required projection (as with the Coyle projections of the elbow, or Clements-Nakayama projection of the hip), the x-ray tube angle may be manipulated to achieve an image similar to that of a standard projection.

Technique Charts

Technique charts, also called *exposure charts*, are predetermined guidelines that aid the radiographer in selecting appropriate exposure factors for a specific examination. Two types of technique charts are fixed kVp / variable mA/s and variable kVp / fixed mA/s; both types of exposure charts will be discussed below. Technique charts serve to maintain consistency of the radiographic images and are used for manual and automatic exposure control (AEC) exposures and also with digital imaging. Technique charts should include the following information:

- Anatomy of interest
- Projection (e.g., anteroposterior [AP], posteroanterior [PA], lateral)
- kVp
- mA/s
- Part thickness (cm)
- Centering point (which will also be the measuring point)
- SID
- Bucky or tabletop
- IR speed
- Grid ratio (if grid used)
- Focal spot

Advantages of technique charts:

- Allow for standardized exposure factors
- Provide consistent image quality and density
- Decrease radiation exposure by reducing the number of repeats due to improper exposure factor selection

Disadvantages of technique charts:

- Technique charts are designed for the average patient, but factors such as build or pathology may affect the resultant image.
- The technique chart may be out of date.
- Technique charts do not consider image processing and equipment fluctuations.

Caliper Measurement

Calipers are measuring devices that are used to accurately determine the thickness of an anatomical area. When using calipers to measure an anatomical part, it is important to measure the exact area where the central ray will be directed, which should be specified on the technique chart. Inaccurate measurements or measurements of the incorrect anatomical area will result in an inappropriate density on the image; technique charts are only as good as the measurements that are taken.

Fixed kVp / Variable mA/s Technique Charts

Fixed kVp / variable mA/s exposure charts use the same kVp, regardless of the thickness of the anatomical area being radiographed. When developing a fixed kVp / variable mA/s technique chart, the highest kVp appropriate for that anatomical part should be used; with screen/film imaging systems, the radiographer must keep in mind the level of contrast that is desired. With these types of technique charts, for every 4- to 5-cm change in part thickness, the mA/s must be doubled or halved accordingly while keeping the kVp the same.

With fixed kVp / variable mA/s technique charts:

- For every 4- to 5-cm increase in part thickness, mA/s should be doubled to maintain density.
- For every 4- to 5-cm decrease in part thickness, mA/s should be halved to maintain density.

Advantages of fixed kVp / variable mA/s technique charts:

- Patient thickness is measured in 4- to 5-cm ranges.
- Compared to variable kVp / fixed mA/s technique charts, exposure factors are easier to memorize.
- Accuracy of measurements is not as crucial as with variable kVp / fixed mA/s technique charts.

Variable kVp / Fixed mA/s Technique Charts

Variable kVp / fixed mA/s technique charts require a change in kVp as the part thickness increases or decreases and are often used when imaging small parts, such as extremities, or pediatric patients. A rule of thumb for these types of exposure charts is that for every 1-cm increase or decrease in part thickness, the kVp must increase or decrease accordingly in order to maintain density.

- For every 1-cm increase in tissue thickness, the kVp should be increased by 2.
- For every 1-cm decrease in tissue thickness, the kVp should be decreased by 2.

Important point to remember with variable kVp / fixed mA/s charts:

- With screen/film imaging systems, contrast will vary.
- Accurate measurement of the anatomy is crucial.
- These types of technique charts are not as effective for extremely large or small patients.

Special Considerations with Technique Charts

Technique charts are produced for average body compositions and without the presence of pathology. The technologist must adjust the exposure factors accordingly with extremely muscular patients, with pediatric patients, when pathology is present, if the patient has a cast or other orthopedic appliance, or when contrast media are used.

Factors requiring an increase in exposure factors:

- Extremely muscular patients
- Patients with additive pathologies (such as ascites)
- Casts (plaster more so than fiberglass)
- After administration of positive contrast agents (barium, iodinated contrast, gadolinium)

Factors requiring a decrease in exposure factors:

- Patients with destructive pathologies (such as osteoporosis)
- After administration of negative contrast agents (air)
- Pediatric patients

Anatomically Preprogrammed Radiography

Some radiographic systems are equipped with anatomically preprogrammed radiography (APR) capabilities. APR allows the radiographer to select an anatomical area from a menu on the control panel that contains preprogrammed exposure factors for that particular anatomy. From those preprogrammed exposure factors, the technologist has the option of changing the kVp or mA/s if necessary, depending on the patient size, presence of pathology, or other circumstances.

Automatic Exposure Control

AEC systems (also called *automatic exposure devices* [AEDs]) are designed to control the amount of radiation that reaches the IR, ensuring the proper density. If used properly, AEC systems will cause the exposure to be terminated once the desired density is reached. When an exposure is made, an electrical charge proportional to the amount of radiation produced travels along a wire. Once a predetermined amount of charge is reached, a timer terminates the exposure. With AEC systems, the length of the exposure is controlled by the system, while the mA, kVp, detector(s), and density setting are selected by the technologist.

In order to achieve the appropriate density when using AEC systems, the technologist must:

- SELECT THE APPROPRIATE DETECTOR(S): If the wrong detector is chosen, the density will either be excessive or insufficient, depending on the anatomy that is positioned over the detector.

- PLACE THE ANATOMY OF INTEREST DIRECTLY OVER THE DETECTOR(S): If the anatomy of interest is not placed directly over the detector, the density will either be excessive or insufficient, depending on the anatomy positioned over the detector. For example, with a hip radiograph, if soft tissue instead of bone is placed over the detector, the exposure will terminate once the soft tissue is adequately exposed and the resulting density will be insufficient.

- TAKE NOTE OF ADDITIVE OR DESTRUCTIVE PATHOLOGIES: Additive pathologies will require an increase in the density setting, while destructive pathologies will require a decrease in the density setting.

- SELECT THE APPROPRIATE DENSITY SETTING: Large patients or those with additive pathologies may require density settings of +1 or +2, while extremely small patients or those with destructive pathologies may require a density setting of −1 or −2.

- COLLIMATE APPROPRIATELY: AEC systems cannot distinguish between primary and scatter radiation. If insufficient collimation is used, the detector(s) will read the excessive scatter as primary radiation and terminate prematurely, resulting in insufficient density.

- USE THE APPROPRIATE SPEED IR: AEC systems cannot distinguish between different speed IRs. If a 100 RSI IR is used in place of a 400, the system will anticipate a 400 RSI and will terminate the exposure prematurely, resulting in insufficient density.

- SELECT THE APPROPRIATE BUCKY (I.E., WALL, TABLE): If the incorrect Bucky is activated, in order to adequately expose those detectors, the exposure time will be excessively long, often triggering the backup timer. The resulting image will exhibit excessive density.

Factors that will not affect density in AEC systems:

- KILOVOLTAGE PEAK: Because the AEC system terminates the exposure once adequate x-ray photons reach the detector(s), the system compensates for changes in kVp according to the 15% rule. As kVp increases, the exposure time, and as a result the mA/s, will decrease.

- SOURCE-TO-IMAGE DISTANCE: As with kVp, the AEC system will terminate the exposure once the desired density is reached. With increases in SID, the exposure time, and as a result the mA/s, will increase.

Digital Imaging Characteristics
Spatial Resolution

Spatial resolution can be defined as the amount of detail in a digital image that is measured in pixels (picture elements). A digital system needs to effectively image small, detailed objects in a pixel matrix, measured as lines per millimeter (lp/mm). Resolution usually displays in lp/mm and will contain a certain amount of memory. The amount of memory of an image will depend of the size of the IP or panel. The acquisition memory will be reduced when smaller-size plates or panels used.

- Spatial resolution—amount of detail in pixels
- Pixels—picture elements
- Resolution—displayed in lp/mm

Sampling Frequency

A digital imaging system needs to match the original image so it will be a direct representation when displayed. Sampling rate determines the width of the pixel, which is measured in pixels per mm. It describes how many times along a scan line the information is sampled in pixels per mm; the more pixels per mm, the higher the resolution. One resulting factor when using a higher sampling rate is that more memory is required. The general rule: The more information, the more memory and the better the detail; the less pixels displayed, the less detailed the image.

- Sampling rate—how many times information is acquired
- More pixels, more memory equals more detail

Detector Element Size

Detector element size or DEL is a term used in digital radiography (DR) to determine the size of the electronic charge detector. The size of these charge collectors determines how fine the image resolution (spatial resolution) is. The finer the element size, the better the spatial resolution. Each size of an element is limited by the electronics of the connectors; therefore, the imaging panel size is limited to the detector size. Detector elements are usually measured in micrometers (μm).

- In DR systems, detector size is limited to the size of the imaging panel.
- The smaller the DEL, the better the spatial resolution.
- DEL is usually measured in μm.

Receptor Size and Matrix

Receptor size determines the matrix size (rows and columns or an array) in CR. A 14″ × 17″ IP will have the most pixels because of its large size. As the size decreases, the number of pixels is reduced. Each pixel has a numerical value and is represented as a brightness level. Spatial resolution is improved with a larger matrix size that includes a greater number of pixels resulting in better resolution. Each pixel in a matrix has a numerical value to determine the brightness of an area in the matrix. The more pixels are in an array, the more memory is required. Table 4-4 shows some common matrix and pixel sizes.

Processing time, network transmission time, and storage space on servers will be increased as the matrix size increases, which can slow down workflow.

A digital monitor also displays images in pixels. Computer monitors come in a variety of pixel displays:

$$1024 \times 1024 = 1,048,576 \text{ pixels}$$

$$2048 \times 2048 = 4,194,304 \text{ pixels}$$

Older monitors used cathode-ray tube (CRT) technology, but they soon were replaced by liquid crystal displays (LCDs). The more pixels on a monitor, the better the displayed resolution. If a high-resolution image is displayed on a high-resolution monitor, the digital image will be more reproducible.

- Matrix size is determined by the number of pixels.
- Spatial resolution is improved with a greater number of pixels, resulting in better resolution.
- Digital display monitors display in pixels.
- The more pixels in a monitor, the better the resolution.

Image Signal Exposure
Quantum Mottle

IPs and panels receive a signal and convert the signal to light energy from an x-ray exposure. Exposure is dose related, depending on the anatomy and how much of the x-ray energy reaches the detector. A numeric value or exposure index (EI) is displayed and

TABLE 4-4 Common Matrix and Pixel Sizes		
IP	**Spatial Resolution**	**Pixel Size**
35 × 42.5 cm (14″ × 17″)	10 pixels/mm	3480 × 4248
25 × 30 cm (10″ × 12″)	10 pixels/mm	2328 × 2928
20 × 25 cm (8″ × 10″)	10 pixels/mm	1728 × 2328
15 × 30 cm (6″ × 12″)	10 pixels/mm	1440 × 2928

can determine if the plate was adequately exposed. The values may be different depending on the manufacturer of the digital system. During processing of an image, these values are averaged out and displayed on the workstation monitor.

Quantum mottle or noise can be the most common issue in DR. This noise depends on the exposure of the IP or panel. Lack of photons reaching the IR will increase quantum mottle and may interfere with image quality. Although the density of the image may be adequate after postprocessing, the image will appear grainy. Increasing the amount of radiation to an exposure will reduce quantum mottle.

- Quantum mottle is a noisy or grainy appearance on an image.
- Lack of photons reaching a detector results in quantum mottle.
- Increasing the amount of radiation to an exposure will reduce quantum mottle.

Signal-to-Noise Ratio

In a digital system, the signal is the resultant exposure displayed on a computer workstation. Along with the exposure will be electronic noise, which may be seen along with the image. Signal-to-noise is expressed as a ratio comparing two components of an image (image and noise). A signal-to-noise ratio of 3:1 will be a better-quality image compared with the same image that has a signal-to-noise ratio of 1:1. The higher the signal-to-noise ratio, the better the image. Another term used in DR is *contrast-to-noise ratio*. These two terms both describe image quality. The contrast of an image should be above the signal noise to create an acceptable diagnostic image. The anatomical part and the exposure will also determine contrast-to-noise ratio. An increase in exposure will increase signal-to-noise.

- Signal-to-noise is expressed as a ratio comparing two components of an image.
- The higher the signal-to-noise ratio, the better the image.

Contrast-to-Noise Ratio

Contrast-to-noise ratio refers to the overall grayscale quality of an image and how an image is perceived by the viewer. Higher-contrast (fewer shades of gray) images help produce a clearer view of image detail. Decreasing the amount of kilovoltage (kV) in an exposure will help improve contrast quality but may increase noise and quantum mottle. Increasing contrast usually results in a type of trade-off and may produce more noise on an image. Using a grid will effectively reduce scatter and improve contrast; other ways of heightening contrast of an image are better columniation and correct patient positioning.

- Contrast-to-noise ratio refers to the overall grayscale quality of an image.
- Decreasing the amount of kV in an exposure will help improve contrast quality but may increase noise and quantum mottle.

IMAGE PROCESSING AND QUALITY ASSURANCE

Image Identification

Photographic

The photographic method requires a film that uses light and exposure time to produce an image. There are a variety of photographic film emulsions, from extremely fine grained to coarse grained, which have a relationship to film speed or light sensitivity. A finer-grained photographic film is slower in speed and requires more light or exposure time. Once an image is exposed on a film and is developed, a second step is required to print the reversed image on another medium. The common medium for image reversal is photographic paper, which is an emulsion-coated paper that is sensitive to light, like film. This paper medium requires another step in processing in a solution to produce a positive image. Another medium that is still in use is a reversal film or slide film. Slide film is similar to photographic film when it is exposed to light, but instead of producing a negative like standard film, when processed in a solution, it produces a positive image.

- Photographic methods use light to expose an image on film.
- Film speed reflects the grain size of photographic film.
- A photographic film once developed needs to be printed a onto a paper medium coated with an emulsion.

Radiographic

A radiographic image utilizes an x-ray source to expose the film medium; the amount of x-ray exposure will determine the density of the image. The film medium is normally a polyester-based material coated with an emulsion that is sensitive to light and when developed in a chemical solution, produces an image. Like a photographic film, there are various film speeds available; all have a finer grain to show better detail. Radiographic films go through a development process for image production. When viewing the film image, a backlighted source is required to pass through the film medium.

- Radiographic films utilize an x-ray source to expose the film.
- Films must go through a processing cycle to develop the exposed image.
- Radiographic films are coated with a light-sensitive emulsion on a polyester base.

Electronic

An electronic image uses no solution, film, or paper medium to produce an image. The images can be both photographic and radiographic. A photographic image is obtained by a CCD or charged-coupled device in a photographic camera; the CCD converts light to an electronic image. The electronic image is called a *digital image*, because the images when passed through a CCD have assigned numeric values for brightness and pixel values for detail.

The process for capturing a digital radiographic image is similar to the digital photographic process where an image is exposed to radiation on a flat plate called a detector. The image is then extracted by a system with a photomultiplier tube (in CR) or is directly connected electronically and converted to a digital image (in DR) and viewed on a monitor. The image will have numeric values for density and pixel values for detail.

- An electronic image in photography uses a CCD to convert light to a digital image.
- Electronic images can be both photographic and radiographic.
- Radiographic images use a detector that converts light or electrical energy to a digital image.

Legal Considerations

The radiologic technologist's role is to provide optimum imaging and care while performing a radiologic exam. In the exam procedure, patient information is available and is entrusted to the radiographer and is kept confidential. This information should be recorded accurately and should be rechecked for any errors. The technologist plays an important role in the patient's right to privacy. Any patient information should not be shared with anyone. Recording patient data incorrectly may be detrimental to workflow and if there is litigation involved.

During the examination process, the radiologic technologist's role is to accurately perform imaging and record quality images. Identification markers should be labeled and placed correctly on the image. Diagnostic information also plays an important role in patient–technologist confidentiality. Providing any diagnostic

interpretation to anyone regarding a patient may cause legal implications to the technologist.

- The radiologic technologist's role is to provide optimum-quality imaging and care and respect the patient's right to privacy.
- A radiologic technologist's role is to accurately perform imaging and record quality images.
- Providing any diagnostic interpretation to anyone regarding a patient may cause legal implications to the technologist.

Film-Screen Processing

Film Storage

Conventional films require proper storage conditions to prevent any premature degradation of the radiographic image. If radiographic films are processed correctly in a film processor with the developer and fixer at the correct temperature, correct processing time, and correct chemical dilution, radiographs should be able to be stored indefinitely in a location that is free of extreme cold and hot temperatures with low humidity. Many hospitals store films for a few years and then scrap the films to recover the silver. Some may archive the films using a digital scanner.

- Proper storage conditions are required to prevent any premature degradation of radiographic films.
- Radiographic films need correct processing parameters and replenishment for proper archiving and storage.
- Radiographic films should be stored in low humidity and kept from extreme temperatures.

Components

Developer

Radiographic film developer is used during processing; the developer turns the silver halide crystals that contain the latent image to black metallic silver. Film developers vary depending on the manufacturer. When diluted to a working solution, the film developer may be a clear or caramel color; each brand of developer will have a specific gravity according to the manufacturer's recommendation. Film developer reacts with the silver halide that is coated on a polyester film. The coating material is called emulsion and has an outer protective layer of gelatin. As the film is immersed in developer, the gelatin swells and allows the emulsion to begin the development process, which turns the emulsion that has been exposed to light or photons into black metallic silver. The unexposed emulsion remains in its normal state during this process.

Fixer

Fixing is the final step in the development process before the image is washed. Fixer is a clear solution and also has a specific gravity depending on the manufacturer; it also may be referred to as *hypo*. In the development process, once the film leaves the developer and is immersed in the fixer tank, the fixer dissolves and removes the unexposed silver halide crystals on the film and stops any further blacking of the black metallic silver exposed to light. This stabilization of the emulsion is commonly called *fixing* or *hardening*.

- Radiographic film developer turns exposed silver halide crystals (latent image) to black metallic silver.
- Fixer stops any further development of the exposed silver halide crystals and hardens the emulsion.
- Fixer dissolves any unexposed silver halide crystals.

Maintenance/Malfunction

Start-up

Film processors comprise solution tanks and a transport system of rollers which carry the film and transport it to the development fix process, after which the film is washed and dried. Film processors need preventive maintenance for trouble-free operation.

When not in use, a film processor contains chemicals that emit vapors, which can deposit on rollers and may cause processing artifacts. In the start-up procedure, all exposed rollers should be cleaned with a damp sponge, especially any crossover rollers that carry the film from one tank to another. Once the rollers are cleaned, the cover should be replaced, making the system lighttight.

The water supply for the processor should be turned on before the film processor. The water supply plays a dual role in the film development process. It is mainly used to wash the film after it comes out of the fixer and also is used to help maintain the proper development temperature. The water temperature of a film processor should be approximately 10°F below the developer temperature. Once the water flow is on and correct, the main breaker of the processor should be turned on, followed by the film processor power switch.

After a few minutes, the processor will come up to the operating temperature. Before processing any diagnostic films, a number of sheets of film should be processed to clear any deposits that may be on the roller transports.

- Exposed rollers should be cleaned with a damp sponge or cloth before processing films.
- Water supply should be turned on before processor start-up.

- The water supply acts as a wash during processing and also helps keep developer at the proper temperature.

Processor Shut-down

Once all films are processed and the processor is ready to be shut down, the power switch should be turned to the off position; then the main breaker should be turned off, if required. Once the power is off, the water supply to the process can be turned off as well. Some newer film processors may have an antialgae system for the wash tank, where a drain opens up automatically to drain the wash water when the unit is shut down. This device prevents any algae buildup. Some processors that do not have this feature may require the drain to be opened manually. If a wash tank sits idly for a long period of time, algae can build up in the tank, which can cause artifacts on the film.

- The power on the processor should be shut down before turning off the main breaker and water supply.
- Wash tanks should be drained if the processor is not used over a long period to prevent algae buildup in the wash tank, which can cause film artifacts.

Malfunction Troubleshooting

The most common problems of film processors come from roller marks on processed films or improper drying or fixing of the film. If roller marks occur, check the crossover rollers and making sure they are clean and free of any solution deposits. Improper drying of films can be a problem caused by the dryer heater, which has heating elements connected to a blower. These elements can burn out over time, causing the films to come out cold and damp. Another problem that can resemble poorly dried films is improper fixing of films.

Film processors are connected to replenishment tanks, which add a small amount of fresh solution to the developer and fixer tanks every time a film is processed. This keeps the solutions at optimum operating strength to develop and fix the films. If the developer is not up to strength, the films will be underdeveloped and look washed out. If films are underfixed, they will feel tacky or damp. In extreme cases, the films will have a milky appearance, indicating diluted fixer or no replenishment at all. The film processor needs to be assessed to see whether the solutions are mixed correctly or there is no replenishment.

Poor water flow or incorrect water temperature can also cause problems. Too cold or too hot incoming water temperature can cause overdevelopment of films. Proper water temperature helps maintain proper development temperature. If the incoming water is too hot, it will override the developer solution temperature, causing dark films. The opposite is true regarding overly cold water. If the water is too cold, films will be underdeveloped and may also be underfixed.

Problems of processor contamination may occur if solutions are not mixed properly. If any fixer get into the developer during mixing of fresh solutions or cleaning of crossover rollers, it will cause contamination. Films will have a dull tint, and the processor will have a smell of ammonia. Proper procedures should be maintained when cleaning rollers or working on the processor with the cover removed. Proper mixing of solutions is required when filling the processor replenishment tanks. Since the developer and fixer tanks are usually close together, there is always a possibility of contamination.

- Processor roller marks are a common problem on films.
- Damp films may indicate a dryer heater problem or may indicate diluted or exhausted fixer.
- Extreme exhaustion of fixer will result in films with a milky appearance.
- Processor contamination is a result of fixer infiltrating into the developer from the processor or replenishment system.

Digital Image Processing

Electronic Collimation (Masking)

Electronic collimation in DR defines a region where x-ray energy will expose a region of interest, reducing scatter and providing optimal exposure to the digital detector. Masking allows better visibility of an image by changing the background of an image. If an image is coned tightly and viewed on a workstation monitor, the brightness of the monitor may interfere with proper viewing. If an image has a white background that may interfere with a region of interest, the background can be turned black, allowing the region of interest to be viewed with less distraction.

- Electronic collimation allows better viewing by blocking the unexposed areas of the image.
- Monitor brightness on an unmasked image may interfere with proper viewing of the image.

Grayscale Rendition (Lookup Table)

Grayscale rendition records all intensity values in a radiographic image; these values form a lookup table (LUT) and are applied by an exposure algorithm of a digital system. These values will vary depending on the anatomical regions being displayed. Imaging technique and size of the anatomical region will have an effect on grayscale values. Thicker areas will have a smaller value compared with thinner regions.

The intensity of the grayscale values is determined by LUTs. Pixels have values of 0 to 255, black being 0 and white being 255, and are used to change or enhance contrast. Each pixel of an image will store a grayscale value and can be altered depending on the contrast desired in an image. The user can choose many different characteristics from the original assigned LUT. In conventional terms, changing an LUT is like varying the slope of an H and D curve to get a desired contrast level. Changing the contrast values for an image is done by changing or substituting a new LUT.

- Grayscale values are determined by LUTs.
- LUTs will vary depending on technique, positioning, and size of the anatomical part.
- Grayscale values can be altered, which is similar to changing the slope of an H and D curve.

Histogram

A histogram is a tool that determines different intensity values on an X Y scale. The horizontal scale translates the image density (gray scale) to the vertical scale, which contains the number of pixels in an image from darkest to lightest. Images produced on a digital system come from an exposure algorithm with assigned values. In digital imaging systems, a histogram can reveal the optical and pixel values anywhere along the scale by moving the cursor along the scale.

A digital imaging system uses a histogram and modifies it, which is called *histogram equalization*. In histogram equalization, the system attempts to normalize the image to help increase the contrast. Histogram normalization, sometimes called *contrast stretching*, helps an image to be more normal to the person viewing the image.

- Algorithms produce images on a digital system, assigning pixel values to an image.
- A histogram determines intensity value along an X Y scale, showing gray scale to pixel values.
- Histogram equalization attempts to normalize an image over a range of grayscale values.

Edge Enhancement

Edge enhancement is an algorithm and a function of postprocessing; it can help increase spatial resolution for better detail within a digital image when the image is refined or sharpened. By increasing the brightness along edges of the pixels, edge enhancement will increase the spatial resolution. Another term for edge enhancement is *high-pass filtering*. Normally when edge enhancement is used, it can increase contrast but it may also increase image noise.

- Edge enhancement can help increase spatial resolution.
- *High-pass filtering* is another term for edge enhancement.

Noise Suppression

Image noise is an undesirable effect on an image. All digital systems have noise and will interfere with image sharpness. Quantum noise is an effect where an underexposed image displays an overall grainy appearance. Noise suppression is also known as *low-pass filtering* or *smoothing*. It takes nearby pixel values and averages them, which can lower the image contrast and reduce noise. Another way to help reduce noise in an image is to increase photon energy.

- Noise suppression is also called *low-pass filtering*.
- Increase in exposure will reduce noise.

Contrast Enhancement

Contrast enhancement is a function that converts the digital signal to an image with increased or decreased contrast. By changing the contrast parameters, the user is changing the curve of the image's contrast scale or changing the dynamic range. The steeper the curve, the more contrast is displayed. The process of changing contrast will alter the number of shades of gray that is displayed. The fewer shades of gray there are, the higher the displayed contrast of the image. A lower-contrast image will have many more shades of gray and a longer scale.

- Changing contrast parameters will reduce or increase the number of shades of gray.
- The steeper the curve on a contrast scale, the higher the contrast.

System Malfunctions

System malfunctions may occur in a digital system. Common problems like dirt and dust can cause problems in the processing or display of an image and can show up as artifacts on an image.

A CR system uses reusable IPs and cassettes; care should be used when storing IPs and cassettes. Although a CR cassette is a closed device that is usually opened internally in a CR reader during processing, the IP is susceptible to dirt and scratches. If a CR cassette is dirty and is being fed into a CR reader, any dirt that is on the surface of the cassette could be deposited on the internal mechanical rollers of the reader.

During the scanning and transport of the IP during the processing sequence, repeated use will begin to deteriorate the IP. Also, any dirt or debris deposited on the rollers can then be deposited to the IP. Over time, this debris can cause imaging artifacts on the image display monitor.

- Dirt and dust can cause problems in processing or in displayed images.
- IPs are susceptible to dirt and scratches.
- IPs on CR systems can transport dirt and dust onto CR scanner rollers.

Ghosting

A ghost image is an effect that occurs when an IP is not completely erased during the erasure cycle. When the IP is exposed again and is processed, a faint image from a previous exam is shown along with a normally exposed image. A second erasure cycle may remove a ghost image. If the image is not fully erased, the IP may have to be discarded.

In DR panels, some ghosting may appear if a trapped charge is carried over to the next image. A ghost image may require a secondary erasure procedure. If the erasure procedure is not adequate, recalibration of the panel may be required.

- *Ghosting* refers to when an image from a previous exposure is not completely erased.
- A secondary erasure may clean a ghost image on a CR IP.
- A DR ghost image can be caused by a trapped charge.

Banding

Banding can occur in both CR and DR. Software problems with the display monitor can cause banding artifacts such as noise artifacts. *Banding* refers to when densities in the form of stripes or wide lines are displayed across an image, which can occur during the digital conversion process. Calibration of monitors and digital imaging systems is essential for optimum performance. Banding artifacts can occur in CR because of problems with the laser scanning process and laser optics. Banding artifacts can be displayed as lines across the display monitor. Since in CR, there are moving parts compared to a DR system, banding artifacts can be caused by a number of issues (e.g., poor roller transport mechanism of the CR plate or a problem with the laser scanner optics).

- Banding is an artifact displaying wide stripes across a monitor display.
- Banding can be caused by issues with the display monitor or the DR or CR system software.
- CR systems are more susceptible to banding than DR because of the transport of the IP, roller transport, and scanning optics.

Erasure Problems

Erasure problems occur in CR systems where the IP is exposed to light to bring the imaging phosphor back to its original state and ready for an exposure. During the processing cycle of a CR plate, the final phase is the erasure cycle. A bank of lamps exposes the IP before it is placed back into the cassette. If some of the lamps are not functioning, the IP my not be fully erased. CR systems determine erasure time, which depends on the dose to the IP. If there is a problem with the erasure lamp, normal erasure time may be extended. Some system software will alert the user on issues and may do a second erasure cycle automatically before the IP is returned to the cassette.

In DR, panels trap charges on the surface of a panel; charges are removed during the erasure cycle. Ghosting of an image can occur if the trapped charges are not removed during the erasure cycle and carry over to the next image.

- CR systems have a bank of lamps that exposes the IP and returns the phosphor to its normal state.
- Erasure cycles in CR can be extended, which may indicate a problem with the erasure lamps.
- Erasure errors occur in a DR system when trapped charges on the surface of a panel are not removed.
- Ghosting can occur if panels are not completely erased.

Dead Pixels

Dead pixels occur only in DR systems.

A digital image is made up of pixels; the more pixels in an image, the finer the detail displayed. In DR systems, some dead pixels occur in images where there is no light value or shades of gray. This happens when the DR panel fails to produce a charge in an area and does not produce an image. Software in DR systems takes dead pixels, averages the surrounding pixels, and electronically fills in the dead areas. Most areas of dead pixels are quite small and may not be seen before averaging.

- Dead pixels occur in DR systems.
- Dead pixels occur where there are no light values displayed in a matrix.
- Software in DR systems will average surrounding pixels and fill in the area where there are dead pixels.

Scratches

Scratches on IPs will cause display artifacts in CR. CR goes through a mechanical transport process where dust and dirt can accumulate in the system and get deposited on the IP and scratch the imaging phosphor. If scratches and dust appear on an image, the appearance of these artifacts will be a lighter density. If an IP is inspected and there are no artifacts or scratches present, further investigation would require a service technician to inspect the laser optics in the system.

- IPs are susceptible to scratch artifacts.
- Dust and dirt may come from dirt on a cassette and can deposit on rollers and guides, which can then scratch the surface of an IP.
- Scratches on IPs will usually display a linear light density across an image.

Computed Radiography Reader Components

CR reader components consist of an IP phosphor in an exposure cassette.

A transport mechanism removes the IP after it is inserted in a CR scanner and transports the image plate to the scanning section.

A laser is projected through an optical scanner and onto the IP, where photostimulable luminescence occurs (the latent image is excited).

A photostimulable tube or light guide records the scanned image from the optical scanner and passes it through an analog-to-digital converter. Certain algorithms apply imaging parameters and the image is then displayed on a workstation.

Once the image has been displayed, the final process for the IP is the erasure. The IP passes through the erasure section, which consists of a bank of lamps where the imaging phosphor is returned to its normal state. The IP is then returned to the exposure cassette.

- In the scanning section of CR, a laser excites an IP; this is called *photostimulable luminescence*.
- A light guide records the scanned image from the optical scanner.
- An analog-to-digital converter changes the luminescent image to a digital image.
- An algorithm applies imaging parameters to the image.

Viewing Conditions for Digital Radiography

The proper viewing conditions for DR are an important part of diagnostic interpretation. Radiologists and radiographers require optimal viewing conditions of the display workstation.

Factors that affect proper viewing conditions are monitor brightness (luminance) and ambient background lighting in the viewing area. High luminance of a monitor can cause eyestrain and fatigue, which may affect proper interpretation by the radiologist who spends a lot of time viewing images. Radiographers who process and view digital images for proper image processing may also have problems with eyestrain and fatigue.

If the ambient lighting is too dark in the viewing area, monitor luminance will be amplified, which can accelerate eyestrain. Proper placement of digital monitors is also an important factor when viewing images. Rear lighting, such as other display monitors or windows, can cause reflections, which can be distracting. In addition, forward lighting, where light distractions are in front of the viewer, can cause problems.

- Proper viewing conditions are an important part of diagnostic interpretation.
- Proper viewing conditions consists of appropriate monitor brightness and ambient background lighting.
- Poor viewing conditions may interfere with the proper interpretation of an image.

Spatial Resolution

Spatial resolution describes the ability to resolve small details in an image. The more pixels in a displayed image, the better the spatial resolution and the finer the detail seen in anatomical structures. To measure spatial resolution, a line pair gauge is used to determine the resolution of a digital system. The more line pairs are seen, the better the resolution. In DR, line pairs usually resolve 2.5 to 5 line pairs per mm (lp/mm); line pairs are a function of the image phosphor in CR and the imaging panel in DR. Line pair resolution is greater in digital imaging compared with conventional film radiography and can resolve up 10 lp/mm depending on the type of film used.

Another factor determining spatial resolution would be the pixel size of the display monitor. Display monitors come in a variety of display sizes. The more pixels in a monitor, the better the display resolution. The optimum spatial resolution of a digital system depends on the spatial resolution of the IR and the display monitor. Factors such as image noise and quantum mottle can affect spatial resolution.

- Spatial resolution is the ability to see small details in an image.
- The more pixels in an image, the better the spatial resolution and the finer the detail seen in anatomical structures.
- DR resolves 2.5 to 5 lp/mm.

Contrast Resolution / Dynamic Range

Contrast resolution is the number of densities or shades of gray of different levels compared in an image. The more separation of densities displayed, the more latitude of an image. The resolution determines the density differences between each density level. The number of these shades or density values determines the dynamic range of an image. Digital radiology allows a wide range of densities displaying minimum and maximum x-ray absorption—significantly more than radiographic film. Contrast resolution and dynamic range may have different responses depending on the different equipment manufacturers.

Digital systems acquire an image and display the image in pixels. Bit depth or number of pixels displayed determines the number of grayscale levels. The more pixels displayed, the more shades of gray in an image and the better the contrast resolution. For example, an 8-bit image will only display 256 shades of gray, whereas a 10-bit image will display 1,024 shades of gray or more dynamic range.

- Contrast resolution describes the number of shades of gray in an image.
- The number of shades or density values determines the dynamic range of an image.
- DR allows a wider dynamic range.
- Bit depth is the number of grayscale levels in an image. The higher the bit depth, the more density levels displayed.

DICOM Grayscale Standard Display Function

Digital Imaging and Communications in Medicine (DICOM)is a standard adopted to be a universal method to transmit images between different digital system manufacturers. Prior to this standard, digital equipment manufacturers processed images differently, which prevented images from being displayed on different systems.

DICOM Grayscale Standard Display Function (GSDF) is a standard within DICOM to derive a common or consistent gray scale that can be used between different manufacturers when viewing images. Since grayscale densities are a measure of light output, the GSDF is defined for a luminance range measured in candelas per square meter (cd/m^2).

Manufacturers of CR and DR systems develop processing algorithms for image optimization; these algorithms involve the use of LUTs for viewing specific body parts or exposure ranges. Manufacturers will use the GSDF standard to calibrate their systems so when images are viewed on a different manufacturer's system, they will have similar contrast displays. Use a photometer to check.

- *DICOM* is an abbreviation of Digital Imaging and Communications in Medicine.
- DICOM is a standard universal method to transmit images between different digital system manufacturers.
- DICOM GSDF is a standard within DICOM for a common gray scale.

- DICOM GSDF uses common LUTs used by algorithms to display image grayscale levels.

Window Level/Width Function

Window leveling is a function of image brightness. The Window Leveling Tool allows the operator to lighten or darken an image to the operator's visual requirements, examining a particular range of grayscale intensity levels and maximizing the ability to see anatomical structures in a defined area. The Window Leveling Tool is useful in diagnostic imaging where there are large anatomical differences, as in chest radiography. Lung tissue may require changing the window level to specific grayscale intensity, whereas visualizing denser areas such as the thoracic spine will require different grayscale intensity.

The Window Leveling Tool does not cause any changes in the original data. It only helps enhance the area of interest during viewing of an image.

Window leveling allows adjustment of gray levels each time, allowing visibility of more specific information on a lower-resolution screen.

An 8-bit image will only display 256 shades of gray, whereas a 10-bit image will display 1,024 shades of gray or more dynamic range. An 8-bit image versus a 10-bit image is a function of bit depth. The more bit depth, the more shades of gray.

Window width is a function of image contrast. Contrast levels within a certain range of densities can be adjusted by the operator to conform to the operator's visual perception. An increase in the width will result in more shades of gray displayed in the image, resulting in lower contrast of the image. If the width of the window is narrowed, a smaller range of densities will result in higher-contrast images. Diagnostic information can be overlooked if window width is too narrow or too wide.

- The Window Leveling Tool does not change the original data.
- The Window Leveling Tool allows the operator to visualize gray intensity scale values (brightness) along the dynamic range of an image.
- Window width is a function of image contrast; increasing window width will result in more shades of gray displayed, whereas narrowing window width will result in fewer shades of gray or higher contrast.

Digital Image Display Informatics

Picture Archiving and Communication System

PACS in radiography is an abbreviation for picture archiving and communication system. A PACS allows digital images, patient data, and other information to be stored and delivered to various sites through a digital network. A PACS will have a local server, usually in the health center radiology department, where the images from all imaging modalities such as CR, DR, and CT are stored. The system is networked so that images and information can be viewed throughout the hospital and be sent through the Internet to outside locations to referring physicians. The PACS uses DICOM for the storage and retrieval of images; other forms of patient information can also be stored using standard documentation formats such as Word, Excel, and PDF. Using a PACS provides multiple workstation accessibility from any location.

- *PACS* is an abbreviation for picture archiving and communication system.
- A PACS is a server to store data and images for retrieval from any location on a network.
- All imaging modalities can be stored on a PACS.

Hospital Information System

HIS is an abbreviation for hospital information system; a HIS provides an efficient way to manage all aspects of patient care. A HIS allows access to clinical information and administration data from all departments in a hospital. A HIS can include information such as medical records, pharmacy, billing, and dietary and is an optimal way to quickly access information from any location. A HIS can be used to manage all aspects of patient care data.

- A HIS manages all aspects of patient care.
- All departments in a hospital use a HIS for administrative, billing, pharmacy, and other administration data from anywhere on a hospital network including outside locations.

Radiology Information System Modality Work List

A radiology information system (RIS) is a computer system that helps manage images and other information in the radiology department. Information can include patient information, reports, schedules, and billing. Procedures can be assigned to radiologists and staff, permitting better workflow through the department to help reduce any backups. A RIS also provides information to radiologists doing group studies, allowing them to access information when compiling patient data on radiologic exams. HISs work together with RISs in order to provide efficient patient care when storing and accessing information.

A modality work list is a server within a RIS. The server receives information from a HIS server; the information can be imported to a RIS from which a staff technologist can request a modality and all data fields are filled in automatically. Staff technologists normally would have to manually enter information on a procedure, which can be time-consuming and also increases the chance of errors. A modality work list can prevent errors and improve workflow.

- A modality work list is a server that works with a RIS.
- A RIS modality work list helps manage images and other information.
- A RIS permits better workflow by automatically assisting in data entry.

Networking

Health Level Seven International DICOM

Health Level Seven International (HL7) is a standard (universal language) that is networked for the exchanging, sharing, and retrieval of electronic health information such as clinical, administrative, and financial information in a medical center. The radiology department uses the integration between RIS, HIS, DICOM, and HL7 to efficiently communicate within the radiology department, other departments in the medical center, and facilities worldwide. HL7 and DICOM integration makes all digital data flow seamlessly through a network where it can be accessed from almost anywhere.

- HL7 is a universal standard used for the sharing and exchange of all aspects of health-care and administration information in a medical center.
- DICOM, HL7, and a HIS work together to share data and medical imaging; the information can be accessed and shared from almost anywhere on a network worldwide.

Workflow

Workflow in the radiology department is a critical process to make sure the patient, patient data, and radiology exams all work together. In a digital world, there is always a chance that there will be a problem with data. Things do occur such as computer errors, lost images, and corrupt data. Proper quality assurance is needed to help reduce issues in a digital environment.

Lost images can occur if they are deleted and not backed up to a PACS system or image data on a digital system get corrupted because of a software error or a lost network. If this occurs, these images may be permanently lost. Some systems have automatic backup of images; should there be a problem where the image is deleted, it can be retrieved from the backup system. If procedures are not in place to back up images or data is completely lost, examination procedures may have to be repeated, causing an increase in radiation dose.

Corrupt data can occur in many areas of a digital imaging system. Network failure, processing software errors, and storage systems all can contribute to data loss from corrupt files.

Mismatched Images

Mismatched images can occur when wrong patient information is entered in a data system. Usually this is a human error where information such as patient information is incorrect. Mismatched information can be time-consuming to correct. As a result, it can interrupt the workflow in the radiology department. Radiology modality work lists can help reduce mismatch errors.

- Workflow is an established method to help maintain a structured procedure in the radiology department for staff to follow.
- Exams, patient data, and clinical data need to flow in the radiology department with minimal or no interruptions.
- Proper quality assurance is needed to help reduce downtime due to computer errors, lost images, or lost patient data.
- Corrupt data, network failure, and mismatched information will interrupt the workflow in the radiology department.
- Loss of imaging data is critical, and the chance of re-examination may be possible.

CRITERIA FOR IMAGE EVALUATION

Image Artifacts

The basic fundamentals of good imaging using film or digital technology are still required in radiography. Even as technology advances, image artifacts still occur in film and DR. Artifacts on film in conventional radiography are due to the fact that radiographic film is handled by loading and unloading a cassette. Films have to be processed and are also subject to artifacts during the processor cycle. Types of artifacts can be fingerprints from moisture and oil from the hands of the technologist, fingernail marks, and roller and scratch marks from film processors. Other factors such as static marks on films can occur in dry (low-moisture) areas. Radiographic films are made from polyester (plastic) and can generate a static charge. This buildup of static can get discharged during the processing cycle, causing a static artifact on the film. Pressure artifacts can occur on films, especially during film processing. Roller transports that carry the film can be too tight, producing high-density marks on the films.

In digital imaging, artifacts can occur especially in CR when the IP is removed from its cassette and is subject to problems on rollers, which can contain dirt and dust that can accumulate on the IP, imaging optics, and guide plates.

Grid line artifacts can occur from table grids in conventional filming and DR. If the x-ray beam is not placed perpendicular to the grid, it will display lines on the image, especially if the focal film distance is not at the correct distance to the grid. Aliasing or moiré patterns is an electronic artifact in the form of wavy or distorted lines displayed on the image. This is due to improper sampling rate of images. A certain range of frequencies are required to record an image. If this frequency does not match the output frequency, aliasing occurs.

Sampling rate when an image is scanned determines the width of the pixel, which is measured in pixels per mm. In other words, sampling rate describes how many times along a scan line the information is sampled or taken in pixels per mm; the more pixels per mm, the higher the resolution. If this rate is incorrect, aliasing is displayed.

- Imaging artifacts occur in both film and DR.
- There is less of a chance for artifacts in DR than in film radiography.
- Film artifacts can be fingerprints, handling and processing scratches, processor roller marks, and static.
- Digital imaging artifacts occur more in CR than DR because of the susceptibility of the IP to dust and dirt accumulation on guides and rollers.
- Aliasing or moiré pattern is an electronic artifact in the form of wavy lines due to improper sampling of pixels.

Fog

Conventional radiographic films are susceptible to a variety of fog artifacts. Radiographic films are manufactured with expiration dates to ensure optimum quality. Expiration dates for film are arbitrary; films can still produce optimum film quality past their expiration dates. Optimum quality film can be determined by base plus fog levels. If image quality is in question, an evaluation process is needed, especially if film densities are high. Processing a blank film with no exposure and reading the base density with a densitometer will produce an optical density. The optical density is then compared to the manufacturer's base plus fog recommendations.

Fog levels can increase if the storage temperature is too high. Films exposed to higher than normal temperatures can increase base plus fog levels to a point that the film is no longer acceptable to use. Fog levels can also increase if processor temperatures are too high, overdeveloping films and producing overall plus densities. Chemical contamination, where a small amount of fixer infiltrated the developer tank or the replenishment tank, can also increase film densities.

Safelights are another source of high fog levels on films. Higher-wattage bulbs in darkroom safelights can produce higher fog levels by producing more light than what the safelight filter is designed for. Higher-wattage bulbs can also burn the coating off the filter, allowing small areas of white light to pass through the filter and cause plus densities on film.

- Radiographic film is susceptible to a variety of fog artifacts.
- Film fog can be from radiation, expired films, high processor temperatures, chemical contamination, and poor safelights.
- An indication of fog will be a high base plus fog level.

Noise

Noise on radiographic films and digital images can be a problem during viewing. As a result, poor-quality images may require repeating the examination procedure if the quality interferes with a proper diagnosis. Noise can be a result of quantum mottle. Quantum mottle can be considered a result of an energy-starved image where not enough photons expose the film, leaving a grainy image. There are other types of noise, such as scatter and electronic noise; signal-to-noise ratio and overprocessing can cause quality issues on images.

- Quantum mottle is a grainy pattern in an image due to low radiation exposure.
- There are various forms of noise, quantum noise, electronic noise, and scatter.
- Noise can cause poor imaging quality and interfere with the proper interpretation of an image.
- Noise can be a result of overprocessing on a digital image.

Acceptable Range of Exposure

In film radiography, an acceptable range of exposures is very small. Once a film is exposed and processed, there can be no further changes to the film. When viewing radiographs, it is easy to discern what is acceptable and not acceptable. Films can be overexposed or underexposed to a certain degree, causing information to be lost. In DR, there is a wider range of acceptability because of the dynamic range. The better the image information is displayed, the better the acceptable range of exposure. Since DR uses image processing, the acceptable range of exposures can be adjusted. Good-quality images will have low noise but a possible trade-off with higher doses of radiation, whereas low-quality images will be lower in dose but with higher noise levels. Lower-dose images, although they may be noisy, may still have diagnostic information and therefore can be in the acceptable range of exposure.

- Film has a very small acceptable range of exposure; when viewing radiographs, it is easier to determine acceptable or unacceptable images.
- Because there is a wider dynamic range and image processing in digital, the acceptable range is much greater.
- A lower-dose image may be noisy but may have diagnostic information.

Exposure Indicator Determination

Exposure indicator determination is an index providing a value that corresponds to the amount of radiation exposure of an anatomical structure to a digital detector. This exposure indicator can vary depending on the equipment manufacturer and how the manufacturer indicates the exposure level. Factors that influence exposure indicators are dose, positioning, and coning. Exposure indicator is a useful tool to determine proper exposure techniques to anatomical structures.

Fuji Computed Radiography S Value

An S value indicates an average exposure value on a particular anatomical part. Ranges for S values are approximately 150 to 200 for a normal exposure. As the S value increases, the radiation exposure to the image detector decreases.

Kodak CR EI uses the EI value of 1,800 to 2,200 to indicate an optimal exposure, whereas Philips uses the same EI term for DR to indicate optimal exposures that are between 200 and 800.

Agfa Computed Radiography

Agfa uses a log system called median exposure (LgM). It compares the exposure level to an established base dose. An optimal exposure is 1.9 to 2.5.

Other manufacturers use other terms, such as *REX*, *EXI*, and *DEI*, to determine exposure levels.

- Manufacturers all have different exposure indicator values.
- Exposure indicators provide information regarding radiation dose to a detector.
- Other factors influencing dose are positioning and coning on anatomical structures.
- Fuji CR uses an S value.

Gross Exposure Error

Gross exposure errors are occurrences of extreme imaging problems. Problems can be caused by mechanical, software, and human errors. Mottle can be a common problem especially due to low exposure to the image detector. Displayed images will lack contrast and spatial resolution, with an overall grayish appearance. A good indicator would be to look at the EI to see the value at the receptor. A high EI value may require a higher imaging technique. Images that are underexposed may lack proper mA values to properly expose images displaying the correct density. With image processing, a good contrast can be possible, but if not enough energy is used, the image will remain noisy. Problems with exposure errors can be human in nature, such as poor positioning, patient movement, and double exposures. Darkening of an image is usually an indicator of overexposure, but there can be other issues such as an uncollimated image or possibly backscatter radiation. Improper beam alignment to the grid can cause exposure errors; images will display grid cutoff. Refer to the EI of a system to determine the saturation level of the detector as a starting point.

In cases of exposure error, it's also important to select the proper imaging algorithm (menu). With DR, a specific algorithm may not detect the correct anatomical part that is being imaged and can result in many types of exposure errors.

- Extreme imaging problems can be categorized as gross exposure errors.
- Gross exposure errors can be mechanical, software, and human.
- Exposure indicators can determine if there is a problem with the image or the software.
- Errors can be from uncollimated images, backscatter radiation, grid cutoff, or wrong image processing algorithms and anatomical positioning.

REVIEW QUESTIONS

1. The term *spatial resolution* refers to:

   a. The amount of memory in a digital image
   b. Resolution measured in lp/cm
   c. The ability to display large objects in a matrix
   d. The amount of detail in a digital image

2. Sampling rate ___.

   a. Requires less memory when increased
   b. Describes how many times information is sampled along a scan line
   c. Shows better detail when the rate is decreased
   d. Varies with patient size

3. DEL _____.

   a. Is a term used in DR
   b. Is used in CR
   c. Is larger for better spatial resolution
   d. All of the answers are correct

4. Which of the following best describes the term *pixel value*?

   a. Is less in a 14″ × 17″ than an 8″ × 10″ image
   b. Is not used in DR
   c. Determines brightness levels on a digital image
   d. The more in an image, the less memory required

5. Quantum mottle is described as:

   a. Noise on an image
   b. A grainy appearance on an image
   c. Caused by a lack of photons reaching the receptor
   d. All of the answers are correct

6. Signal-to-noise refers to:

   a. The higher the signal-to-noise, the better the image
   b. The lower the signal-to-noise, the better the image
   c. Is better at 1:1 than 3:1 ratio
   d. Is only used in DR panels

7. The term *contrast-to-noise ratio* can be explained by which of the following?

   a. Quality increases with an increase of kV levels
   b. Refers to the brightness of an image
   c. Is determined by matrix size
   d. Refers to grayscale quality of an image

8. Which of the following regarding film is true?

   a. Finer-grained films are more sensitive to light
   b. Finer-grained films show less detail
   c. Radiographic films are coated on an acrylic base
   d. Film grain reflects film speed (sensitivity)

9. The following is true regarding electronic images:

   a. Digital x-ray images are exposed directly in a DR system or through a photomultiplier tube in CR
   b. Are exposed through a photomultiplier tube in DR or directly on CR
   c. CR uses a CCD to produce an image
   d. Digital photographic images do not use pixel values for image display

10. When performing a radiographic exam on a patient, a technologist:

    a. Can provide diagnostic interpretation to family members
    b. Plays an important role in the patient right to privacy
    c. Provides diagnostic results to the patient
    d. Cannot be liable for incorrect exam information or giving out patient information

11. Radiographs should be able to be stored indefinitely if:

    a. Films are developed in the correct temperature solution
    b. Chemistry is at the correct dilution
    c. Films are stored in correct humidity
    d. All of the answers are correct

12. What is the function of film developer?

    a. Dissolves and removes the unexposed silver halide crystals on the film
    b. Fixes and stabilizes the emulsion
    c. Turns silver halide crystals of a latent image to black metallic silver
    d. Turns silver halide crystals back into film emulsion

13. In most film processors, wash water plays a dual role during the processing cycle. This role includes which of the following?

    a. Film washing and fixing
    b. Film washing and solution temperature control
    c. Temperature and dryer regulation
    d. None of the answers are correct

14. Intensity of grayscale values is determined by:

    a. LUTs
    b. Detector size
    c. Monitor brightness
    d. Spatial resolution

15. What is the purpose of histogram equalization?

    a. It helps to increase system brightness
    b. It assigns equal pixel values to an image
    c. It attempts to normalize an image
    d. It is also called *contrast reduction*

16. The function of edge enhancement is which of the following?

    a. Decreases brightness along the edges of pixels
    b. Helps increase spatial resolution
    c. Is another term for low-pass filtering
    d. All of the answers are correct

17. Noise suppression, which is also known as low-pass filtering, is explained by which of the following statements?

    a. Averages nearby pixel values, which also can lower image contrast and reduce noise
    b. Averages nearby pixel values, which also can increase image contrast and reduce noise
    c. Can be reduced by lowering photon energy
    d. Has no effect on a digital image

18. Increasing the contrast of a digital image:

    a. Increases the number of shades of gray
    b. Decreases the number of shades of gray on an image
    c. Decreases the exposure curve
    d. Increases the detector size

19. Ghosting:

    a. Is dependent on detector size
    b. Can only occur in CR
    c. Can only occur in DR
    d. Can occur in both CR and DR

20. DICOM GSDF is defined as:

    a. A standard within DICOM to derive a common grayscale standard between different viewers
    b. A standard within DICOM to derive a common attenuation standard between different manufacturers
    c. A standard within DICOM to derive a common spatial resolution standard between different manufacturers
    d. A standard within DICOM to derive a common grayscale standard between different manufacturers

21. PACS in radiography is:

    a. A system where digital images, patient data, and other information can be stored and delivered to various sites through a digital network
    b. A system where only CR digital images, patient data, and other information can be stored and delivered to various sites through a digital network
    c. A system where only DR digital images, patient data, and other information can be stored and delivered to various sites through a digital network
    d. A system where digital images, patient data, and other information can be used only in the radiology department of a hospital

22. *HL7* is a term describing:

    a. A standard that is not integrated by the radiology department's DICOM
    b. A standard that is networked for the exchanging, sharing, and retrieval of electronic health information
    c. A standard that is limited only to a hospital for the sharing and retrieval of electronic health information
    d. A standard that is not compatible with HIS

23. Image artifacts can occur in DR and conventional radiography as a result of:

    a. Static
    b. Scratches
    c. Dirt and dust
    d. All of the answers are correct

24. The following is true regarding acceptable range of exposure:

    a. CR and DR have a narrow acceptable range of exposure
    b. DR has a narrow acceptable range of exposure
    c. Film has a narrow acceptable range of exposure
    d. High-quality images will be lower in dose but with higher noise levels

REFERENCES

1. American Registry of Radiologic Technologists. Content specifications for the examination in radiography. http://www.arrt.org/pdfs/Disciplines/Content-Specification/RAD-content-specification.pdf. Published 2010. Accessed May 14, 2013.

2. Fauber T. *Radiographic Imaging & Exposure.* 4th ed. St. Louis, MO: Elsevier; 2013.

3. Fosbinder R, Orth D. Grids and scatter reduction. In: Fosbinder R, Orth D, eds. *Essentials of Radiologic Science.* Baltimore, MD: Lippincott Williams & Wilkins; 2011:179. http://books.google.com/books?id=jRVg5iIM1UEC&pg=PA179&lpg=PA179&dq=how+much+air+gap+is+needed+to+reduce+scatter?&source=bl&ots=Jx4QEqSANJ&sig=l0WL4MXd5_VCCoRz6yBsrmZQcdY&hl=en&sa=X&ei=saqaUZH4K7be4AObh4CoCg&ved=0CD8Q6AEwAw#v=onepage&q=how%20much%20air%20gap%20is%20needed%20to%20reduce%20scatter%3F&f=false. Accessed May 21, 2013.

4. Fauber T. *Radiographic Imaging & Exposure.* 2nd ed. St. Louis, MO: Mosby Elsevier; 2004:79.

5. Fauber T. *Radiographic Imaging & Exposure.* 2nd ed. St. Louis, MO: Mosby Elsevier; 2004:84.

6. Fauber T. *Radiographic Imaging & Exposure.* 2nd ed. St. Louis, MO: Mosby Elsevier; 2004:103-104.

7. Conference of Radiation Control Program Directors, Inc. A brief overview of computed radiography. http://www.crcpd.org/Pubs/QAC/Oct08QAC.pdf. Published 2008. Accessed May 21, 2013.

CHAPTER 5

Imaging Procedures

THORAX

Chest
Posteroanterior Upright
Positioning Criteria

- Patient erect, posteroanterior (PA), and shielded
- Place 14″ × 17″ (35 × 42.5 centimeter [cm]) image receptor (IR) in Bucky
- Instruct patient to stand, placing chest as close to IR as possible
- Patient should roll shoulders forward and down, resting hands on hips palm up
- Central ray is perpendicular to the Bucky and directed to thoracic vertebra T6 or T7
- Collimate to skin margins; include all pertinent anatomy
- Place appropriate side marker within light field; it is suggested to place the left marker on the left side in order to be prepared for the left lateral
- Minimum source-to-image distance (SID): 72″ (180 cm)
- Respiration: double inhalation

Evaluation Criteria

- Sternoclavicular joints should be symmetrical bilaterally
- All pertinent anatomy demonstrated
- Appropriate collimation to reduce dose to patient
- Long-scale contrast for optimal exposure
- Heart shadow without excessive magnification
- Chin lifted up and out of the way
- Scapula moved out laterally away from chest anatomy
- Distance from lateral rib margins to vertebral column equal
- No motion evident by sharp lung markings in the hilar region

Demonstrates

- Bilateral lungs, apices, bases, costophrenic angles, cardiophrenic angle, air-filled trachea, hilum, great vessels, and bony thorax
- Full inspiration allows visualization of at least 10 posterior ribs

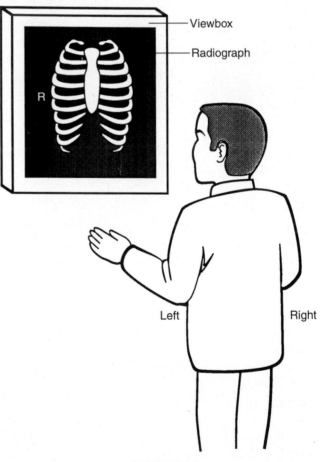

FIGURE 5-1

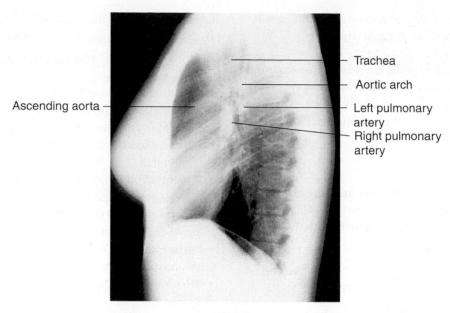

Trachea

Aortic arch

Ascending aorta

Left pulmonary artery

Right pulmonary artery

FIGURE 5-2

Lateral

Positioning Criteria

- Patient erect, PA, and shielded
- Place 14″ × 17″ (35 × 42.5 cm) IR lengthwise in Bucky
- Instruct patient to stand 90 degrees with the left aspect of the body against the IR (unless radiologist states right lateral to better demonstrate pathology to the right lung field)
- Central ray is perpendicular, directed to the midthorax at the level of T6–T7
- Patient should be instructed to raise arms up out of the way of the thorax
- Collimate to skin margins; include all pertinent anatomy
- Place appropriate side marker within light field
- Minimum SID: 72″ (180 cm)
- Respiration: double inhalation

Evaluation Criteria

- No rotation evident by superimposition of posterior ribs
- Hilar region should be centered to the image
- All pertinent anatomy demonstrated
- Appropriate collimation to reduce dose to patient
- Long-scale contrast for optimal exposure allowing visualization of heart, vascular markings, air, potential fluid, and bone
- Heart shadow without excessive magnification
- Chin lifted up and out of the way
- No motion evident by sharp lung markings in the hilar region

Demonstrates

- Bilateral lungs, apices, bases, costophrenic angles, sternum anteriorly, and thoracic vertebrae posteriorly
- Full inspiration allows visualization of at least 10 posterior ribs
- Potential pathology present posterior to heart

Anteroposterior Lordotic

Positioning Criteria

- Patient erect, anteroposterior (AP), and shielded
- Place 14″ × 17″ (35 × 42.5 cm) IR crosswise in Bucky
- Instruct patient to start off placing back as close to IR as possible
- Then instruct the patient to move the feet approximately 12″ (30 cm) from the upright radiographic unit, maintaining the back and shoulders against the unit
- Patient should roll the shoulders forward and rest hands on hips
- Central ray is perpendicular to the Bucky and directed 2 (5 cm) below the jugular notch
- Patient's midsagittal plane (MSP) should be centered to the Bucky
- Collimate to lung field
- Place appropriate side marker within light field
- Minimum SID: 72″ (180 cm)
- Respiration: double inhalation

Evaluation Criteria

- Sternoclavicular joints should be symmetrical bilaterally
- All pertinent anatomy demonstrated

- Appropriate collimation to reduce dose to patient
- Long-scale contrast for optimal exposure
- Chin lifted up and out of the way
- Scapula moved out laterally away from chest anatomy
- Distance from lateral rib margins to vertebral column should be equal
- No motion evident by sharp lung markings in the hilar region

Demonstrates

- Apices without superimposition from the clavicles
- Posterior ribs should superimpose over anterior ribs
- Potential calcifications and masses beneath the clavicles

Anteroposterior Supine

Positioning Criteria

- Performed for patients who are unable to assume an erect or decubitus position
- Patient recumbent, supine, and shielded
- Place 14″ × 17″ (35 × 42.5 cm) IR lengthwise in Bucky
- Central ray angled 3 degrees to 5 degrees caudal, preventing clavicles from obscuring apices of the lungs
- Patient's MSP should be centered to the Bucky
- Collimate to skin margins
- Place appropriate side marker within light field
- Minimum SID: 48″ to 72″ (120 to 180 cm)
- Respiration: double inhalation

Evaluation Criteria

- Sternoclavicular joints should be symmetrical bilaterally
- All pertinent anatomy demonstrated
- Appropriate collimation to reduce dose to patient
- Long-scale contrast for optimal exposure
- Chin lifted up and out of the way
- Distance from lateral rib margins to vertebral column should be equal
- No motion evident by sharp lung markings in the hilar region

Demonstrates

- Bilateral lungs, apices, bases, costophrenic angles, cardiophrenic angle, air-filled trachea, hilum, great vessels, and bony thorax
- Heart will appear magnified because of object-to-image distance (OID) and inability to maintain 72″ (120 cm) SID
- Full inspiration allows visualization of at least 10 posterior ribs

Lateral Decubitus

Positioning Criteria

- 14″ × 17″ (35 × 42.5 cm) IR with a stationary grid placed crosswise
- Patient placed in left lateral decubitus position (unless there is known fluid/pathology in the right aspect of the lung field), PA is preferred
- Patient should remain in this position for 10 to 20 minutes
- Patient should be propped up onto a radiolucent sponge so the chest side down is not clipped
- Central ray is perpendicular, directed to the midthorax at the level of T7
- Patient should be instructed to raise arms up out of the way of the thorax
- Move the IR so that the central ray is exiting through its center
- Collimate to skin margins; include all pertinent anatomy
- Place appropriate side marker within light field on the side up
- Minimum SID: 48″ to 72″ (120 to 180 cm)
- Respiration: double inhalation

Evaluation Criteria

- All pertinent anatomy demonstrated
- Appropriate collimation to reduce dose to patient
- Long-scale contrast for optimal exposure, allowing visualization of heart, vascular markings, air, potential fluid, and bone
- Heart shadow without excessive magnification
- Chin lifted up and out of the way
- No motion evident by sharp lung markings in the hilar region

Demonstrates

- Bilateral lungs, apices, bases, costophrenic angles, and lateral borders of ribs
- Full inspiration allows visualization of at least 10 posterior ribs
- Air-fluid levels, small pleural effusions
- Pathology of chest

Anterior/Posterior Obliques

Done to rule out superimposed opacities or pulmonary nodes

Positioning Criteria

- Patient erect and shielded
- Place 14″ × 17″ (35 × 42.5 cm) IR in Bucky lengthwise
- Instruct patient to stand, placing chest as close to IR as possible

- Various degrees of obliquity may be performed, depending on purpose of the oblique
- The patient should be instructed to raise the arm closest to the IR up, resting on radiographic unit, and the arm away from the IR bent, resting on the hip
- 10 degrees to 15 degrees oblique sufficient for superimposition
- 45 degrees oblique; right anterior oblique (RAO) or left anterior oblique (LAO) preferred for pathology in lung field
- 60 degrees LAO for heart studies and air-filled trachea
- Central ray is perpendicular to the Bucky and directed to T6 or T7
- The vertical beam will have to be centered in order for the entire thorax to be demonstrated
- Anterior obliques demonstrate the side of interest that is furthest from the IR; for example, the LAO position will demonstrate the right lung field because the thoracic spine (T-spine) moves to the left aspect
- Posterior obliques demonstrate the side of interest closest to the IR; however, will demonstrate magnification of the heart and great vessels
- Collimate to skin margins; include all pertinent anatomy
- Place appropriate side marker within light field
- Minimum SID: 72″ (180 cm)
- Respiration: double inhalation

Evaluation Criteria
- All pertinent anatomy demonstrated
- Appropriate collimation to reduce dose to patient
- Long-scale contrast for optimal exposure
- Chin lifted up and out of the way
- No motion evident by sharp lung markings in the hilar region

Demonstrates
- Bilateral lungs, apices, bases, costophrenic angles, cardiophrenic angle, air-filled trachea, hilum, great vessels, and bony thorax
- Full inspiration allows visualization of at least 10 posterior ribs

Ribs
Anteroposterior
Evaluation Criteria
- Patient AP, recumbent or erect, and shielded
- Place 14″ × 17″ (35 × 42.5 cm) IR lengthwise in Bucky
- Central ray perpendicular to the IR, directed 4″ inferior to jugular notch, and midway between the lateral border of the affected ribs and sternum
- Collimate to affected ribs

- Place appropriate side marker within light field
- Minimum SID: 40″ (100 cm)
- Respiration: inhalation if area of interest is above diaphragm
- Respiration: exhalation if ribs below diaphragm are the area of interest

Evaluation Criteria
- Affected ribs above the diaphragm I to X should be visualized; if affected ribs below the diaphragm, ribs VIII to XII present
- No rotation

Demonstrates
- Posterior ribs
- Optimal exposure factors
- Fractures

Posteroanterior Ribs

All factors remain the same with the exception that the anterior ribs are best demonstrated.

Anterior Obliques
Positioning Criteria
- Patient AP, recumbent or erect, and shielded
- Place 14″ × 17″ (35 × 42.5 cm) IR lengthwise in Bucky
- Patient rotated 45 degrees toward affected side
- Instruct patient to raise arm closest to Bucky and rest it over the radiographic unit and place arm away from the IR on hip
- Central ray perpendicular to the IR, directed 4″ (10 cm) inferior to jugular notch, and midway between the lateral border of the affected ribs and sternum
- Collimate to affected ribs
- Place appropriate side marker within light field
- Minimum SID: 40″ (100 cm)
- Respiration: inhalation if area of interest is above diaphragm
- Respiration: exhalation if ribs below diaphragm are the area of interest

Evaluation Criteria
- Affected ribs above the diaphragm I to X should be visualized; if affected ribs are below the diaphragm, ribs VIII to XII should be present
- Coned-down image of lower ribs may be done using a 10″ × 12″ (25 × 30 cm) IR, placing the bottom of the IR approximately 1″ (2.5 cm) superior to iliac crest, then centering to the Bucky
- Spine should move toward the unaffected side of the ribs, allowing the elongation of ribs closest to the IR

Demonstrates

- Axillary portion of posterior ribs
- Optimal exposure factors
- Fractures

Posterior Oblique Ribs

Positioning Criteria

- Patient PA, recumbent or erect, and shielded
- Place 14″ × 17″ (35 × 4.5 cm) IR lengthwise in Bucky
- Patient rotated 45 degrees away from affected side
- Instruct patient to raise arm closest to IR, and place arm away from the IR on hip
- Central ray perpendicular to the IR, directed 4″ inferior to jugular notch, and midway between the lateral border of the affected ribs and sternum
- Collimate to affected ribs
- Place appropriate side marker within light field
- Minimum SID: 40″ (100 cm)
- Respiration: inhalation if area of interest is above diaphragm
- Respiration: exhalation if ribs below diaphragm are the area of interest

Evaluation Criteria

- Affected ribs above the diaphragm I to X should be visualized; if affected ribs below the diaphragm, ribs VIII to XII present
- Follow guidelines for a cone-down of the lower ribs from the AP oblique guidelines
- Spine should move toward the unaffected side of the ribs, allowing the elongation of ribs closest to the IR

Demonstrates

- Axillary portion of the anterior ribs
- Optimal exposure factors
- Fractures

Sternum
Lateral

Positioning Criteria

- Patient erect and shielded
- Place 10″ × 12″ (25 × 30 cm) IR lengthwise in Bucky
- Instruct patient to stand 90 degrees with the left aspect of the body against the IR (unless radiologist states right lateral to better demonstrate pathology to the right lung field)
- Patient may instead assume the left lateral recumbent position or a cross-table lateral image may be performed in the supine position

- Central ray is perpendicular, directed to the midsternum (jugular notch and xiphoid)
- Patient should be instructed to arch back, allowing chest to be pushed forward, and grasp arms behind back
- Collimate close to sternum
- Place appropriate left marker within light field
- Minimum SID: 72″ (180 cm)
- Respiration: inhalation

Evaluation Criteria

- No rotation evident
- All pertinent anatomy demonstrated
- Appropriate collimation to reduce dose to patient
- Chin lifted up and out of the way
- Arms and vertebrae should not be superimposed over the sternum
- No motion evident

Demonstrates

- Sternum over heart shadow
- Fractures and pathologies

Right Anterior Oblique

Positioning Criteria

- Patient erect and shielded
- Place 10″ × 12″ (25 × 30 cm) IR lengthwise in Bucky
- Patient should be RAO 15 degrees to 20 degrees; hypersthenic patients may require less obliquity and asthenic patients more obliquity
- Place the top of the IR approximately 1½″ (4 cm) superior to the jugular notch and the central ray centered to the IR and 1″ (2.5 cm) to the left of midline
- Appropriate marker placed within collimated field
- Minimum SID: 40″ (100 cm)
- Respiration: autotomography to blur out vascular/pulmonary markings or, if the patient is unable to perform the breathing technique, patient should suspend respiration on exhalation

Evaluation Criteria

Sternum should be visualized within the heart shadow and centered to the IR.

Demonstrates

- Sternum superimposed over heart shadow
- Optimal contrast and density
- Fractures
- Pathologies such as pectus excavatum and pectus carinatum

Left Anterior Oblique

- All criteria from RAO remain the same except the patient is rotated 15 degrees to 20 degrees toward the left side in LAO position.
- The heart will not act as a filter as it would with the RAO; therefore, the ribs will appear more prominent than the sternum.

Posteroanterior Sternoclavicular Joints
Positioning Criteria

- Patient PA and shielded
- Place 10″ × 12″ (25 × 30 cm) IR in the Bucky crosswise
- Central ray directed approximately 3″ (7.5 cm) inferior to vertebral prominence and along the midline of the vertebrae
- MSP parallel to midline of grid
- Appropriate marker placed within collimated field
- Minimum SID: 40″ (100 cm)
- Respiration: suspend at the end of exhalation

Evaluation Criteria
No rotation present

Demonstrates

- Bilateral sternoclavicular joints through superimposed vertebral and rib shadows

Anterior Oblique Sternoclavicular Joints
Positioning Criteria

- Patient PA and shielded
- Place 10″ × 12″ (25 × 30 cm) IR in the Bucky crosswise
- All factors remain the same as the PA sternoclavicular joints, except the patient is obliqued 15 degrees to 20 degrees
- RAO demonstrates right sternoclavicular joint and the LAO demonstrates the left sternoclavicular joint
- Side closest to IR is demonstrated
- Central ray is perpendicular to the sternoclavicular joint closest to the IR
- Central ray enters at the level of T2–T3, which is approximately 3″ (7.5 cm) from the vertebral prominence and 1″ to 2″ (2.5 to 5 cm) lateral from MSP
- Appropriate marker placed within collimated field
- Minimum SID: 40″ (100 cm)
- Respiration: suspend at the end of exhalation

Evaluation Criteria

- Proper exposure factors allowing the visualization of the sternoclavicular joint of interest

Demonstrates

- Sternoclavicular joint of interest open and adjacent to vertebral column with minimal obliquity through superimposing vertebral and rib shadows
- Joint separation or other pathology

SOFT TISSUE NECK

Anteroposterior Upper Airway

Positioning Criteria

- Patient AP and erect if possible
- Place a 10″ × 12″ (25 × 30 cm) IR in the Bucky lengthwise
- MSP aligned to grid
- Instruct patient to raise chin, bringing the acanthomeatal line perpendicular to the IR
- Central ray perpendicular to the IR and directed to T1 or T2, about 1″ (2.5 cm) above the jugular notch
- Shield patient
- Minimum SID: 40″ (100 cm)
- Collimate from mentum to approximately an inch below the jugular notch and to the soft tissue margins laterally
- Respiration: performed during a slow, deep inspiration

Evaluation Criteria

- Air-filled trachea and upper airway
- Symmetric sternoclavicular joints evident if there is no rotation

Demonstrates

- Larynx to trachea, C3 to T4 filled with air
- Proximal cervical vertebrae to midthoracic region should be included

Lateral Upper Airway

Positioning Criteria

- Patient in a 90-degree lateral position and erect if possible (right or left lateral does not matter)
- Place a 10″ × 12″ (25 × 30 cm) IR in the Bucky lengthwise
- Midaxillary plane aligned to grid
- Instruct patient to raise chin and rotate shoulders posteriorly, clasping hands behind back
- Central ray perpendicular to the IR and directed to C6 or C7
- Collimate from mentum to approximately an inch below the jugular notch and to the soft tissue margins laterally
- Minimum SID: 72″ (180 cm)
- Respiration: performed during a slow, deep inspiration

Evaluation Criteria

- Air-filled trachea and larynx
- Shoulders moved away from trachea

Demonstrates

- Larynx to trachea filled with air, including region of thyroid and thymus gland
- External auditory meatus (EAM) to T2 or T3, unless distal larynx is of interest, in which case, centering should be lower to include C3–T5
- Proximal cervical vertebrae to midthoracic region should be included
- Rule out epiglottitis
- Potential foreign body

ABDOMEN AND GASTROINTESTINAL STUDIES

Abdomen Projections
Anteroposterior Supine Abdomen
Positioning Criteria

- Patient supine with legs fully extended; gonadal shield for male patients; breast shield for females
- Place 14″ × 17″ (35 × 42.5 cm) IR in Bucky aligned with iliac crest at midpoint of receptor
- Central ray directed perpendicular to midpoint of IR and MSP
- Collimate to all sides to include all pertinent anatomy
- Place appropriate side marker in light field at lower lateral aspect of image
- Minimum SID: 40″ (100 cm)
- Image taken on full expiration

Evaluation Criteria

- Anatomy from kidneys to bladder is visualized
- No evidence of rotation
- Iliac wings and obturators (if visible) are symmetrical
- Spinous processes centered on vertebrae; transverse processes equidistant to vertebrae

Demonstrates

- Scout view of abdomen
- Outline of liver, spleen, kidneys
- Air-filled stomach and bowel
- Psoas muscle on asthenic patients
- Symphysis pubis for bladder region
- Pathologies including but not limited to: obstruction, choleliths, renal calculi

Anteroposterior Upright/Erect Abdomen
Positioning Criteria

- Patient should be placed in an AP erect position against the upright Bucky; gonadal region shielded
- Place 14″ × 17″ (35 × 42.5 cm) IR in Bucky with midpoint aligned at 2″ (5 cm) above iliac crest
- Central ray directed perpendicular to midpoint of IR and MSP
- Collimate to all sides to include all pertinent anatomy
- Place appropriate side marker in light field at lower lateral aspect of image

- Minimum SID: 40″ (100 cm)
- Image taken on full expiration

Evaluation Criteria

- Anatomy from diaphragm and lower is included
- No evidence of rotation
- Iliac wings and obturators (if visible) are symmetrical
- Spinous processes centered on vertebrae, transverse processes equidistant to vertebrae

Demonstrates

- Air-fluid levels in the gastrointestinal (GI) tract
- Pathologies including but not limited to: retroperitoneal air, abnormal masses

Lateral Decubitus Abdomen
Positioning Criteria

- Patient should be placed in a PA left lateral position elevated off tabletop with radiolucent sponge; patient should remain in this position for minimum of 5 minutes prior to exposure (10 minutes is preferred)
- Utilize 14″ × 17″ (35 × 42.5 cm) gridded IR with midpoint aligned at 2″ (5 cm) above iliac crest; gonadal region shielded
- Central ray directed horizontally to midpoint of IR and MSP
- Collimate to all sides to include all pertinent anatomy
- Place appropriate side marker in light field at lower lateral aspect of image
- Minimum SID: 40″ (100 cm)
- Image taken on full expiration

Evaluation Criteria

- Anatomy from diaphragm and lower is included
- No evidence of rotation
- Iliac wings and obturators (if visible) are symmetrical
- Spinous processes centered on vertebrae, transverse processes equidistant to vertebrae

Demonstrates

- Air-fluid levels in the GI tract
- Pathologies including but not limited to: retroperitoneal air, abnormal masses

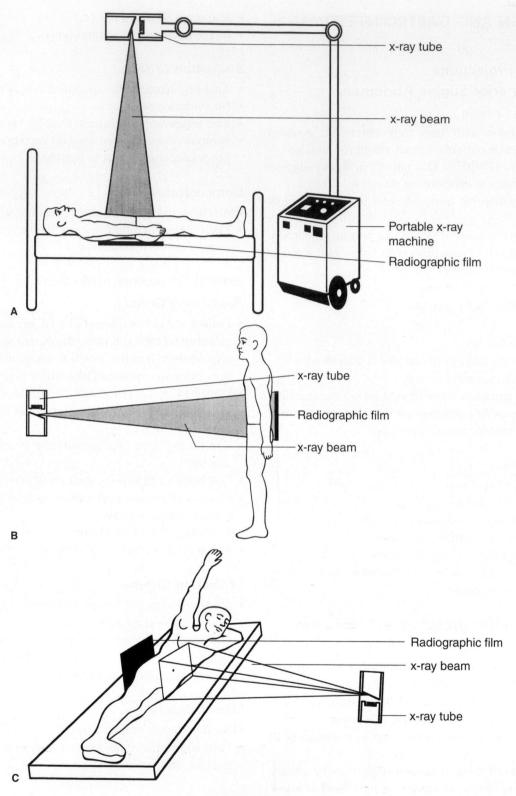

A

- x-ray tube
- x-ray beam
- Portable x-ray machine
- Radiographic film

B

- x-ray tube
- Radiographic film
- x-ray beam

C

- Radiographic film
- x-ray beam
- x-ray tube

FIGURE 5-3

Dorsal Decubitus Abdomen

Positioning Criteria

- Patient is placed supine on radiolucent sponge
- Utilize 14″ × 17″ (35 × 42.5 cm) gridded IR with midpoint aligned at 2″ (5 cm) above iliac crest; gonadal region shielded
- Central ray directed horizontally to midpoint of IR and midcoronal plane
- Collimate to all sides to include all pertinent anatomy
- Place appropriate side marker in light field at lower lateral aspect of image
- Minimum SID: 40″ (100 cm)
- Image taken on full expiration

Evaluation Criteria

- Anatomy from diaphragm and lower is included
- No evidence of rotation
- Demonstrates superimposition of anterior superior iliac spine (ASIS), iliac crests, and posterior ribs

Demonstrates

- Air-fluid levels in the GI tract
- Anterior abdominal soft tissue anatomy and prevertebral region
- Pathologies including but not limited to: retroperitoneal air, abnormal masses, aneurysms, aortic calcifications

BARIUM STUDIES

For all upper gastrointestinal (UGI) studies, small bowel series (SBS), and barium enemas (BEs), a scout view of the abdomen is performed. The entire abdomen must be demonstrated prior to contrast administration.

Esophagus Projections

Patient Preparation

No special preparation is necessary unless the patient is also having a UGI exam.

Right Anterior Oblique Esophagus

Positioning Criteria

- Place patient in an RAO 35 degrees to 40 degrees; shield the gonadal region
- Place top of 14″ × 17″ (35 × 42.5 cm) IR 2″ (5 cm) above shoulder
- Cup of barium in patient's left hand with straw in mouth
- Central ray perpendicular to IR centered at approximately T5–T6 and 2″ (5 cm) anterior to the spine (up side)
- Collimate crosswise to create a band of 5″ to 6″ (12.5 to 15 cm)
- Patient is instructed to drink barium; on third/fourth swallow, image is taken

Evaluation Criteria

- Entire esophagus visualized
- Seen between the spine and heart

Demonstrates

- Entire esophagus filled with barium
- Visualized between spine and heart
- Pathologies including but not limited to: anatomic anomalies, dysphagia, varices, diverticulum

Right Lateral Esophagus

Positioning Criteria

- Place patient in a right lateral with arms anterior to body, elbows flexed; shield gonadal region
- Place top of 14″ × 17″ (35 × 42.5 cm) IR 2″ (5 cm) above shoulder
- Cup of barium against patient's flexed elbows, straw in mouth
- Central ray perpendicular to IR centered at approximately T5–T6 and at midcoronal plane
- Collimate crosswise to create a band of 5″ to 6″ (12.5 to 15 cm)
- Patient is instructed to drink barium; on third/fourth swallow, image is taken

Evaluation Criteria

- True lateral position with posterior ribs superimposed
- Entire esophagus visualized
- Seen between T-spine and heart

Demonstrates

- Entire esophagus filled with barium
- Visualized between spine and heart
- Pathologies including but not limited to: anatomic anomalies, dysphagia, varices, diverticulum

Anteroposterior/Posteroanterior Esophagus

Positioning Criteria

- Place patient supine on the table; shield gonadal region
- Place top of 14″ × 17″ (35 × 42.5 cm) IR 2″ (5 cm) above shoulder
- Use either arm to hold cup; place straw in mouth
- Central ray perpendicular to IR centered at approximately T5–T6 and at MSP
- Collimate crosswise to create a band of 5″ to 6″ (12.5 to 15 cm)
- Minimum SID: 40″ (100 cm)
- Patient is instructed to drink barium; on third/fourth swallow, image is taken

Evaluation Criteria

No rotation as noted by sternoclavicular joints

Demonstrates

- Barium-filled esophagus
- Alternate PA can be performed in the prone position with same positioning, centering, and collimation
- Pathologies including but not limited to: anatomic anomalies, dysphagia, varices, diverticulum

Left Anterior Oblique Esophagus

Positioning Criteria

- Place patient in an LAO 35 degrees to 40 degrees; shield gonadal region
- Place top of 14″ × 17″ (35 × 42.5 cm) IR 2″ (5 cm) above shoulder
- Cup of barium in patient's right hand with straw in mouth
- Central ray perpendicular to IR centered at approximately T5–T6 and 2″ (5 cm) anterior to the spine (up side)
- Collimate crosswise to create a band of 5″ to 6″ (12.5 to 15 cm)
- Minimum SID: 40″ (100 cm)
- Patient is instructed to drink barium; on third/fourth swallow, image is taken

Evaluation Criteria
- Entire esophagus visualized
- Seen between the spine and hilar region of lungs

Demonstrates
- Entire esophagus filled with barium
- Visualized between spine and hilar region of lungs
- Pathologies including but not limited to: anatomic anomalies, dysphagia, varices, diverticulum

Swallowing Dysfunction Study (Modified Barium Swallow)[1]
- Exam performed by the physician initially
- Utilizes fluoroscopy in the AP and lateral positions to assess patient's swallowing function
- Spot radiographs are taken to document
- Technologist may perform an esophagram series postprocedure (see above section)

Upper Gastrointestinal Projections
Patient Preparation
- Patient should have nothing by mouth (be NPO) for 8 hours for stomach to be empty
- No smoking or chewing gum during this time

Right Anterior Oblique Upper Gastrointestinal
Positioning Criteria
- Place patient in a 40-degree to 70-degree RAO; shield gonadal region
- Utilize a 10″ × 12″ (25 × 30 cm) IR placed lengthwise in the Bucky
- Central ray perpendicular to IR centered at level of duodenal bulb
- Level of duodenal bulb varies based on body habitus:
  Asthenic patient: lumbar vertebrae L2–L3
  Sthenic patient: L1
  Hypersthenic patient: T12
- Collimate to size of IR or smaller
- Minimum SID: 40″ (100 cm)
- Image taken on full exhalation

Evaluation Criteria
- Entire stomach and C-loop of duodenum are visualized
- Duodenal bulb in profile

Demonstrates
- Fundus of stomach filled with air
- Body and pylorus of stomach filled with barium
- Pathologies including but not limited to: polyps, ulcers

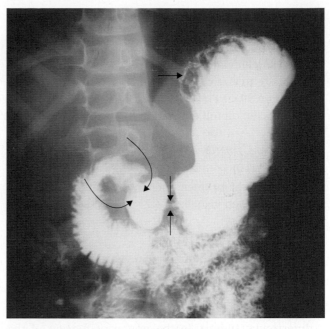

FIGURE 5-4

Posteroanterior Upper Gastrointestinal
Positioning Criteria
- Patient placed in a prone position on the table; shield the gonadal region
- Central ray perpendicular to IR centered at level of duodenal bulb
- Level of duodenal bulb varies based on body habitus
  Asthenic patient: L2–L3
  Sthenic patient: L1
  Hypersthenic patient: T12
- Collimate to size of IR or smaller
- Minimum SID: 40″ (100 cm)
- Image taken on full exhalation

Evaluation Criteria
- Entire stomach and duodenum are visualized

Demonstrates
- Entire stomach and duodenum barium filled
- Pathologies including but not limited to: polyps, diverticula, bezoars, gastritis

Right Lateral Upper Gastrointestinal
Positioning Criteria
- Place patient in a left lateral with arms anterior to body, elbows flexed; shield gonadal region
- Utilize a 10″ × 12″ (25 × 30 cm) IR placed in the Bucky
- Central ray perpendicular to IR centered at level of duodenal bulb

- Level of duodenal bulb varies based on body habitus
  Asthenic patient: L2–L3
  Sthenic patient: L1
  Hypersthenic patient: T12
- Collimate to size of IR or smaller
- Minimum SID: 40″ (100 cm)
- Image taken on full exhalation

Evaluation Criteria

- Vertebral bodies in lateral position
- Intervertebral foramen open in true lateral position
- Entire stomach visualized

Demonstrates

- Entire stomach and duodenum visualized
- Retrogastric space
- Pylorus and C-loop demonstrated
- Pathologies including but not limited to: polyps, diverticula, tumors in the posterior margin of the stomach

Left Posterior Oblique Upper Gastrointestinal

Positioning Criteria

- Place patient in a 30-degree to 60-degree left posterior oblique (LPO); shield gonadal region
- Utilize a 10″ × 12″ (25 × 30 cm) IR placed in the Bucky aligned with central ray
- Central ray perpendicular to IR centered at level of duodenal bulb and midway between MSP and lateral margin
- Approximate level of duodenal bulb varies based on body habitus
  Asthenic patient: L2
  Sthenic patient: L1
  Hypersthenic patient: T12
- Collimate to size of IR or smaller
- Minimum SID: 40″ (100 cm)
- Image taken on full exhalation

Evaluation Criteria

- Entire stomach and C-loop of duodenum are visualized
- Duodenal bulb in profile

Demonstrates

- Fundus of stomach filled with barium
- Body and pylorus of stomach filled with air for a double-contrast study
- Pathologies including but not limited to: gastritis and ulcers during a double-contrast study

Anteroposterior Upper Gastrointestinal

Positioning Criteria

- Place patient supine on the table; shield gonadal region
- Utilize a 10″ × 12″ (25 × 30 cm) IR placed in the Bucky
- Central ray perpendicular to IR centered at level of duodenal bulb and midway between MSP and lateral margin
- Approximate level of duodenal bulb varies based on body habitus
  Asthenic patient: L2
  Sthenic patient: L1
  Hypersthenic patient: T12
- Collimate to size of IR or smaller
- Minimum SID: 40″ (100 cm)
- Image taken on full exhalation

Evaluation Criteria

- Entire stomach and duodenum are visualized
- Lower lung field included

Demonstrates

- Fundus of stomach filled with barium
- Pathologies including but not limited to: hiatal hernia

Small Bowel Series Projections

Types of Small Bowel Series

Performed in combination with UGI, SBS only, or enteroclysis

Patient Preparation

- Patient should be NPO for 8 hours for stomach to be empty
- No smoking or chewing gum during this time

Posteroanterior (Follow-through) Small Bowel Series

- Several images are taken in the PA projection to follow the barium through the small intestine
- Place the patient prone on the imaging table
- First image taken at 15 to 30 minutes after barium ingested centered 2″ (5 cm) above iliac crest; all other images centered at iliac crest
- Utilize shield providing it does not cover pertinent anatomy
- Place appropriate side marker in light field at lower lateral aspect of image
- Minimum SID: 40″ (100 cm)
- Image taken on full expiration

Evaluation Criteria

- Anatomy from stomach and inferior is visualized
- No evidence of rotation
- Iliac wings and obturators (if visible) are symmetrical
- Spinous processes centered on vertebrae; transverse processes equidistant to vertebrae

Demonstrates

- PA view of abdomen
- Documentation of entire stomach and small bowel barium filled with series of pictures
- Study complete when barium reaches the ileocecal valve

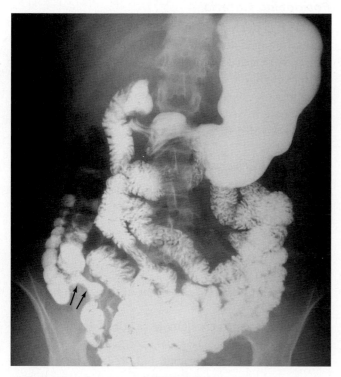

FIGURE 5-5

- Pathologies including but not limited to: enteritis, Meckel diverticulum, Whipple disease, and Crohn disease

Ileocecal Spots Small Bowel Series

Physician will image the ileocecal valve under fluoroscopic guidance using compression.

Enteroclysis Small Bowel Series

Indicated for patients with clinical history of Crohn disease, small bowel ileus, or malabsorption syndrome. Under fluoroscopic guidance, a duodenojejunal tube is placed into the terminal duodenum. During this double-contrast procedure, barium is injected through the duodenojejunal tube and the patient is imaged in the same manner as a traditional SBS. Then air or methylcellulose is injected to distend the bowel. Catheter is removed when study is complete. The study provides increased detail from the standard SBS procedure; however, there is increased risk of perforation owing to catheter placement.

Barium Enema Procedure

Patient Preparation

Patient preparation may vary from facility to facility; however, it typically includes the following:

- If time permits, the patient should be on a light diet for 2 to 3 days prior to the exam
- Clear liquid diet for the immediate 24 hours before the study
- Increased fluid intake, two glasses per hour from 12 pm until 12 am
- 10 ounces of magnesium citrate or equivalent night before
- NPO 8 to 12 hours prior to exam
- Cleansing enema morning of exam

Preparation for Tip Insertion

- Patient is placed in the Sims position (LAO) on the table after changing
- Patient is instructed prior to tube placement to:

    Keep sphincter contracted to hold tube in place
    Concentrate on breathing to keep abdominal muscles relaxed to reduce spasms
- Lubricated enema tip is inserted 1″ to 1½″ (2.5 to 4 cm) anterior toward the umbilicus, then superior and slightly anterior
- Total insertion should not exceed 1″ to 1½″ (2.5 to 4 cm)
- Hang barium bag no more than 24″ (60 cm) above the table

Left Lateral Rectum Barium Enema

Positioning Criteria

- Patient is placed in a left lateral position on the table
- Central ray is directed to the level of ASIS and midcoronal plane
- Utilize a 10″ × 12″ (25 × 30 cm) IR lengthwise centered to the central ray
- Collimate to the size of the IR
- Minimum SID: 40″ (100 cm)
- Image taken on expiration

Evaluation Criteria

- No rotation
- Femoral heads are superimposed
- Visualize rectum barium filled

Demonstrates

- Barium-filled rectum in a lateral projection
- Pathologies including but not limited to: polyps, diverticulum, strictures, and fistulas between rectum and bladder/uterus

For double-contrast study, IR is taken utilizing a horizontal central ray with the patient in a ventral decubitus position. Centering is the same. Demonstration in this view also includes air-fluid level in the rectum.

Left Lateral Decubitus Barium Enema Projection

Positioning Criteria

- Performed as part of a double-contrast BE study only
- Can be performed with the patient AP or PA (PA preferred to reduce gonadal dose)
- Patient is placed in a left lateral position against the 14″ × 17″ (35 × 42.5 cm) gridded IR
- Central ray is directed horizontally to MSP and iliac crest
- Minimum SID: 40″ (100 cm)
- Image taken on expiration

Evaluation Criteria

- No rotation as evident by appearance of pelvis and spine
- Entire large intestine is included

Demonstrates

- Provides detail of the air-filled structures of the large intestine, lateral aspect of the ascending colon, and medial aspect of the descending colon
- Entire colon with air-fluid levels
- Pathologies including but not limited to: presence of polyps, diverticula

Right Lateral Decubitus Barium Enema Projection

Positioning Criteria

- Performed as part of a double-contrast BE study only
- Can be performed with the patient AP or PA (PA preferred to reduce gonadal dose)
- Patient is placed in a right lateral position against the 14″ × 17″ (35 × 42.5 cm) gridded IR
- Central ray is directed horizontally to MSP and iliac crest
- Minimum SID: 40″ (100 cm)
- Image taken on expiration

Evaluation Criteria

- No rotation as evident by appearance of pelvis and spine
- Entire large intestine is included

Demonstrates

- Provides detail of the air-filled structures of the large intestine, medial aspect of the ascending colon, and lateral aspect of the descending colon
- Entire colon with air-fluid levels
- Pathologies including but not limited to: presence of polyps, diverticula

Left Posterior Oblique Barium Enema Projection

Positioning Criteria

- Patient is positioned in a 35-degree to 45-degree LPO
- Central ray is directed to the level of iliac crest and 1″ (2.5 cm) medial to the elevated ASIS
- Utilize a 14″ × 17″ (35 × 42.5 cm) IR in table Bucky lengthwise centered to central ray
- Collimate to size of IR
- Minimum SID: 40″ (100 cm)

Evaluation Criteria

- Ala of left ilium will be elongated; right will be foreshortened
- No tilt is present
- Entire large intestine visualized

Demonstrates

- Right colic flexure seen open and free of superimposition
- Ascending and rectosigmoid portions should appear open
- Pathologies including but not limited to: obstructions, volvulus, ileus, diverticula, and polyps during a double-contrast study

This projection can also be performed in the PA RAO position to demonstrate the same anatomy free of superimposition.

Right Posterior Oblique Barium Enema Projection

Positioning Criteria

- Patient is positioned in a 35-degree to 45-degree right posterior oblique (RPO)
- Utilize a 14″ × 17″ (35 × 42.5 cm) IR in table Bucky lengthwise aligned with central ray
- Central ray is directed 1″ to 2″ (2.5 to 5 cm) superior to iliac crest and 1″ (2.5 cm) medial to the elevated ASIS

- Collimate to size of IR
- Minimum SID: 40″ (100 cm)

Evaluation Criteria

- Ala of right ilium will be elongated; left will be fore-shortened
- No tilt is present
- Entire large intestine visualized

Demonstrates

- Left colic flexure seen open and free of superimposition
- Ascending and rectosigmoid portions should appear open
- Pathologies including but not limited to: obstructions, volvulus, ileus, diverticula, and polyps during a double-contrast study

This projection can also be performed in the PA LAO position to demonstrate the same anatomy free of superimposition.

Posteroanterior Barium Enema Projection

Positioning Criteria

- Patient is placed in the prone position on the table
- Central ray is directed at iliac crest and MSP
- 14″ × 17″ (35 × 42.5 cm) IR in table Bucky lengthwise aligned with central ray
- Collimate to size of IR
- Minimum SID: 40″ (100 cm)

Evaluation Criteria

- No rotation visible
- Spine is centered and in middle of image (unless patient has scoliosis)
- Iliac wings are even and symmetrical

Demonstrates

- Entire colon
- For double-contrast study, air will be in the rectum and ascending and descending portions of the colon

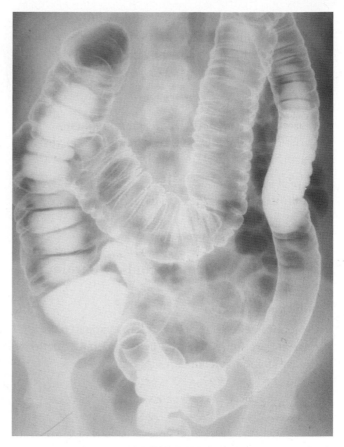

FIGURE 5-6

This projection can also be performed in the AP position to demonstrate the same anatomy. During a double-contrast study, the air will now be in the transverse and loops of the sigmoid colon.

Anteroposterior Axial (Butterfly) Projection

Positioning Criteria

- Place patient in the supine position on the table
- Central ray is directed 30 degrees to 40 degrees cephalic at MSP and 2″ (5 cm) below ASIS
- Collimate to area of interest
- Alternate position: Patient can be placed in the LPO position if the sigmoid is tortuous; centering is then adjusted to 2″ (5 cm) inferior to ASIS and 2″ (5 cm) medial to the right ASIS

Evaluation Criteria

- Rectosigmoid junction seen free of superimposition
- Adequate tube angle noted by elongation of rectosigmoid junction

Demonstrates

- Less overlapping of the rectosigmoid junction
- Pathologies including but not limited to: polyps, neoplasm, colitis

This projection can also be performed in the PA RAO position with a 30-degree to 40-degree tube angle centered at iliac crest and MSP. Same anatomy is demonstrated with reduced gonadal dose.

Posteroanterior Postevacuation Barium Enema Projection

Positioning Criteria

- Projection taken after patient has evacuated barium
- Patient prone; gonadal shield for male patients; breast shield for females

- Place 14″ × 17″ (35 × 42.5 cm) IR in Bucky aligned with iliac crest at midpoint of receptor
- Central ray directed perpendicular to midpoint of IR and MSP
- Collimate to all sides to include all pertinent anatomy
- Place appropriate side marker in light field at lower lateral aspect of image
- Minimum SID: 40″ (100 cm)
- Image taken on full expiration

Evaluation Criteria

- Anatomy from kidneys to bladder is visualized
- Colon visualized
- No evidence of rotation
- Iliac wings and obturators (if visible) are symmetrical
- Spinous processes centered on vertebrae; transverse processes equidistant to vertebrae

Demonstrates

- Residual barium in colon
- Small polyps and defects can be noted

SURGICAL CHOLANGIOGRAPHY

This exam is performed in the operating room with the C-arm. The technologist must be able to manipulate the C-arm to image the biliary ductal system. A picture in the AP projection is obtained either before or following surgical removal of the gallbladder. A contrast medium is injected into the biliary system to check for residual stones and proper drainage into the duodenum.

ENDOSCOPIC RETROGRADE CHOLANGIOPANCREATOGRAPHY

Endoscopic retrograde cholangiopancreatography (or ERCP) is performed to view the biliary and pancreatic ducts. The procedure can be diagnostic or therapeutic in nature. This procedure is performed by the gastroenterologist assisted by a team including the technologist.

Under fluoroscopy, a cannula is inserted into the common bile duct or the pancreatic duct. Retrograde injection of contrast media into the ducts is followed by fluoroscopy. The technologist on occasion may be asked to perform AP/PA or oblique images of the right upper quadrant postprocedure for documentation.

UROLOGICAL STUDIES

All urological studies utilize an AP abdomen as a scout projection.

Cystography
Anteroposterior Projection
Positioning Criteria

- Patient is placed in the supine position with legs fully extended
- Place a 10″ × 12″ (25 × 30 cm) IR lengthwise in table Bucky
- Central ray is directed 10 degrees to 15 degrees caudal at 2″ (5 cm) superior to pubic symphysis and MSP

Evaluation Criteria

- Entire bladder visualized superior to the pubic symphysis

Demonstrates

- Entire bladder free from superimposition
- Pathology including but not limited to: cystitis, obstruction, vesicoureteral reflux, and calculi

Left Posterior Oblique/Right Posterior Oblique 60-Degree Projection
Positioning Criteria

- Patient placed in a 60-degree posterior oblique position on the table Bucky; keep patient's legs fully extended to not obscure the bladder
- Place a 10″ × 12″ (25 × 30 cm) IR lengthwise in the table Bucky
- Central ray is directed perpendicular to 2″ (5 cm) superior to the symphysis pubis and 2″ (5 cm) medial to the up ASIS

Evaluation Criteria

- Urinary bladder free of superimposition

Demonstrates

- Entire bladder free from superimposition
- Visualization of posterolateral aspect of bladder and vesicoureteral junction
- Pathology including but not limited to: cystitis, obstruction, vesicoureteral reflux, and calculi

Lateral Projection
Positioning Criteria

- Patient placed in the true left lateral position
- Place a 10″ × 12″ (25 × 30 cm) IR lengthwise in the table Bucky aligned with central ray
- Central ray is directed perpendicular to a point 2″ (5 cm) superior and posterior to pubic symphysis

Evaluation Criteria

- Urinary bladder free of superimposition

Demonstrates

- Entire bladder free from superimposition
- Visualization of posterolateral aspect of bladder and vesicoureteral junction
- Pathology including but not limited to: cystitis, obstruction, vesicoureteral reflux, and calculi

Cystourethrography
Anteroposterior Voiding Cystourethrogram, Female
Positioning Criteria

- Patient is placed supine on the table or upright against the Bucky
- Place a 10″ × 12″ (25 × 30 cm) IR lengthwise in the Bucky
- Central ray is directed perpendicular to pubic symphysis and MSP

Evaluation Criteria

- Contrast-filled urethra and bladder

Demonstrates

- Urethra seen inferior to bladder
- Functional study of the urinary bladder and urethra
- Pathology including but not limited to: urinary retention, vesicoureteral reflux

Right Posterior Oblique 30-Degree Voiding Cystourethrogram, Male
Positioning Criteria

- Patient is placed in a 30-degree RPO on the table or against the upright Bucky
- Superimpose urethra over soft tissue of right thigh

- Place a 10″ × 12″ (25 × 30 cm) IR lengthwise in the Bucky
- Central ray is directed perpendicular to pubic symphysis and 2″ (5 cm) medial to up ASIS

Evaluation Criteria

- Contrast-filled urethra and bladder

Demonstrates

- Urethra seen inferior to bladder
- Functional study of the urinary bladder and urethra
- Pathology including but not limited to: urinary retention, vesicoureteral reflux

Intravenous Urography

All images are taken at timed intervals from the start of contrast injection. Images at each time interval may vary by department protocol. If performing a hypertensive urogram, images are taken at 1, 2, and 3 minutes with additional radiographs at similar short intervals to assess this pathology appropriately.

Anteroposterior Abdomen Projection, Scout and Series

Positioning Criteria

- Patient supine with legs fully extended; gonadal shield for male patients; breast shield for females
- Place 14″ × 17″ (35 × 42.5 cm) IR in Bucky aligned with iliac crest at midpoint of receptor
- Central ray directed perpendicular to midpoint of IR and MSP
- Collimate to all sides to include all pertinent anatomy
- Place appropriate side marker in light field at lower lateral aspect of image
- Minimum SID: 40″ (100 cm)
- Image taken on full expiration

Evaluation Criteria

- Anatomy from kidneys to bladder is visualized
- No evidence of rotation
- Iliac wings and obturators (if visible) are symmetrical
- Spinous processes centered on vertebrae; transverse processes equidistant to vertebrae

Demonstrates

- Scout view of abdomen
- Outline of liver, spleen, and kidneys
- Air-filled stomach and bowel
- Psoas muscle on asthenic patients
- Symphysis pubis for bladder region
- Pathologies including but not limited to: obstruction, choleliths, renal calculi

Right and Left Posterior Oblique 30 Degrees

Positioning Criteria

- Patient is supine with legs extended
- Patient is rotated 30 degrees toward the right or left side; elevated knee is bent slightly for stability and elevated arm is crossed over upper chest
- Place a 14″ × 17″ (35 × 42.5 cm) IR in the table Bucky
- Central ray directed perpendicular to the level of iliac crest and 1″ to 2″ (2.5 to 5 cm) off MSP toward the up side
- Exposure is made on full expiration
- Minimum SID: 40″ (100 cm)

Evaluation Criteria

- Entire abdomen included from kidneys to bladder
- Elevated kidney is parallel to IR and in view
- Down ureter is free from superimposition from spine

Demonstrates

- Elevated kidney in profile/parallel to the IR
- Down ureter is filled with contrast and free from superimposition
- Pathology including but not limited to: infections, trauma, obstruction, renal calculi

Posteroanterior Postvoid

Positioning Criteria

- Patient prone on the table; gonadal shield for male patients; breast shield for females
- Place 14″ × 17″ (35 × 42.5 cm) IR in Bucky aligned with iliac crest at midpoint of receptor
- Central ray directed perpendicular to midpoint of IR and MSP

- Collimate to all sides to include all pertinent anatomy
- Place appropriate side marker in light field at lower lateral aspect of image
- Minimum SID: 40″ (100 cm)
- Image taken on full expiration

Evaluation Criteria

- Anatomy from kidneys to bladder is visualized
- No evidence of rotation
- Iliac wings and obturators (if visible) are symmetrical
- Spinous processes centered on vertebrae; transverse processes equidistant to vertebrae

Demonstrates

- Residual contrast present in the urinary system
- Outline of liver, spleen, kidneys
- Air-filled stomach and bowel
- Psoas muscle on asthenic patients
- Symphysis pubis for bladder region
- Pathologies including but not limited to: obstruction, choleliths, renal calculi

The above projection can be performed in the upright position against the wall Bucky. All centering is the same. The erect position will also demonstrate nephroptosis, benign prostatic hyperplasia, and prolapse of bladder.

Nephrotomography

Positioning Criteria

- Patient supine with legs fully extended; gonadal shield for all patients
- Place 10″ × 12″ (25 × 30 cm) IR crosswise in Bucky
- Central ray directed perpendicular to a point midway between xiphoid and iliac crest (angle of the ribs and MSP)
- Collimate to all sides to include all pertinent anatomy
- Measure patient thickness to indicate appropriate slice with tomography
  If the patient thickness is measured including a mat on the table, use thickness minus 2 divided by 3 for the first slice
  If measuring the patient with no mat, use thickness divided by 3 for the first slice
- Place appropriate side marker within light field at lower lateral aspect of IR; include marker for cm
- Tomography exposure angle typically 10 degrees or less to minimize number of slices necessary to image entire kidneys
- Minimum SID: 40″ (100 cm)
- Image taken on full expiration

Evaluation Criteria

- Renal parenchyma of kidneys
- No evidence of rotation
- Spinous processes centered on vertebrae; transverse processes equidistant to vertebrae

Demonstrates

- Contrast-filled kidneys unobstructed
- Pathologies including but not limited to: renal cysts, adrenal masses, calculi, obstructions

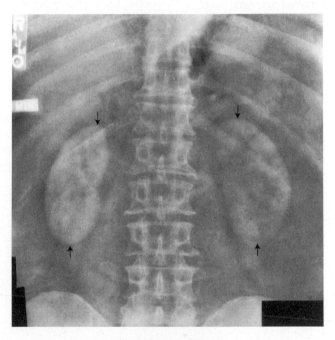

FIGURE 5-7

Projection can be performed using a perpendicular central ray with same centering. This is referred to as a *nephrogram* when taken within 60 seconds of contrast injection.

Anteroposterior Uretic Compression

Uretic compression may be applied prior to contrast injection to allow for imaging of the proximal urinary system. Positioning and centering is the same as for the AP abdomen.

Retrograde Pyelography

Procedure is a nonfunctional study of the urinary system performed in the surgical suite. Under sterile conditions, the urologist places a catheter directly into the patient's renal pelvis. This is followed by contrast injection, and images are taken via a special cystoscopic-radiographic table, mobile unit, or C-arm. AP abdomen scout image is taken after catheter placement for positioning and technique. Contrast is injected, and the AP pyelogram is taken immediately. Following this projection, the urologist may remove the catheter(s) from the renal pelvis and place directly in the ureter. Again, contrast is injected into one or both ureters, and a ureterogram is taken.

Anteroposterior Pyelogram/Anteroposterior Ureterogram

Positioning Criteria

- Patient is on the surgical table in the supine position; breast shield when possible for female patients
- Place a 14″ × 17″ (35 × 42.5 cm) IR beneath the patient
- Centering is at iliac crest and MSP

- Wait for instruction for urologist on completion of injection to expose
- Patient should be instructed to suspend respiration on expiration

Evaluation Criteria

- AP projection of abdomen
- Contrast present in kidney injected
- No rotation, symmetrical transverse processes and iliac wings

Demonstrates

- Pyelogram: renal pelvis and contrast-filled major and minor calyces, presence of catheter
- Ureterogram: ureter filled with contrast
- Pathology including but not limited to: renal calculi and obstructions

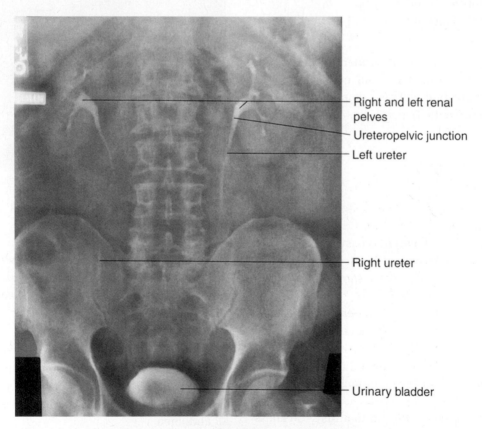

Right and left renal pelves
Ureteropelvic junction
Left ureter
Right ureter
Urinary bladder

FIGURE 5-8

SPINE AND PELVIS

Cervical Spine
Anteroposterior Angled Cephalad Cervical Spine

Positioning Criteria

- Patient placed AP erect (or supine) against the Bucky; gonadal shielding used
- Central ray angled 15 degrees to 20 degrees cephalic
- Place an 8″ × 10″ (20 × 25 cm) IR in the Bucky and center to central ray
- Central ray directed at C3–C4 and MSP
- Collimate on all four sides
- Place appropriate side marker within light field on lateral aspect of image
- Minimum SID: 40″ (100 cm)
- Suspended respiration

Evaluation Criteria

- No rotation of spine
- Entire cervical spine is included
- No evidence of motion

Demonstrates

- Presence of cervical ribs
- Medial/lateral alignment of cervical spine

- Pathology including but not limited to: cervical ribs, clay shoveler's fracture, compression fractures, and herniated nucleus pulposus

Anteroposterior Open Mouth

Positioning Criteria

- Patient placed AP erect (or supine) against the Bucky; gonadal shielding used
- Place an 8″ × 10″ (20 × 25 cm) IR in the Bucky and center to central ray
- Central ray directed to canthus of lips and MSP
- Instruct patient to open mouth; adjust baseline of mastoid tip and lower margin of upper teeth to be perpendicular to receptor
- Collimate on all four sides
- Place appropriate side marker within light field on lateral aspect of image
- Minimum SID: 40″ (100 cm)
- Suspended respiration

Evaluation Criteria

- Unobstructed view of the dens

Demonstrates

- Entire C2 vertebra and lateral masses of C1 free of superimposition

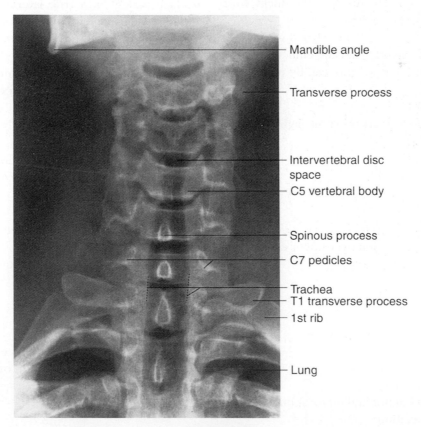

Mandible angle

Transverse process

Intervertebral disc space
C5 vertebral body

Spinous process

C7 pedicles

Trachea
T1 transverse process
1st rib

Lung

FIGURE 5-9

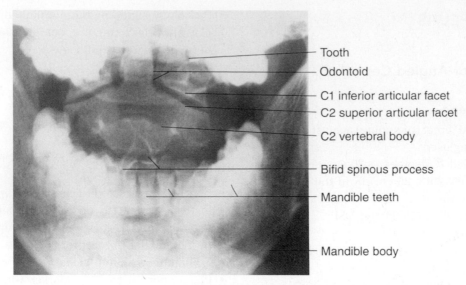

Tooth
Odontoid
C1 inferior articular facet
C2 superior articular facet
C2 vertebral body
Bifid spinous process
Mandible teeth
Mandible body

FIGURE 5-10

- Pathology including but not limited to: odontoid fractures, Jefferson fracture, pathologies associated with C1–C2

Lateral Cervical Spine

Positioning Criteria

- Place patient in a true lateral position against the Bucky, typically left lateral; gonadal shielding used
- Place an 8″ × 10″ (20 × 25 cm) IR in the Bucky with top of IR aligned with top of ear
- Central ray directed to C3–C4 and aligned with EAM
- Instruct patient to slightly elevate chin and relax shoulders; 5- to 10-pound weights can be used if patient can tolerate
- Collimate on all sides
- Place appropriate side marker within light field on lateral aspect of image
- Minimum SID: 72″ (180 cm)
- Take image on full expiration

Evaluation Criteria

- Cervical spine visualized in its entirety
- No superimposition of gonion over upper cervical
- No evidence of rotation

Demonstrates

- C1–C7
- Zygapophyseal joints of cervical spine
- Spinous process
- Intervertebral disc spaces
- Vertebral body alignment
- Pathology including but not limited to: spondylolysis, osteoarthritis, subluxation

This projection can also be performed with hyperflexion and hyperextension. Instruct patient to flex or extend as much as tolerated. These views are done to assess vertebral mobility status after trauma or surgical fusion.

Cross-Table Lateral

Positioning Criteria

- Place patient in a true lateral position against the Bucky, typically left lateral; gonadal shielding used
- Place an 8″ × 10″ (20 × 25 cm) or 10″ × 12″ (25 × 30 cm) IR with top of IR aligned with top of ear supported vertically against shoulder of patient centered to the central ray; no grid is necessary because of use of air-gap technique
- Central ray directed horizontally to C3–C4 and aligned with EAM
- Instruct patient to relax shoulders by reaching toward feet; traction on arms can be done by a qualified physician
- Collimate on all sides
- Place appropriate side marker within light field on lateral aspect of image
- Minimum SID: 72″ (180 cm) to offset large OID and decrease magnification
- Take image on full expiration

Evaluation Criteria

- Cervical spine visualized in its entirety
- No superimposition of gonion over upper cervical
- No evidence of rotation

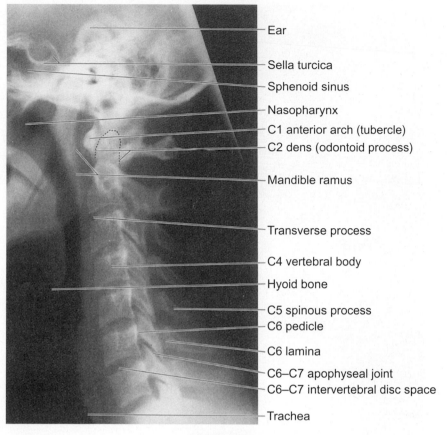

Ear
Sella turcica
Sphenoid sinus
Nasopharynx
C1 anterior arch (tubercle)
C2 dens (odontoid process)
Mandible ramus
Transverse process
C4 vertebral body
Hyoid bone
C5 spinous process
C6 pedicle
C6 lamina
C6–C7 apophyseal joint
C6–C7 intervertebral disc space
Trachea

FIGURE 5-11

Demonstrates

- C1–C7
- Zygapophyseal joints of cervical spine
- Spinous process
- Intervertebral disc spaces
- Vertebral body alignment
- Pathology including but not limited to: clay shoveler's fracture, compression fracture, hangman's fracture, odontoid fracture, teardrop burst fracture, or subluxation

Anterior and Posterior Oblique Cervical Spine

Positioning Criteria

- Patient is rotated 45 degrees, keeping head and neck aligned and centered to the upright Bucky; gonadal shielding used
- Place an 8″ × 10″ (20 × 25 cm) IR in the Bucky lengthwise and aligned with the central ray
- Anterior obliques: Central ray is angled 15 degrees caudal, centered to C4 and midline of neck
- Posterior obliques: Central ray is angled 15 degrees cephalic, centered to C4 and midline of neck

- Instruct patient to slightly elevate chin to reduce superimposition of mandible
- Collimate on all four sides
- SID of 72″ (180 cm) to reduce magnification from OID
- Exposure made on suspended expiration

Evaluation Criteria

- Correct rotation and angulation
- Intervertebral spaces and foramina are open
- Pedicles in profile

Demonstrates

- Anterior obliques: intervertebral foramina and pedicle on the side of the patient closest to the IR (e.g., RAO: right foramina and pedicles)
- Posterior obliques: intervertebral foramina and pedicles on the side of the patient farthest from the IR (e.g., LPO: right foramina and pedicles)
- Pathology including but not limited to: stenosis involving the intervertebral foramen

Projections can be performed recumbent with the patient on the table.

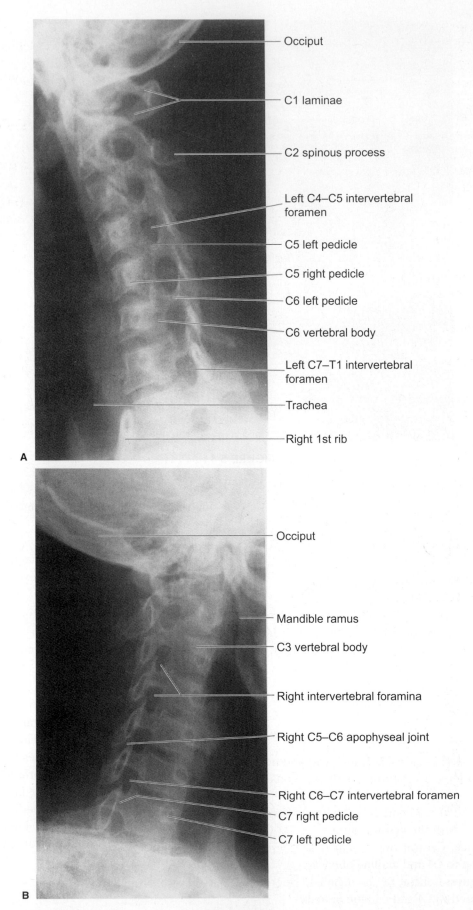

FIGURE 5-12

Lateral Swimmer's Projection (Cervicothoracic Lateral)

Performed when C7–T1 is not seen well on routine cervical lateral projection

Positioning Criteria

- Erect is preferred, but can be performed supine
- Elevate patient's arm and shoulder nearest the IR; arm and shoulder farthest from IR should be relaxed and down; gonadal shielding used
- Place 10″ × 12″ (25 × 30 cm) IR in upright Bucky aligned with central ray
- Central ray perpendicular to T1, level of jugular notch, and level of vertebra prominens posteriorly; a 3-degree to 5-degree caudal angle can be used on patients with limited flexibility of the upper extremities
- Minimum SID: 72″ (180 cm)
- Exposure taken on full expiration; if patient can cooperate, a breathing technique can be employed to improve visibility of the cervicothoracic junction

Evaluation Criteria

- Vertebral rotation should be minimal
- Humeral heads should be separated vertically

Demonstrates

- Vertebral bodies and intervertebral disc spaces of C4–T3 are shown
- Pathology including but not limited to: fractures, subluxation, osteoarthritis

Anteroposterior Dens (Fuchs) Projection

Positioning Criteria

- Place patient AP against the upright Bucky or supine on the table; gonadal shielding used
- Place an 8″ × 10″ (20 × 25 cm) IR in the Bucky
- Adjust patient so that the mentomeatal line (MML) is perpendicular to the IR with no rotation of the head; if patient is status post head and neck trauma, do not attempt movement: Central ray can be angled as needed to be parallel to MML
- Central ray is directed parallel to the MML at MSP and inferior to the tip of mentum
- Four-sided collimation appropriate for anatomy
- Minimum SID: 40″ (100 cm)
- Exposure is made on suspended respiration

Evaluation Criteria

- Symmetrical appearance of mandibular arch over foramen magnum
- Dens in foramen magnum

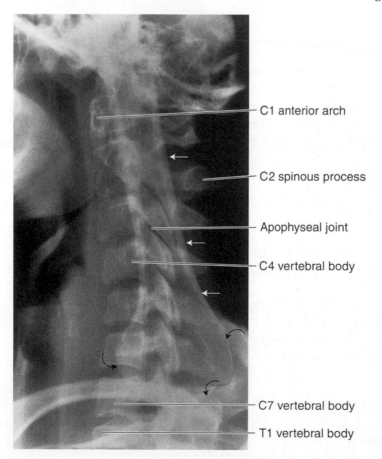

C1 anterior arch

C2 spinous process

Apophyseal joint

C4 vertebral body

C7 vertebral body

T1 vertebral body

FIGURE 5-13

Demonstrates

- Dens through the foramen magnum free of superimposition of mandible
- Demonstration of the superior portion of the dens when not well seen on the AP open mouth projection
- Pathology including but not limited to: fractures of C1 and C2

Posteroanterior Dens (Judd) Projection

Positioning Criteria

- Place patient PA against the upright Bucky or prone on the table; gonadal shielding used
- Place an 8″ × 10″ (20 × 25 cm) IR in the Bucky
- Adjust patient so that the MML is perpendicular to the IR with no rotation of the head; central ray can be angled as needed to be parallel to MML
- Central ray is directed parallel to the MML at MSP and 1″ (2.5 cm) inferoposterior to mastoid tips through midoccipital bone
- Four-sided collimation appropriate for anatomy
- Minimum SID: 40″ (100 cm)
- Exposure is made on suspended respiration

Evaluation Criteria

- Symmetrical appearance of mandibular arch over foramen magnum
- Dens in foramen magnum

Demonstrates

- Dens through the foramen magnum free of superimposition of mandible
- Demonstration of the superior portion of the dens when not well seen on the AP open mouth projection
- Pathology including but not limited to: fractures of C1 and C2

Thoracic Spine

Anteroposterior Thoracic Spine

Positioning Criteria

- Place the patient AP against the Bucky; if supine, flex knees and hips to reduce thoracic curvature; gonadal shielding used
- Place a 14″ × 17″ (35 × 42.5 cm) IR in the Bucky lengthwise centered to central ray
- Utilize anode heel effect to create a more uniform density
- Central ray directed to T6–T7, 3″ to 4″ (7.5 to 10 cm) below jugular notch, and MSP
- Minimum SID: 40″ (100 cm)
- Collimate on lateral margins to about 5″ to 6″ (12.5 to 15 cm)
- Exposure taken on full expiration

Evaluation Criteria

- Vertebral column visualized from C7–L1
- No rotation as evident by symmetrical sternoclavicular notches

Demonstrates

- Entire T-spine, intervertebral joint spaces, and spinous and transverse processes visualized
- Posterior ribs and costovertebral articulations

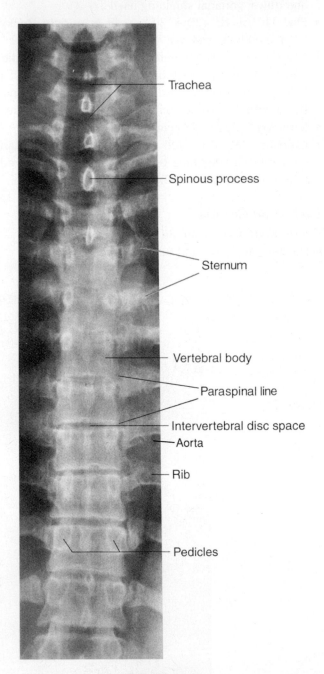

Trachea

Spinous process

Sternum

Vertebral body

Paraspinal line

Intervertebral disc space

Aorta

Rib

Pedicles

FIGURE 5-14

- Pathology including but not limited to: compression fractures, scoliosis

Lateral Thoracic Spine

Positioning Criteria

- Place the patient in a left lateral position with arms bent and one on top of the other anteriorly against the Bucky; if recumbent, flex knees and hips to create a wider base for patient to maintain position; gonadal shielding used
- Provide support of patient's waist to ensure entire T-spine is parallel with IR; patients with broad shoulders will require support in the lower thoracic region; patients with large hips may require support in the upper thoracic region
- Place a 14″ × 17″ (35 × 42.5 cm) IR in the Bucky lengthwise centered to central ray
- Central ray directed to T6–T7, 3″ to 4″ (7.5 to 10 cm) below jugular notch and the long axis of the T-spine
- Minimum SID: 40″ (100 cm)
- Collimate on lateral margins to about 5″ to 6″ (12.5 to 15 cm); additional lead shielding should also be placed posterior to the spine out of the field of view to absorb scatter
- Exposure taken on full expiration or utilize a breathing technique to blur lungs and ribs overlying vertebrae

Evaluation Criteria

- Vertebral column visualized from T1–L1 (T1–T3 not well visualized)
- No rotation as evident by superimposed posterior aspects of vertebrae

Demonstrates

- Entire T-spine seen
- Open intervertebral foramina and intervertebral joint spaces
- Pathology including but not limited to: compression fractures, kyphosis, subluxation

Scoliosis Series

Anteroposterior/Posteroanterior Scoliosis Series (Ferguson Method)

Two-view series

Positioning Criteria

- Patient is positioned standing or seated in the AP or PA position with arms at sides against the upright Bucky; PA is preferred to reduce gonadal dose
- Place a 14″ × 17″ (35 × 42.5 cm) or 14″ × 36″ (35 × 90 cm) IR in the Bucky; place bottom of IR 1″ to 2″ (2.5 to 5 cm) below iliac crests
- Central ray directed perpendicular to MSP and centered to IR
- Utilize a compensating filter to create a uniform density on the image
- Collimate to area of interest
- SID 40″ to 60″ (100 to 150 cm); use longer SID if using a 14″ × 36″ (35 × 90 cm) IR
- Exposure taken on full expiration
- For second image, positioning and centering is same; add a 3″ to 4″ (7.5 to 10 cm) block under the foot or hip if seated on the convex side of the curve

Evaluation Criteria

- All thoracic and lumbar vertebrae should be visualized
- A minimum of 1″ (2.5 cm) of iliac crest should be seen

Demonstrates

- Entire thoracic and lumbar spine in a true AP or PA projection
- Pathology including but not limited to: scoliosis, differentiating primary versus compensatory curve

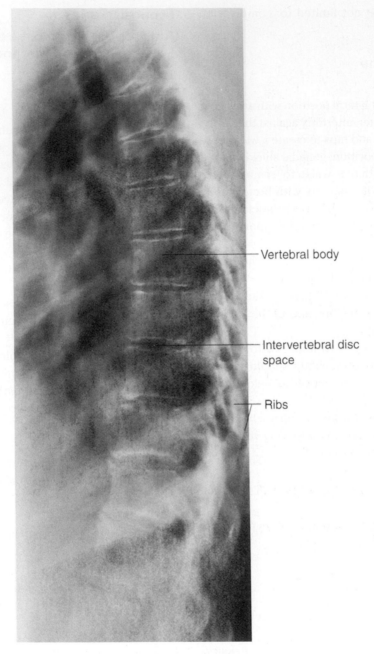

Vertebral body

Intervertebral disc space

Ribs

FIGURE 5-15

Lumbar Spine
Anteroposterior Projection

Positioning Criteria

- Patient is placed supine on the table with knees flexed to reduce lordotic curve of the spine; gonadal shielding
- Utilize a 14″ × 17″ (35 × 42.5 cm) IR lengthwise centered to the central ray
- Central ray directed to the iliac crest and MSP
- Minimum SID: 40″ (100 cm)
- Collimate on all four sides
- Exposure taken on full expiration

Evaluation Criteria

- Entire lumbar spine seen
- No patient rotation as indicated by: symmetrical transverse processes, spinous processes centered on vertebrae

Demonstrates

- Lumbar vertebrae, intervertebral joints, transverse processes, sacroiliac (SI) joints

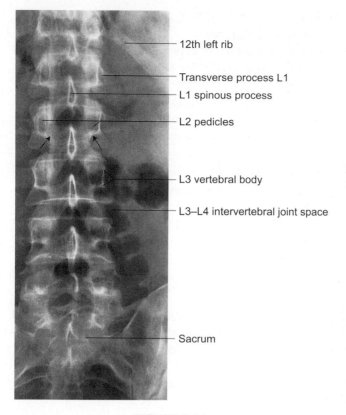

12th left rib

Transverse process L1

L1 spinous process

L2 pedicles

L3 vertebral body

L3–L4 intervertebral joint space

Sacrum

FIGURE 5-16

- Pathology including but not limited to: fractures, scoliosis, Marie-Strümpell disease

Projection can also be performed in the PA and erect positions with same centering.

If desired, smaller IR (11″ × 14″ [27.5 to 35 cm]) can be used; centering needs to be adjusted to 2″ (5 cm) superior to iliac crest.

Lateral Projection

Positioning Criteria

- Place patient in a left lateral position on the table with the knees bent and the arms flexed and placed anterior to the body; gonadal shielding
- Utilize a 14″ × 17″ (35 × 42.5 cm) IR lengthwise in the Bucky aligned with the central ray
- Central ray is directed perpendicular to iliac crest and midcoronal plane
- Minimum SID: 40″ (100 cm)
- Collimate on all four sides
- Exposure taken on full expiration

Evaluation Criteria

- Entire lumbar spine seen
- No patient rotation as indicated by: symmetrical transverse processes, spinous processes centered on vertebrae

Demonstrates

- Lumbar vertebrae, intervertebral joints, transverse processes, SI joints

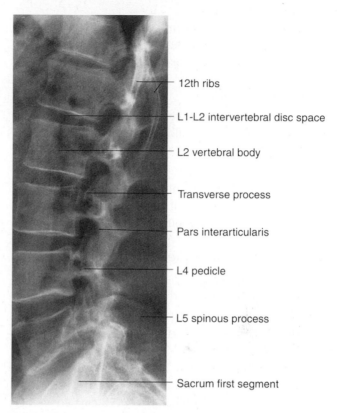

12th ribs

L1-L2 intervertebral disc space

L2 vertebral body

Transverse process

Pars interarticularis

L4 pedicle

L5 spinous process

Sacrum first segment

FIGURE 5-17

- Pathology including but not limited to: fractures, scoliosis, Marie-Strümpell disease, spondylolisthesis, spondylolysis, spinal fusion

Projection can also be performed in the PA and erect positions with same centering.

If desired, smaller IR (11″ × 14″ [27.5 to 35 cm]) can be used; centering needs to be adjusted to 2″ (5 cm) superior to iliac crest.

Lateral hyperflexion and hyperextension can also be performed. Patients are instructed to keep pelvis still and bend forward (hyperflexion) or backward (hyperextension) as much as possible. Centering for these projections is 2″ (5 cm) above iliac crest.

L5–S1 Spot Projection

Positioning Criteria

- Place patient in a left lateral position on the table with the knees bent and the arms flexed and placed anterior to the body; gonadal shielding
- Utilize an 8″ × 10″ (20 × 25 cm) IR lengthwise in the Bucky aligned with the central ray

- Central ray is directed perpendicular to 1½″ (4 cm) inferior to iliac crest and 2″ (5 cm) posterior to ASIS
- Central ray can be angled 5 degrees to 8 degrees caudal to be parallel to the interiliac line (imaginary line between iliac crests)
- Minimum SID: 40″ (100 cm)
- Collimate on all four sides
- Exposure taken on full expiration

Evaluation Criteria

- L5–S1 seen free of superimposition
- No patient rotation as indicated by open joint space

Demonstrates

- L5–S1 intervertebral joint
- Pathology including but not limited to: fractures, spondylolysis, spondylolisthesis

Lumbar Spine Obliques

Positioning Criteria

Obliques can be performed in either the AP or PA position. Both obliques must be performed.

- Patient is placed in a 45-degree oblique either recumbent or erect; gonadal shielding
- Utilize a 10″ × 12″ (25 × 30 cm) IR placed lengthwise aligned with central ray
- Central ray is perpendicular to 2″ (5 cm) above iliac crest and 2″ (5 cm) medial to ASIS
- Minimum SID: 40″ (100 cm)
- Collimate on all four sides to area of interest
- Exposure taken on full expiration

Evaluation Criteria

- L1–L5 vertebrae are seen
- Presence of "scotty dog"
- Spine down center of image and straight

Demonstrates

- RPO/LAO: left zygapophyseal joints
- LPO/RAO: right zygapophyseal joints
- Pathology including but not limited to: defects in pars interarticularis (spondylolysis)

Anteroposterior L5–S1, 30 Degrees to 35 Degrees Cephalic

Positioning Criteria

- Patient is placed recumbent in the supine position with knees bent to reduce lordosis of lumbar spine; gonadal shielding

- Utilize an 8″ × 10″ (20 × 25 cm) IR crosswise aligned with the central ray
- Central ray directed 30 degrees cephalic for male and 35 degrees cephalic for female patients, entering at the level of ASIS and MSP
- Collimate on all four sides as appropriate for anatomy
- Minimum SID: 40″ (100 cm)
- Exposure taken on suspended respiration

Evaluation Criteria

- L5–S1 joint space is open and centered in the collimated field
- SI joints are symmetrical from spine

Demonstrates

- Open L5–S1 junction
- SI joints are open
- This projection can be performed PA using a caudal angle centered slightly above iliac crest; PA projection increases OID and decreases gonadal dose

Anteroposterior/Posteroanterior Right and Left Bending

Positioning Criteria

- Patient can be placed in the AP or PA position, erect or recumbent; gonadal shielding
- Utilize a 14″ × 17″ (35 × 42.5 cm) IR with the bottom placed 2″ (5 cm) below iliac crest
- Central ray is directed perpendicular to IR and midline of patient
- Instruct patient to lean from waist holding pelvis still; two images are taken: right and left
- Collimate to size of IR and crosswise as appropriate for anatomy
- Minimum SID: 40″ (100 cm)
- Exposure taken on full expiration

Evaluation Criteria

- Lumbar vertebrae visualized in lateral flexion
- No rotation of pelvis
- L5 to iliac crests visualized

Demonstrates

- Range of motion of the lumbar spine

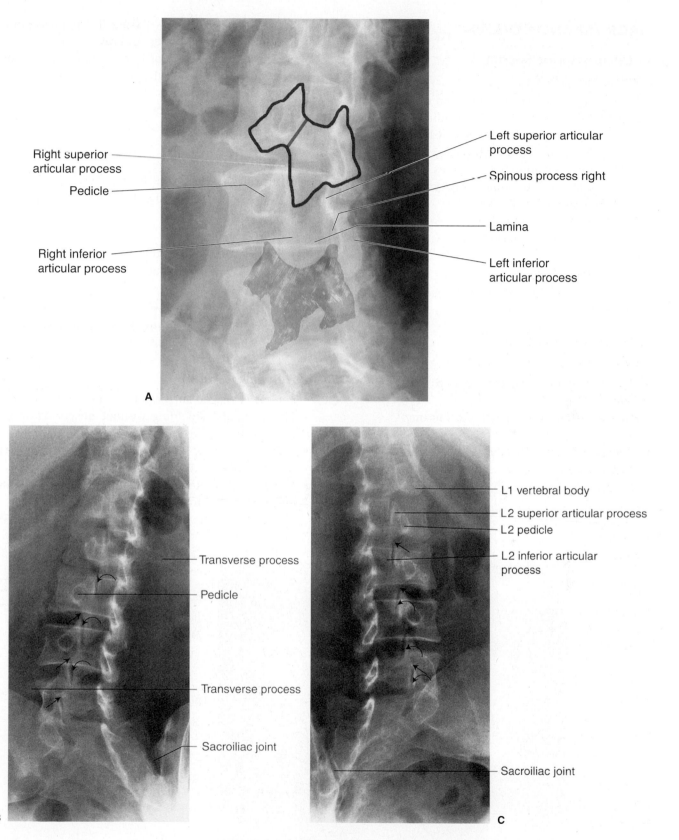

Right superior
articular process

Pedicle

Right inferior
articular process

Left superior articular
process

Spinous process right

Lamina

Left inferior
articular process

Transverse process

Pedicle

Transverse process

Sacroiliac joint

L1 vertebral body

L2 superior articular process

L2 pedicle

L2 inferior articular
process

Sacroiliac joint

A

B

C

FIGURE 5-18

SACRUM AND COCCYX

Anteroposterior Sacrum

Positioning Criteria

- Patient is positioned AP recumbent on the table with legs slightly elevated; breast shielding for females
- Utilize a 10″ × 12″ (25 × 30 cm) IR lengthwise in the Bucky aligned with the central ray
- Central ray angulation of 15 degrees cephalic to enter 2″ (5 cm) superior to pubic symphysis
- Collimation on all four sides
- Minimum SID: 40″ (100 cm)
- Exposure taken on full expiration

Evaluation Criteria

- Sacrum centered in pelvic inlet, free of foreshortening, centered on image
- Symmetrical SI joints

Demonstrates

- AP projection of the sacrum, L5–S1 junction, and SI joints
- Pathologies associated with the sacrum

Anteroposterior Coccyx

Positioning Criteria

- Patient is positioned AP recumbent on the table with legs slightly elevated; breast shielding for females
- Utilize an 8″ × 10″ (20 × 25 cm) IR lengthwise in the Bucky aligned with the central ray
- Central ray angulation of 10 degrees caudal to enter 2″ (5 cm) superior to pubic symphysis
- Collimation on all four sides
- Minimum SID: 40″ (100 cm)
- Exposure taken on full expiration

Evaluation Criteria

- Coccyx centered in pelvic inlet and centered on image
- Coccyx seen superior to pubic symphysis

Demonstrates

- AP projection of the coccyx
- Pathologies associated with the coccyx

Lateral Sacrum and Coccyx

It is recommended to perform a combined lateral of this anatomy to reduce gonadal dose.

Positioning Criteria

- Patient is placed in the left lateral position on the table; gonadal shielding without obscuring area of interest
- Utilize a 10″ × 12″ (25 × 30 cm) IR lengthwise in the Bucky aligned with the central ray
- Central ray directed perpendicular at the level of ASIS and 3″ to 4″ (7.5 to 10 cm) posterior

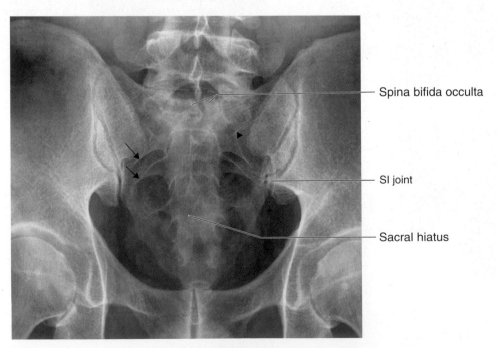

Spina bifida occulta

SI joint

Sacral hiatus

FIGURE 5-19

- Collimation on all four sides; use an additional shield posterior to the patient to absorb scatter
- Minimum SID: 40″ (100 cm)
- Exposure made on suspended expiration

Evaluation Criteria

- Sacrum and coccyx seen in entirety
- Posterior margins of pelvis are superimposed, no rotation

Demonstrates

- Lateral of sacrum and coccyx, L5–S1 joint
- Pathology including but not limited to: anterior/posterior displacement of fractures

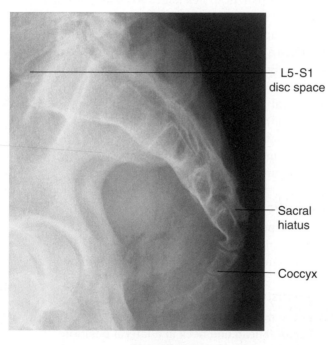

L5-S1 disc space

Sacral hiatus

Coccyx

FIGURE 5-20

Sacroiliac Joints
Anteroposterior Axial Sacroiliac Joints
Positioning Criteria

- Patient is placed recumbent in the supine position with knees bent to reduce lordosis of lumbar spine; gonadal shielding
- Utilize a 10″ × 12″ (25 × 30 cm) IR lengthwise aligned with the central ray

- Central ray directed 30 degrees cephalic for male and 35 degrees cephalic for female patients, entering 2″ (5 cm) below level of ASIS and MSP
- Collimate on all four sides as appropriate for anatomy
- Minimum SID: 40″ (100 cm)
- Exposure taken on suspended respiration

Evaluation Criteria

- L5–S1 joint space is open and centered in the collimated field
- SI joints are symmetrical from spine

Demonstrates

- Open L5–S1 junction
- SI joints are open

This projection can be performed in the PA position using a caudal angle and centered slightly above iliac crest. PA projection increases OID and decreases gonadal dose.

Sacroiliac Joint Obliques

Obliques can be performed in the AP or PA position. Both obliques are performed for comparison.

Positioning Criteria

- Patient is recumbent on the table and rotated 25 degrees to 30 degrees; gonadal shielding
- Utilize a 10″ × 12″ (25 × 30 cm) IR lengthwise aligned to the central ray
- Central ray is perpendicular to a point 1″ medial to up side ASIS for posterior obliques; center to down SI joint for anterior obliques
- Collimation on all four sides
- Minimum SID: 40″ (100 cm)
- Exposure made on full expiration

Evaluation Criteria

- Joint space appears open and is centered on the image

Demonstrates

- LPO/RAO: right SI joint
- RPO/LAO: left SI joint
- Dislocation or subluxation of the joint

PELVIS AND HIP

Anteroposterior Pelvis

Positioning Criteria

- Patient is placed supine on the table with arms at sides; gonadal shield for males, breast shield for females
- Instruct patient to separate legs 8″ to 10″ (20 to 25 cm) and medially rotate the entire lower extremity 15 degrees to 20 degrees; DO NOT DO THIS IF THERE IS SUSPECTED FRACTURE OR DISLOCATION
- Utilize a 14″ × 17″ (35 × 42.5 cm) IR placed crosswise in the Bucky, positioned so that the upper edge of the IR is 1″ (2.5 cm) superior to iliac crest
- Central ray perpendicular to midpoint of IR, 2″ (5 cm) inferior to ASIS and MSP
- Collimate on all four sides
- Minimum SID: 40″ (100 cm)
- Exposure taken on suspended respiration

Evaluation Criteria

- Entire pelvis is visualized
- Iliac wings are symmetrical
- Obturator foramen are symmetrical and open

Demonstrates

- Entire pelvis and proximal femora
- Femoral necks elongated, greater trochanter in profile

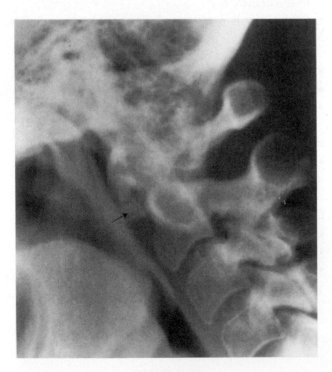

FIGURE 5-21

- Pathology including but not limited to: fractures including Malgaigne and Duverney, degenerative disease, bone lesions

Anteroposterior Pelvis Bilateral Frog-Leg Projection (Modified Cleaves Method)

Projection typically performed on younger patients to assess congenital hip dysplasia.

Positioning Criteria

- Patient is placed supine on the table with arms at sides
- Gonadal shielding for both male and female patients with care to not obscure the hip joints
- Instruct patient to flex knees to 90 degrees, place the plantar surfaces of the feet together, and abduct the knees approximately 45 degrees from vertical
- Utilize a 14″ × 17″ (35 × 42.5 cm) IR placed crosswise in the Bucky, positioned so that the upper edge of the IR is at iliac crest
- Central ray perpendicular to midpoint of IR, 3″ (7.5 cm) inferior to ASIS and MSP
- Collimate on all four sides
- Minimum SID: 40″ (100 cm)
- Exposure taken on suspended respiration

Evaluation Criteria

- Entire pelvis is visualized
- Iliac wings are symmetrical
- Obturator foramen are symmetrical and open

Demonstrates

- Entire pelvis and proximal femora
- Femoral head and neck in a lateral position
- Acetabulum and trochanteric areas seen well
- Pathology including but not limited to: congenital hip dysplasia, degenerative disease, bone lesions

Anteroposterior Axial Pelvis Inlet Projection

- Patient is placed supine on the table with arms at sides; gonadal shield for males, breast shield for females
- Utilize a 14″ × 17″ (35 × 42.5 cm) IR placed crosswise in the Bucky aligned with central ray
- Central ray angled 40 degrees caudal at the level of ASIS and MSP
- Collimate on all four sides
- Minimum SID: 40″ (100 cm)
- Exposure taken on suspended respiration

Evaluation Criteria
- Unobstructed view of the pelvic ring
- No rotation of pelvis
- Ischial spines are symmetrical
- Collimation laterally extends to include femoral heads and acetabula; superiorly includes the iliac wing and inferiorly includes the symphysis pubis

Demonstrates
- Pelvic inlet (superior aperture) seen free of superimposition
- Ischial spines
- Pathology including but not limited to: trauma assessment, posterior displacement, inward or outward rotation of anterior pelvis

Anteroposterior Axial Pelvis Outlet Projection
Positioning Criteria
- Patient is placed supine on the table with arms at sides; gonadal shield for males; breast shield for females
- Utilize a 10″ × 12″ (25 × 30 cm) IR placed crosswise in the Bucky aligned with central ray
- Central ray angled 20 degrees to 35 degrees for males, 30 degrees to 45 degrees for females, cephalic at a point 1″ to 2″ (2.5 to 5 cm) below pubic symphysis and MSP
- Collimate on all four sides
- Minimum SID: 40″ (100 cm)
- Exposure taken on suspended respiration

Evaluation Criteria
- Unobstructed view of the pelvic outlet
- No rotation of pelvis
- Obturator and ischia are open and equal in size
- Collimation laterally extends to include femoral heads and acetabula; superiorly includes body and superior pubic rami and inferiorly includes the ischial tuberosities

Demonstrates
- Superior and inferior rami of pubes and body and ramus of ischium
- Pathology including but not limited to: trauma assessment for fractures and displacement

Anteroposterior Oblique Pelvis: Judet Method
Positioning Criteria
- Place patient in the supine position on the table; gonadal shielding

- Rotate patient into a 45-degree oblique depending on what anatomy is of interest
- RPO: Right anterior rim and posterior ilioischial column and left posterior rim and anterior ilioischial column are demonstrated
- LPO: Left anterior rim and posterior ilioischial column and right posterior rim and anterior ilioischial column are demonstrated
- Central ray directed perpendicular
- Up side: 2″ (5 cm) distal to up side ASIS
- Down side: 2″ (5 cm) distal and 2″ (5 cm) medial to down side ASIS
- Collimate on all four sides
- Minimum SID: 40″ (100 cm)
- Exposure taken on suspended expiration

Evaluation Criteria
- Hip joint of interest centered in image
- Four-sided collimation
- Obturator foramen of up side is open and closed on down side if obliqued correctly

Demonstrates
- Acetabulum with minimal superimposition of structures and in profile
- Ilioischial column
- Pathology including but not limited to: acetabular fractures and hip dislocation

Anteroposterior Unilateral Hip Projection
Positioning Criteria
- Patient is supine on the table with arms at the sides; gonadal shielding
- Place a 10″ × 12″ (25 × 30 cm) IR lengthwise in the Bucky aligned to the central ray
- Central ray is directed perpendicular to the femoral neck located 1″ to 2″ (2.5 to 5 cm) medial and 3″ to 4″ (7.5 to 10 cm) inferior to ASIS
- Instruct patient to internally rotate lower extremity 15 degrees to 20 degrees unless fracture or dislocation is suspected
- Collimate on all four sides
- Minimum SID: 40″ (100 cm)

Evaluation Criteria
- Greater trochanter, femoral neck and head seen in profile without foreshortening
- If after joint replacement, entire orthopedic appliance must be included
- Sufficient internal rotation noted by minimal visualization of lesser trochanter medially

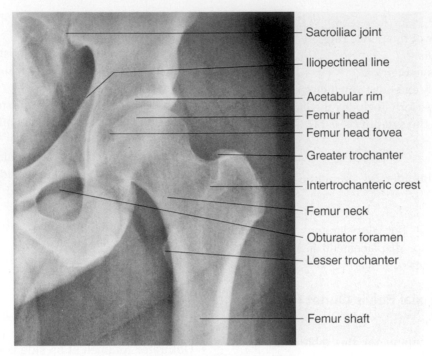

FIGURE 5-22

Demonstrates

- Proximal femur, acetabulum, and adjacent parts of the pelvis
- Condition and placement of any existing orthopedic appliance
- Pathology including but not limited to: intertrochanteric fracture, femoral neck fracture, pathological fractures due to stress or low bone mass

Unilateral Frog-Leg Projection (Modified Cleaves Method)

Positioning Criteria

- Patient supine; position affected hip area to be centered to the midline of table and/or IR; gonadal region shielded
- Place 10″ × 12″ (25 × 30 cm) IR in table Bucky lengthwise
- Flex knee and hip of affected side; rest sole of foot against the inside of the opposite leg, near knee
- Abduct femur 45 degrees from vertical to demonstrate the proximal femur region
- Center affected femoral neck to central ray, which is 3″ to 4″ (7.5 to 10 cm) distal to ASIS

- Collimate to four sides to include all pertinent anatomy
- Place appropriate side marker within light field on lateral aspect of image
- Minimum SID: 40″ (100 cm)

Evaluation Criteria

- Lateral views of acetabulum and femoral head and neck, trochanteric area, and proximal one-third of femur are visible
- Proper abduction of femur indicated by visualization of femoral neck profile and its superimposition by greater trochanter
- Femoral neck in center of collimated field indicates proper centering
- Optimal exposure

Demonstrates

- Lateral view of hip joint and proximal femur to midfemur

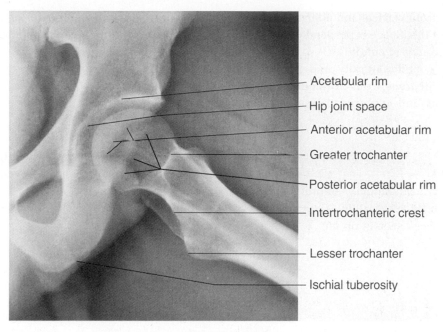

Acetabular rim
Hip joint space
Anterior acetabular rim
Greater trochanter
Posterior acetabular rim
Intertrochanteric crest
Lesser trochanter
Ischial tuberosity

FIGURE 5-23

Axiolateral Inferosuperior (Danelius-Miller Method)

Positioning Criteria

- Patient is supine/dorsal decubitus on stretcher, bedside, or radiographic table; elevate pelvis 1″ to 2″ (2.5 to 5 cm)
- Flex and elevate unaffected leg (for assistance, place foot on step stool or lower leg on leg lift positioning device) so that thigh is near vertical position and outside collimation
- To ensure no rotation of pelvis, ASIS to tabletop distance should be equal on both sides
- Place top of 10″ × 12″ (25 × 30 cm) IR in stationary grid in crease above iliac crest on affected side and adjust so that IR is parallel to the femoral neck
- Direct central ray so that it is perpendicular to the IR and exiting femoral neck
- If not contraindicated by possible fracture or other pathologic process, internal rotation of the affected leg by 15 degrees to 20 degrees is recommended
- Close collimation to four sides to femoral head and neck region
- Place appropriate side marker within light field on lateral aspect of image
- Minimum SID: 40″ (100 cm)

Evaluation Criteria

- Entire femoral head and neck, trochanter, and acetabulum should be visible on image

- With inversion, lesser trochanter should be seen
- Distal aspect of femoral neck superimposed by greater trochanter
- No superimposition of soft tissue from raised unaffected leg
- No grid lines visible indicate proper central ray–IR alignment
- Optimal exposure

Demonstrates

- Lateral view of proximal femur to midfemur
- Anterior/posterior dislocation of proximal femur to midfemur
- Detection of fractures when affected leg is not able to be moved

Modified Axiolateral: Clements-Nakayama Method

Used in cases of bilateral lower limb immobility.

Positioning Criteria

- Patient supine; position affected side near edge of table with legs fully extended and arms across chest; gonadal regions shielded as much as possible
- Rest 8″ × 10″ (20 × 25 cm) stationary grid IR on extended Bucky tray, placing bottom edge of IR 2″ (5 cm) below the level of the tabletop
- Maintain neutral (anatomic) position of leg

- Tilt IR 15 degrees from vertical and adjust alignment of IR to ensure that the IR face is perpendicular to the central ray to prevent grid cutoff
- Direct central ray mediolaterally and posteriorly 15 degrees to 20 degrees from horizontal so that it is perpendicular and centered to femoral neck and IR
- Minimum SID: 40″ (100 cm)

Evaluation Criteria

- Lateral oblique of acetabulum, femoral head and neck, and trochanteric area visible
- Femoral head and neck seen in profile

- Lesser trochanter seen posterior to femoral shaft
- Greater trochanter is superimposed by femoral head and neck
- No visible grid lines indicate proper central ray–IR alignment
- Optimal exposure

Demonstrates

- Lateral of proximal femur and hip for patients with limited bilateral lower limb movement due to trauma or arthroplasty
- Anterior/posterior dislocation of proximal femur and hip

HEAD

Skull

Anteroposterior Axial (Towne)

Positioning Criteria

- Patient AP; sitting, erect, or supine; and shielded
- 10″ × 12″ (25 × 30 cm) IR lengthwise
- Central ray angled 30 degrees caudal if orbitomeatal line (OML) is perpendicular to the IR
- Central ray is angled 37 degrees caudal if the infraorbitomeatal line (IOML) is perpendicular
- Central ray is directed 2½″ (6 cm) superior to the glabella and will exit ¾″ (2 cm) superior to the EAM, through the foramen magnum
- Collimate to four sides to include all pertinent anatomy
- Place appropriate side marker within light field on lateral aspect of the image
- Minimum SID: 40″ (100 cm)

Evaluation Criteria

- No rotation is evident when distance from foramen magnum to lateral aspect of skull is equal on both sides of skull
- Petrous ridges should be symmetric

Demonstrates

- Occipital bone, petrous pyramids, and foramen magnum
- Dorsum sellae and posterior clinoids visualized through the foramen magnum
- Underangulation projects the dorsum sella superior to foramen magnum
- Overangulation will push the anterior arch of C1 into the foramen magnum
- Petrous ridges superior to mastoid process
- Fractures, neoplastic processes, and Paget disease

Lateral Skull

Positioning Criteria

- Patient erect or prone, and shielded
- 10″ × 12″ (25 × 30 cm) IR crosswise in Bucky
- Place side of interest closest to IR
- Palpate occipital protuberance and nasion in order to determine rotation
- MSP should be parallel to IR
- The interpupillary line should be perpendicular
- Adjust head so the IOML is perpendicular to the front edge of the IR
- Central ray perpendicular to IR and directed 2″ (5 cm) superior to the EAM

- Collimate to four sides to include all pertinent anatomy
- Place appropriate side marker within light field on lateral aspect of the side down
- Minimum SID: 40″ (100 cm)

Evaluation Criteria

- No rotation or tilt of the cranium is evident
- Rotation evident by separation of EAMs, mandibular rami, and greater wings of sphenoid
- Tilt evident by orbital roofs, EAMs, and lesser wings of sphenoid

Demonstrates

- Superimposition of cranial halves
- Sella turcica and clivus in profile
- Sella turcica, anterior/posterior clinoids, and dorsum sellae

Posteroanterior Caldwell Skull

Positioning Criteria

- Patient PA and shielded
- 10″ × 12″ (25 × 30 cm) IR lengthwise placed in Bucky
- OML perpendicular to IR
- Central ray angled 15 degrees caudal, directed to exit the nasion
- Collimate to four sides to include all pertinent anatomy
- Place appropriate side marker within light field on lateral aspect of image
- Minimum SID: 40″ (100 cm)

Evaluation Criteria

- No rotation evident by lateral orbit and lateral skull symmetric on each side

Demonstrates

- Petrous pyramids in lower one-third of orbit
- Superior orbital ridge free of superimposition
- Greater/lesser sphenoid wing, frontal bone, superior orbital fissures, frontal and anterior ethmoid sinuses, superior orbital margins, and crista galli
- Skull fractures, neoplastic processes, and Paget disease

Posteroanterior (No Angle)

Positioning Criteria

- Patient PA and shielded
- 10″ × 12″ (25 × 30 cm) IR lengthwise placed in Bucky
- OML perpendicular to IR
- MSP perpendicular to table
- Central ray perpendicular and directed to exit glabella

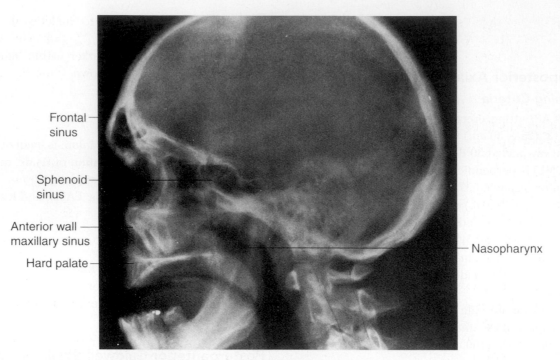

Frontal sinus

Sphenoid sinus

Anterior wall maxillary sinus

Hard palate

Nasopharynx

FIGURE 5-24

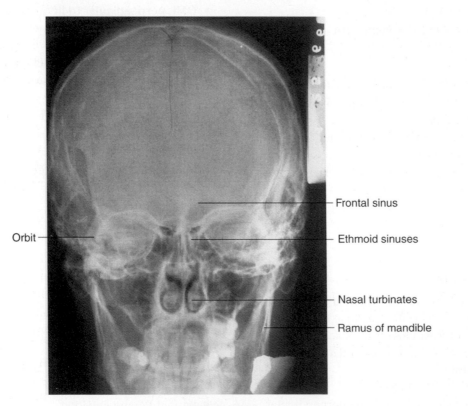

Orbit

Frontal sinus

Ethmoid sinuses

Nasal turbinates

Ramus of mandible

FIGURE 5-25

- Collimate to four sides to include all pertinent anatomy
- Place appropriate side marker within light field on lateral aspect of image
- Minimum SID: 40″ (100 cm)

Evaluation Criteria

- No rotation evident by lateral orbit and lateral skull symmetric on each side

Demonstrates

- Petrous pyramids fill orbit
- Superior orbital ridge superimposed by petrous ridges
- Posterior/anterior clinoids superior to ethmoid sinuses
- Greater/lesser sphenoid wing, frontal bone, frontal and anterior ethmoid sinuses, superior orbital margins, internal auditory canals, dorsum sellae, and crista galli
- Skull fractures, neoplastic processes, and Paget disease

Submentovertical (Full Basal)

Positioning Criteria

- Patient AP erect and shielded
- 10″ × 12″ (25 × 30 cm) IR lengthwise placed in Bucky
- Patient's IOML is parallel to IR
- MSP is perpendicular to the IR
- Central ray perpendicular and directed 1″ (2.5 cm) anterior to EAMs
- Collimate to four sides to include all pertinent anatomy
- Place appropriate side marker within light field on lateral aspect of image
- Minimum SID: 40″ (100 cm)

Evaluation Criteria

- No rotation or tilt evident by equal distance bilaterally from mandibular condyles to lateral border of skull
- Foramen magnum in center of image

Demonstrates

- Foramen ovale, spinosum, mandible, sphenoid, posterior ethmoid sinus, mastoid processes, petrous ridges, foramen magnum, and (of course) occipital
- Basal skull fractures
- Advanced bony pathology of inner temporal structures

Posteroanterior 25 Degrees to 30 Degrees (Haas)

Positioning Criteria

- Patient PA and shielded
- 10″ × 12″ (25 × 30 cm) IR lengthwise placed in Bucky
- OML and MSP perpendicular to IR

- Central ray angled 25 degrees to 30 degrees cephalic, directed to enter 1½″ (4 cm) inferior to inion
- Collimate to four sides to include all pertinent anatomy
- Place appropriate side marker within light field on lateral aspect of image
- Minimum SID: 40″ (100 cm)

Evaluation Criteria

- No rotation is evident when distance from foramen magnum to lateral aspect of skull is equal on both sides of skull
- Petrous ridges should be symmetric

Demonstrates

- Occipital bone, petrous pyramids, and foramen magnum
- Dorsum sellae and posterior clinoids visualized through the foramen magnum
- Petrous ridges superior to mastoid process
- Fractures, neoplastic processes, and Paget disease

Trauma Cross-Table Lateral Skull

Positioning Criteria

- Patient supine on stretcher or imaging table and shielded
- 10″ × 12″ (25 × 30 cm) grid IR vertical lengthwise
- Carefully place radiolucent sponge under patient's head if possible; if patient's head cannot be manipulated, place grid IR at least 1″ below the inferior aspect of the patient's skull
- Bring patient as close to IR as possible
- MSP should be parallel to IR
- The interpupillary line should be perpendicular
- Adjust head so the IOML is perpendicular to the front edge of the IR
- Horizontal beam is directed perpendicular to IR and 2″ (5 cm) superior to the EAM
- Collimate to four sides to include all pertinent anatomy
- Place appropriate side marker within light field according to side closest to IR
- Minimum SID: 40″ (100 cm)

Evaluation Criteria

- No rotation or tilt of the cranium is evident
- Rotation evident by separation of EAMs, mandibular rami, and greater wings of sphenoid
- Tilt evident by orbital roofs, EAMs, and lesser wings of sphenoid

Demonstrates

- Superimposition of cranial halves
- Sellae turcica and clivus in profile
- Sellae turcica, anterior/posterior clinoids, and dorsum sellae
- Intracranial trauma indicated by sphenoidal effusion

Trauma Anteroposterior (No Angle)

Positioning Criteria

- Patient AP and shielded
- 10″ × 12″ (25 × 30 cm) IR lengthwise placed in Bucky
- OML should be perpendicular to IR; however, if the head cannot be manipulated because of trauma, angle the central ray parallel to the patient's OML
- MSP perpendicular to table
- Central ray directed to glabella
- Collimate to four sides to include all pertinent anatomy
- Place appropriate side marker within light field on lateral aspect of image
- Minimum SID: 40″ (100 cm)

Evaluation Criteria

- No rotation evident by lateral orbit and lateral skull symmetric on each side

Demonstrates

- Petrous pyramids fill orbit
- Superior orbital ridge superimposed by petrous ridges
- Posterior/anterior clinoids superior to ethmoid sinuses
- Greater/lesser sphenoid wing, frontal bone, frontal and anterior ethmoid sinuses, superior orbital margins, internal auditory canals, dorsum sellae, and crista galli
- Skull fractures, neoplastic processes, and Paget disease

Anteroposterior Axial Trauma

Positioning Criteria

- Patient AP on stretcher or radiographic table and shielded
- 10″ × 12″ (25 × 30 cm) IR lengthwise placed in Bucky
- OML should be perpendicular to IR; however, if the head cannot be manipulated because of trauma, angle the central ray parallel to the patient's OML
- Central ray angled 15 degrees cephalic to OML, directed to exit the nasion
- Collimate to four sides to include all pertinent anatomy
- Place appropriate side marker within light field on lateral aspect of image
- Minimum SID: 40″ (100 cm)

Evaluation Criteria

- No rotation evident by lateral orbit and lateral skull symmetric on each side
- AP evident by magnified orbits due to OID

Demonstrates

- Petrous pyramids in lower one-third of orbit
- Superior orbital ridge free of superimposition
- Greater/lesser sphenoid wing, frontal bone, superior orbital fissures, frontal and anterior ethmoid sinuses, superior orbital margins, and crista galli
- Skull fractures, neoplastic processes, and Paget disease

FACIAL BONES

Lateral Facial Bones

Positioning Criteria

- Patient erect or prone
- 8″ × 10″ (20 × 25 cm) IR crosswise in Bucky
- Place side of interest closest to IR
- Palpate occipital protuberance and nasion in order to determinc rotation
- MSP should be parallel to IR
- The interpupillary line should be perpendicular
- Adjust head so the IOML is perpendicular to the front edge of the IR
- Central ray perpendicular to IR and directed 1″ (2.5 cm) inferior and 1″ (2.5 cm) posterior to outer canthus to include mandible 2″ (5 cm) superior to the EAM
- Collimate to four sides to include all pertinent anatomy
- Place appropriate side marker within light field on lateral aspect of the side down
- Minimum SID: 40″ (100 cm)

Evaluation Criteria

- No rotation evident by superimposed mandibular rami
- No tilt evident by respective superimposition of orbital roofs and greater wings of sphenoid

Demonstrates

- Superimposition of facial bones
- Greater wings of sphenoid, sellae turcica, sigma, and mandible
- Fractures of facial bones
- Inflammation

Parietoacanthial (Waters): Facial Bones

Positioning Criteria

- Patient PA erect or recumbent, shielded
- 10″ × 12″ (25 × 30 cm) IR lengthwise placed in Bucky
- MML perpendicular to IR
- OML 37 degrees to IR and MSP perpendicular to midline of Bucky
- Central ray perpendicular and exits acanthion
- Collimate to four sides to include all pertinent anatomy
- Place appropriate side marker within light field
- Minimum SID: 40″ (100 cm)

Evaluation Criteria

- No rotation evident by nasal septum to outer skull margin
- Acanthion centered to image

Demonstrates

- Maxillae, inferior orbital rim, nasal septum, anterior nasal spine, and zygomatic arches
- Petrous ridges inferior to maxillary sinus
- Entire skull demonstrated
- Best demonstrates blow-out and tripod fractures and deviation of nasal septum
- Foreign body of orbit also demonstrated

Posteroanterior (Modified Waters): Facial Bones

Positioning Criteria

- Patient PA erect or recumbent and shielded
- 10″ × 12″ (25 × 30 cm) IR lengthwise placed in Bucky
- Canthus of lips and meatal line are perpendicular to Bucky
- OML forms a 55-degree angle with the IR
- Central ray exits acanthion
- MSP perpendicular to midline of grid
- Collimate to four sides to include all pertinent anatomy
- Place appropriate side marker within light field
- Minimum SID: 40″ (100 cm)

Evaluation Criteria

- No rotation evident by nasal septum to outer skull margin
- Inferior orbital rims on center or image

Demonstrates

- Orbital floors and less distortion of orbital rims
- Petrous ridges in inferior half of maxillary sinus, inferior orbital rim, nasal septum, anterior nasal spine, and zygomatic arches
- Entire skull
- Foreign body of orbit
- Orbital fractures

Posteroanterior Caldwell: Facial Bones

Positioning Criteria

- Patient PA and shielded
- 10″ × 12″ (25 × 30 cm) IR lengthwise placed in Bucky
- OML perpendicular to IR
- Central ray angled 15 degrees caudal, directed to exit the nasion
- Collimate to four sides to include all pertinent anatomy
- Place appropriate side marker within light field on lateral aspect of image
- Minimum SID: 40″ (100 cm)

Evaluation Criteria

- No rotation evident by lateral orbit and lateral skull symmetric on each side

Demonstrates

- Petrous pyramids in lower one-third of orbit
- Orbital rim, maxillae, nasal septum, zygomatic bones, and anterior nasal
- Fractures, neoplastic processes, and inflammatory conditions

MANDIBLE

Posteroanterior (No Angle)

Positioning Criteria

- Patient PA and shielded
- 10″ × 12″ (25 × 30 cm) IR lengthwise placed in Bucky
- OML perpendicular to IR
- MSP perpendicular to table
- Central ray perpendicular and directed to lips
- Collimate to four sides to include all pertinent anatomy
- Place appropriate side marker within light field on lateral aspect of image
- Minimum SID: 40″ (100 cm)

Evaluation Criteria

- No rotation evident by symmetry of mandibular rami
- Mandibular rami in center of image

Demonstrates

- Mandibular rami and lateral portion of body
- Midbody and mentum slightly superimposed over cervical spine
- Fractures and neoplastic pathology

Posteroanterior Axial Mandible

Positioning Criteria

- Patient PA and shielded
- 10″ × 12″ (25 × 30 cm) IR lengthwise placed in Bucky
- OML perpendicular to IR
- MSP perpendicular to table
- Central ray angled 20 degrees to 25 degrees cephalic and directed to exit acanthion
- Collimate to four sides to include all pertinent anatomy
- Place appropriate side marker within light field on lateral aspect of image
- Minimum SID: 40″ (100 cm)

Evaluation Criteria

- No rotation evident by symmetry of mandibular rami
- Mandibular rami in center of image

Demonstrates

- Temporomandibular joint (TMJ) and condyles are evident through the mastoid process
- Condyloid processes are elongated
- Fractures and neoplastic pathology

Posteroanterior Modified Waters: Mandible

Positioning Criteria

- Patient PA, erect or recumbent, and shielded
- 10″ × 12″ (25 × 30 cm) IR lengthwise placed in Bucky
- Canthus of lips and meatal line are perpendicular to Bucky
- OML forms a 55-degree angle with the IR
- Central ray exits acanthion
- MSP perpendicular to midline of grid
- Collimate to four sides to include all pertinent anatomy
- Place appropriate side marker within light field
- Minimum SID: 40″ (100 cm)

Evaluation Criteria

- No rotation evident by symmetrical mandibular rami

Demonstrates

- True PA of mandible
- 1″ (2.5 cm) superior to TMJ down to mentum of mandible

Anteroposterior Axial Towne: Mandible

Positioning Criteria

- Patient AP and shielded
- 10″ × 12″ (25 × 30 cm) IR lengthwise
- Central ray angled 35 degrees to 40 degrees caudal if OML is perpendicular to the IR
- Central ray is angled 7 degrees more caudal if the IOML is perpendicular
- Central ray is directed to the glabella and midway between EAMs and angles of mandible
- Collimate to four sides to include all pertinent anatomy
- Place appropriate side marker within light field on lateral aspect of the image
- Minimum SID: 40″ (100 cm)

Evaluation Criteria

- Distance from mandibular rami on each side should be equal if there is no rotation

Demonstrates

- Condyles of mandible and temporomandibular (TM) fossae
- Minimum superimposition of TM fossae and mastoid process
- Includes condyloid processes and TM fossae
- Fractures, neoplastic processes, and Paget disease

Submentovertical (Full Basal) Mandible

Positioning Criteria

- Patient AP erect and shielded
- 10″ × 12″ (25 × 30 cm) IR lengthwise placed in Bucky
- Patient's IOML is parallel to IR
- MSP is perpendicular to the IR
- Central ray perpendicular and directed midway between mandible angles and 1½″ (4 cm) inferior to mandibular symphysis
- Collimate to four sides to include all pertinent anatomy
- Place appropriate side marker within light field on lateral aspect of image
- Minimum SID: 40″ (100 cm)

Evaluation Criteria

- No rotation or tilt evident by equal distance from mandible to lateral border of skull

Demonstrates

- Coronoid and condylar process of mandible
- Fractures

Axiolateral Obliques Mandible

Positioning Criteria

- Perform imaging on tabletop with a 15-degree inclined positioning sponge or, if patient may stand, use Bucky
- Interpupillary line perpendicular to IR
- MSP parallel to IR and IOML parallel to the horizontal aspect of IR
- Head will be rotated 30 degrees toward receptor; patient positioning dependent on area of concern
- Central ray will be angled 20 degrees to 25 degrees cephalic and 2″ (5 cm) inferior to up gonion
- This best demonstrates mandibular body

Evaluation Criteria

- Must include: mentum to coronoid, mandibular fossa, and condyle
- Done bilaterally for comparison
- Side closest to IR/Bucky is the side of interest

Demonstrates

- Body best demonstrated with 30-degree rotation
- Mentum best demonstrated with 45 degrees of rotation
- Rami best demonstrated when head in true lateral

Temporomandibular Joints
Axiolateral: Law's Method

Positioning Criteria

- Patient placed in a true lateral position erect or prone (erect preferred) with affected side closest
- Place an 8″ × 10″ (20 × 25 cm) IR lengthwise in the Bucky aligned with the central ray
- Adjust IOML to be perpendicular to front edge of IR
- Rotate patient's head 15 degrees toward the IR
- Central ray directed 15 degrees caudal and 2″ (5 cm) superior to EAM, exiting the down TMJ
- A series of two projections are taken: one with the mouth closed and one with it open
- Collimate on all four sides
- Minimum SID: 40″ (100 cm)

Evaluation Criteria

- Down TMJ seen free of superimposition of contralateral side
- TMJ of interest is centered on image

Demonstrates

- Range of motion between TM fossa and mandibular condyle
- Closed-mouth image shows mandibular condyle in fossa, open mouth demonstrates movement of condyle to anterior margin of the fossa

Axiolateral: Schüller Method

Positioning Criteria

- Patient placed in a true lateral position erect or prone (erect preferred) with affected side closest to IR; full lead apron provided
- Place an 8″ × 10″ (20 × 25 cm) IR lengthwise in the Bucky aligned with the central ray
- Adjust IOML to be perpendicular to front edge of IR, interpupillary line parallel to IR, and MSP parallel to IR
- Central ray directed 25 degrees to 30 degrees caudal at a point 2″ (5 cm) superior to EAM, exiting the down TMJ
- A series of two projections are taken: one with the mouth closed and one with it open
- Collimate on all four sides
- Minimum SID: 40″ (100 cm)

Evaluation Criteria

- Down TMJ seen free of superimposition of contra-lateral side
- TMJ of interest is centered on image

Demonstrates

- Range of motion between TM fossa and mandibular condyle
- Closed-mouth image shows mandibular condyle in fossa; open mouth demonstrates movement of condyle to anterior margin of the fossa

Anteroposterior Axial: Modified Towne

Positioning Criteria

- Patient in the AP position erect or supine; full-body lead shielding
- Position the OML line perpendicular to IR
- Utilize a 10″ × 12″ (25 × 30 cm) IR lengthwise in the Bucky aligned with the central ray
- Central ray is directed 30 degrees caudal at a point 2″ (5 cm) anterior to EAM
- A series of two projections are taken: one with the mouth closed and one with it open
- Collimate on all four sides
- Minimum SID: 40″ (100 cm)

Evaluation Criteria

- Down TMJ seen free of superimposition of contra-lateral side
- TMJ of interest is centered on image

Demonstrates

- Range of motion between TM fossa and mandibular condyle
- Closed-mouth image shows mandibular condyle in fossa; open mouth demonstrates movement of con-dyle to anterior margin of the fossa

Nasal Bones
Parietoacanthial Projection for Nasal Bones

Positioning Criteria

- Patient positioned PA either erect or prone; full-body shielding
- Adjust the patient's head to bring the MML perpen-dicular to the IR (OML forms a 37-degree angle to IR)
- Utilize an 8″ × 10″ (20 × 25 cm) IR lengthwise in Bucky aligned with central ray
- Central ray directed perpendicular to MSP and exit-ing at the level of acanthion
- Collimate on all four sides appropriate to the anatomy of interest
- Minimum SID: 40″ (100 cm)

Evaluation Criteria

- No rotation noted by symmetrical appearance of right and left sinuses
- Proper extension of head noted by position of pars petrosa

Demonstrates

- Nasal septum
- Maxillary sinus free of superimposition from petrous ridge
- Pathology including but not limited to: displacement of nasal septum, sinusitis

Lateral Projection: Nasal Bones

Positioning Criteria

- Performed bilaterally
- Patient in an anterior oblique position
- Utilize an 8″ × 10″ (20 × 25 cm) IR crosswise, nongrid; divide IR in half to expose one lateral on each side; full lead apron
- Adjust the interpupillary line to be perpendicular to the IR
- Central ray perpendicular to a point ½″ (1 cm) infe-rior to the nasion
- Use exposure similar to that for a finger
- Minimum SID: 40″ (100 cm)

Evaluation Criteria

- Must include nasofrontal suture, all soft tissue, and anterior nasal spine

Demonstrates

- Fracture of the nasal bones
- Anterior/posterior dislocation of nasal bone

Posteroanterior Caldwell 30 Degrees

Positioning Criteria

- Patient positioned PA against the upright Bucky
- Align OML and MSP perpendicular to IR
- Utilize an 8″ × 10″ (20 × 25 cm) IR lengthwise aligned with the central ray
- Central ray is directed 30 degrees caudal to exit nasion
- Minimum SID: 40″ (100 cm)

Evaluation Criteria

- No rotation of head
- Baseline is correct when petrous ridge is seen below the inferior margin of the orbit

Demonstrates

- Nasal septum free of superimposition
- Floor of the orbit

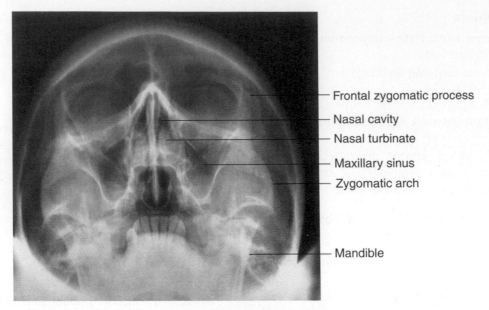

Frontal zygomatic process
Nasal cavity
Nasal turbinate
Maxillary sinus
Zygomatic arch

Mandible

FIGURE 5-26

- Frontal sinus is seen (because of angle, cannot assess air-fluid level)
- Frontal and ethmoid sinus

Paranasal Sinuses

Sinuses function as resonation chambers for the voice, decrease cranial weight by containing air, and warm and moisten inhaled air. In order to detect fluid levels, all sinuses imaging must be performed with a horizontal beam. Sinuses develop in the following manner:

Maxillary sinus: largest; well aerated at birth; antra of Highmore

Sphenoidal sinus (can be single) and frontal sinus: develop at ages 6 to 7 years

Ethmoid sinus: develops at ages 17 to 18 years

Parietoacanthial Projections (Water Projection)
Positioning Criteria

- Patient is positioned PA against the upright Bucky
- Adjust the MML to be perpendicular to IR and aligned with the central ray (OML forms a 37-degree angle to IR)
- Central ray directed perpendicular to MSP and exiting at the level of acanthion
- Collimate on all four sides appropriate to the anatomy of interest
- Minimum SID: 40″ (100 cm)

Evaluation Criteria

- No rotation noted by symmetrical appearance of right and left sinuses
- Proper extension of head noted by position of pars petrosa

Demonstrates
- Nasal septum
- Maxillary sinus free of superimposition from petrous ridge
- Pathology including but not limited to: displacement of nasal septum, sinusitis

A transoral open mouth Water projection can be performed with the same positioning. Prior to exposure, patient is instructed to open mouth. This will additionally demonstrate the sphenoid sinus through the mouth.

Posteroanterior Caldwell: 15-Degree Projection
Positioning Criteria

- Patient positioned PA against the upright Bucky
- Align MSP perpendicular to IR and OML 15 degrees from horizontal; a radiolucent support between forehead and upright Bucky may be used to maintain this position
- Central ray is directed perpendicular to exit nasion
- ALTERNATE METHOD: If the Bucky can be tilted 15 degrees, the patient's forehead and nose can be supported directly against the Bucky with the OML perpendicular to the Bucky surface and 15 degrees to the horizontal central ray

Evaluation Criteria

- No rotation of head
- Baseline is correct when petrous ridge is seen in the inferior one-third of the orbit

Demonstrates

- Air-fluid levels in the frontal and anterior ethmoid sinuses (see Figure 5-25)

Lateral Projection Sinuses

Positioning Criteria

- Patient in an anterior oblique position with the side of interest closest to IR; full lead apron
- Align the interpupillary line to be perpendicular and MSP parallel to the IR
- IOML is parallel to the floor
- Utilize 8" × 10" (20 × 25 cm) IR lengthwise in upright Bucky aligned with central ray
- Central ray perpendicular to a point 1" (2.5 cm) posterior to outer canthus of the eye
- Collimate from the EAM forward and from the bottom lip to the top of the skull
- Minimum SID: 40" (100 cm)

Evaluation Criteria

- No rotation evident noted by superimposition of the anterior and posterior clinoid processes as well as the infraorbital margins

Demonstrates

- All four sinuses: frontal, ethmoid, maxillary, and sphenoid

Submental Vertex (SMV/Basilar) Projection

Positioning Criteria

- Patient positioned AP against the upright Bucky
- Instruct patient to hyperextend to a point that brings the IOML parallel and MSP perpendicular to IR
- Utilize an 8" × 10" (20 × 25 cm) IR lengthwise in the Bucky aligned to the central ray
- Central ray is directed perpendicular to IOML at a point 1" (2.5 cm) anterior to EAMs

Evaluation Criteria

- No rotation noted by symmetrical petrous pyramids
- Mandibular condyles projected anterior to petrous ridges

Demonstrates

- Ethmoid, sphenoid, and maxillary sinuses and nasal fossae

Orbits

A series of projections are taken to demonstrate the orbits, including a parietoacanthial projection. The positioning for this projection is the same as for sinuses.

Parietoorbital Oblique Projection: Optic Foramina (Rhese Method)

Positioning Criteria

- Patient positioned PA against the Bucky; full lead apron
- Align acanthiomeatal line perpendicular to the IR
- Rotate head 37 degrees; use three-point landing technique: place chin, cheek, and nose against unit; MSP 53 degrees to IR
- Utilize an 8" × 10" (20 × 25 cm) IR in the Bucky aligned to the central ray
- Central ray directed perpendicular to 1" (2.5 cm) superior and 1" (2.5 cm) posterior to top of ear attachment (TEA) through affected orbit
- Collimate on all four sides
- Minimum SID: 40" (100 cm)

Evaluation Criteria

- Optic canal visualized in the lower inner quadrant of the orbit seen in profile

Demonstrates

- Optical canal and optical foramen
- Bony abnormalities of the optic foramen

Anteroposterior Toes

Positioning Criteria

- Instruct the patient to flex the knee and place the plantar surface of the foot in contact with the IR
- Long axis of the anatomy of interest should be aligned with the long axis of the IR
- Center the metatarsophalangeal joint of the digit of interest to the IR
- A sandbag may be used to prevent the IR from sliding
- In order to ensure that the anatomy of interest is parallel to the IR, either:
  Direct the central ray 15 degrees caudal to enter at the metatarsophalangeal joint OR
  Elevate the foot 15 degrees on a wedge-shaped radiolucent positioning sponge
- Collimate to include from the distal phalanx to at least the distal half of the metatarsal; include a portion of the adjacent digits as well

Evaluation Criteria

- Digit of interest visualized in an AP view with a portion of the adjacent digits and no superimposition of adjacent structures
- No rotation of the foot (equal concavity on both sides of the phalanges and metatarsals)

Demonstrates

- Digit of interest from the distal phalanx to at least the distal half of the metatarsal
- Open interphalangeal and metatarsophalangeal joints

Anteroposterior Oblique Toes (Medial Rotation)

Positioning Criteria

- Medial rotation is performed for the 1st, 2nd, and 3rd digits
- Instruct the patient to flex the knee and place the plantar surface of the foot in contact with the IR
- Long axis of the anatomy of interest should be aligned with the long axis of the IR
- Center the metatarsophalangeal joint of the digit of interest to the IR
- Oblique the foot 30 degrees to 45 degrees medially (a radiolucent angle sponge may be used to minimize patient motion)
- A sandbag may be used to prevent the IR from sliding
- Central ray directed perpendicular to metatarsophalangeal joint of the digit of interest
- Collimate to include from the distal phalanx to at least the distal half of the metatarsal; include a portion of the adjacent digits as well

Evaluation Criteria

- Digit of interest visualized in an oblique view with a portion of the adjacent digits and minimal superimposition of adjacent structures
- Increased concavity on one side of each phalanx and metatarsal

Demonstrates

- Digit of interest from the distal phalanx to at least the distal half of the metatarsal
- Open interphalangeal and metatarsophalangeal joints

Anteroposterior Oblique Toes (Lateral Rotation)

Positioning Criteria

- Lateral rotation is performed for the 4th and 5th digits
- Instruct the patient to flex the knee and place the plantar surface of the foot in contact with the IR
- Long axis of the anatomy of interest should be aligned with the long axis of the IR
- Center the metatarsophalangeal joint of the digit of interest to the IR
- Oblique the foot 30 degrees to 45 degrees laterally (a radiolucent angle sponge may be used to minimize patient motion)

- A sandbag may be used to prevent the IR from sliding
- Central ray directed perpendicular to metatarsophalangeal joint of the digit of interest
- Collimate to include from the distal phalanx to at least the distal half of the metatarsal; include a portion of the adjacent digits as well

Evaluation Criteria

- Digit of interest visualized in an oblique view with a portion of the adjacent digits and minimal superimposition of adjacent structures
- Increased concavity on one side of each phalanx and metatarsal

Demonstrates

- Digit of interest from the distal phalanx to at least the distal half of the metatarsal
- Open interphalangeal and metatarsophalangeal joints

Lateral Toes

Positioning Criteria

- Rotate the affected lower extremity medially for the 1st, 2nd, or 3rd digit and laterally for the 4th or 5th digit
- Long axis of the anatomy of interest should be aligned with the long axis of the IR
- Center the interphalangeal joint (for 1st digit) or proximal interphalangeal joint (for 2nd to 5th digits) to the IR
- Gauze or tape may be used to separate the toes and minimize superimposition
- A sandbag may be used to prevent the IR from sliding
- Direct the central ray to the interphalangeal joint (for 1st digit) or proximal interphalangeal joint (for 2nd to 5th digits) of the digit of interest
- Collimate close to the digit of interest; include from the distal phalanx to the distal portion of the metatarsal

Evaluation Criteria

- The digit of interest visualized in a lateral view with no superimposition
- No superimposition of the phalanges
- Metatarsophalangeal joint must be demonstrated, even if superimposition exists

Demonstrates

- Digit of interest from the distal phalanx to the distal portion of the metatarsal
- Open interphalangeal joints and possible slight superimposition of the metatarsophalangeal joint
- Anterior/posterior displacement of fracture fragments would be demonstrated in the lateral projection

Anteroposterior Foot

Positioning Criteria

- Instruct the patient to flex the knee and place the plantar surface of the foot in contact with the IR
- Long axis of the foot should be aligned with the long axis of the IR
- Center the base of the 3rd metatarsal to the center of the IR
- A sandbag may be used to prevent the IR from sliding
- Direct the central ray 10 degrees posteriorly to enter at the base of the 3rd metatarsal
- Patients with pes cavus (high arches) may require a larger angle (approximately 15 degrees)
- Patients with pes planus (flat feet) may require a smaller angle (approximately 5 degrees)
- Collimate close to the anatomy to include the entire foot

Evaluation Criteria

- No rotation of the foot
- Bases of the 1st and 2nd metatarsals are free of superimposition
- Bases of the 3rd to 5th metatarsals superimposed

- Open joint space between the 1st and 2nd cuneiforms (medial and intermediate cuneiforms)

Demonstrates

- All phalanges, interphalangeal joints, metatarsophalangeal joints, metatarsals, and cuneiforms are demonstrated in addition to the cuboid and navicular
- Because of superimposition, the talus and calcaneus are not visualized well in this projection

Anteroposterior Oblique Foot (Medial Rotation)

Positioning Criteria

- Instruct the patient to flex the knee and place the plantar surface of the foot in contact with the IR
- Long axis of the anatomy of interest should be aligned with the long axis of the IR
- Center the foot to the IR
- Oblique the foot 30 degrees to 40 degrees medially (a radiolucent angle sponge may be used to minimize patient motion)
- A sandbag may be used to prevent the IR from sliding

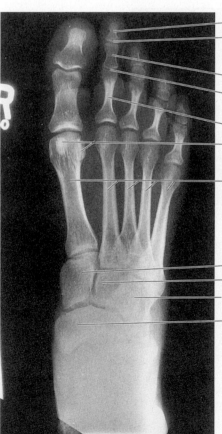

Distal phalanx
Distal interphalangeal joint (DIP)
Middle phalanx
Proximal interphalangeal joint (PIP)
Proximal phalanx
Sesamoid bones
1st, 2nd, 3rd, 4th, 5th metatarsals
1st (medial) cuneiform
2nd (intermediate) cuneiform
3rd (lateral) cuneiform
Navicular

FIGURE 5-27

- Central ray directed perpendicular to enter the base of the 3rd metatarsal
- Collimate close to the anatomy to include the entire foot

Evaluation Criteria

- Base of the 1st and 2nd metatarsals are superimposed
- Entire 3rd to 5th metatarsals free of superimposition

Demonstrates

- The entire foot, including all phalanges, interphalangeal joints, metatarsophalangeal joints, metatarsals, and tarsals
- The cuboid, 3rd (lateral) cuneiform, sinus tarsi, and base of the 5th metatarsal are well visualized in this projection

Anteroposterior Oblique Foot (Lateral Rotation)

Positioning Criteria

- Instruct the patient to flex the knee and place the plantar surface of the foot in contact with the IR

- Long axis of the anatomy of interest should be aligned with the long axis of the IR
- Center the foot to the IR
- Oblique the foot 30 degrees laterally (a radiolucent angle sponge may be used to minimize patient motion)
- Sandbags may be used to prevent the IR from sliding
- Central ray directed perpendicular to enter the base of the 3rd metatarsal
- Collimate close to the anatomy to include the entire foot

Evaluation Criteria

- The entire foot is demonstrated with slight superimposition of the digits
- Superimposition at the bases of the 1st to 5th metatarsals

Demonstrates

- The medial portions of the 1st cuneiform and navicular are demonstrated

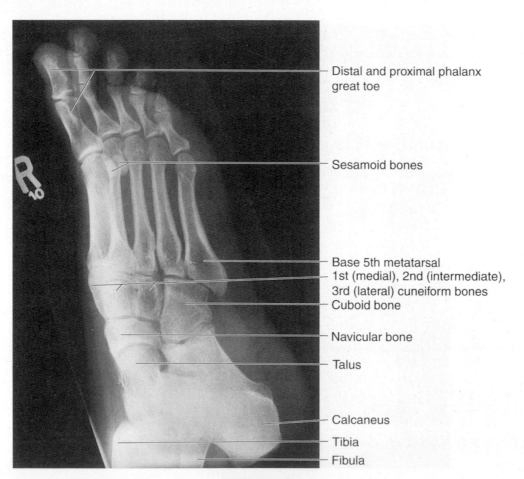

Distal and proximal phalanx great toe

Sesamoid bones

Base 5th metatarsal
1st (medial), 2nd (intermediate), 3rd (lateral) cuneiform bones
Cuboid bone

Navicular bone

Talus

Calcaneus

Tibia

Fibula

FIGURE 5-28

Lateral Foot (Lateromedial)

Positioning Criteria

- Patient is positioned lateral recumbent onto unaffected side
- Flex knee and place medial portion of the foot in contact with the IR
- Adjust the long axis of the foot in line with the long axis of the IR and center the foot to the IR
- The plantar surface of the foot should be perpendicular to the IR
- Instruct the patient to slightly dorsiflex the foot if possible
- Direct the central ray perpendicular to the midportion of the foot at the level of the base of the 3rd metatarsal
- Collimate close to the anatomy to include the entire foot and approximately 1″ (2.5 cm) of the distal tibia

Evaluation Criteria

- As compared to the mediolateral lateral projection of the foot, this projection enables a more true lateral view of the foot
- The entire foot from the superimposed phalanges to the calcaneus is demonstrated
- The distal fibula is superimposed by the posterior portion of the tibia, and the tibiotalar joint space is open

Demonstrates

- The calcaneus and talus and tuberosity of the 5th metatarsal are well visualized
- The navicular is partially superimposed over the cuboid and the cuneiforms; metatarsals and phalanges are superimposed

Lateral Foot (Mediolateral)

Positioning Criteria

- Patient is positioned lateral recumbent onto affected side
- Flex knee and place lateral portion of the foot in contact with the IR
- Adjust the long axis of the foot in line with the long axis of the IR and center the foot to the IR
- The plantar surface of the foot should be perpendicular to the IR
- Instruct the patient to slightly dorsiflex the foot if possible
- Direct the central ray perpendicular to the midportion of the foot at the level of the base of the 3rd metatarsal
- Collimate close to the anatomy to include the entire foot and approximately 1″ (2.5 cm) of the distal tibia

Evaluation Criteria

- As compared to the lateromedial lateral projection of the foot, this projection is easier for the patient to attain
- The entire foot from the superimposed phalanges to the calcaneus is demonstrated
- The distal fibula is superimposed by the posterior portion of the tibia and the tibiotalar joint space is open

Demonstrates

- The calcaneus and talus and tuberosity of the 5th metatarsal are well visualized
- The navicular is partially superimposed over the cuboid and the cuneiforms; metatarsals and phalanges are superimposed

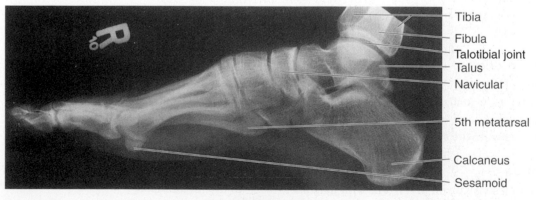

Tibia
Fibula
Talotibial joint
Talus
Navicular

5th metatarsal

Calcaneus
Sesamoid

FIGURE 5-29

Sesamoid Bones (Lewis Method)

Positioning Criteria

- Position the patient prone and instruct the patient to dorsiflex the foot and 1st toe, placing the 1st toe in contact with the center of the IR
- Adjust the plantar surface of the foot so that it is 15 degrees to 20 degrees from vertical (calcaneus not superimposed over metatarsal head)
- Ensure that there is no rotation of the foot
- Direct the central ray in tangent to the 1st metatarsophalangeal joint
- Collimate close to the anatomy to include the 1st to 2nd metatarsals

Evaluation Criteria

- No rotation of the foot
- Sesamoid bones visualized free of metatarsal superimposition
- Open space between the sesamoids and the metatarsals

Demonstrates

- Sesamoid bones visualized in tangent with minimal magnification

Sesamoid Bones (Holly Method)

Positioning Criteria

- Position the patient supine or seated and instruct the patient to slightly dorsiflex the foot and attain maximum dorsiflexion of the 1st toe
- Adjust the plantar surface of the foot so that it is 15 degrees to 20 degrees from vertical (calcaneus not superimposed over metatarsal head)
- Gauze or strong tape may be used to assist in dorsiflexion of the toes and to minimize patient motion
- Ensure that there is no rotation of the foot
- Direct the central ray in tangent to the 1st metatarsophalangeal joint
- Collimate close to the anatomy to include the 1st to 2nd metatarsals

Evaluation Criteria

- No rotation of the foot
- Sesamoid bones visualized free of metatarsal superimposition
- Open space between the sesamoids and the metatarsals

Demonstrates

- Sesamoid bones visualized in tangent with magnification due to the increased OID

Anteroposterior Weight-Bearing Feet

Positioning Criteria

- Instruct the patient to stand on the IR and evenly distribute weight on both feet
- Adjust the feet so that they are pointing forward and are centered to each half of the IR
- Central ray is directed 15 degrees posteriorly midway between both feet to enter at the level of the base of the metatarsals
- Collimate to include both feet in their entirety

Evaluation Criteria

- No rotation of the feet
- Bases of the 1st and 2nd metatarsals are free of superimposition
- Bases of the 3rd to 5th metatarsals superimposed
- Open joint space between the 1st and 2nd cuneiforms (medial and intermediate cuneiforms)

Demonstrates

- Both feet, including phalanges, metatarsals, and tarsals
- The presence of hallux valgus is best demonstrated in this projection

Lateral Weight-Bearing Feet

Positioning Criteria

- Instruct the patient to stand on wood blocks or a special positioning device designed for weight-bearing feet
- Ensure that the x-ray tube is able to be lowered enough to be centered to the foot; otherwise, the platform that the patient is standing on must be elevated
- Place the IR between the feet with the medial aspect of the foot in contact with the IR
- Ensure that the foot is not rotated
- Lower the x-ray tube and direct the central ray horizontally to the level of the base of the 3rd metatarsal
- Collimate to include the entire foot and ankle joint
- Turn the patient toward the opposite direction and repeat for the other foot

Evaluation Criteria

- The foot is visualized in a lateral position with no rotation
- The ankle joint is visualized

Demonstrates

- The entire foot is demonstrated from the phalanges to the metatarsals
- Pes planus (flat feet) and pes cavus (high arches) are demonstrated in the lateral projections

Anteroposterior Ankle

Positioning Criteria

- Dorsiflex foot in order to create a 90-degree angle with the plantar portion of the foot and the distal leg
- Ensure toes are not superimposed over ankle
- Entire lower leg must be parallel with the longitudinal axis of the IR
- Central ray directed perpendicular to midpoint of malleoli
- Collimate to include distal one-third of tibia and fibula proximally and the talus distally

Evaluation Criteria

- Distal tibia and fibula will be slightly superimposed
- Distal anterior view of tibia, fibula, lateral and medial malleoli, tibiotalar joint, and talus should be visualized
- The navicular, cuboid, and cuneiforms will display the shadow of the dorsiflexed foot, therefore will not be optimally visualized
- Long axis of distal leg should run parallel with the IR
- Distal 5th metatarsal should be within the collimated field because this area is a common site of fracture
- Collimation should be four sided, but open enough to include the soft tissue of the ankle

Demonstrates

- AP view of ankle, talus, medial and lateral malleoli, and distal one-third of tibia and fibula
- Talofibular articulation will not appear open; with proper AP alignment, this is an indication there are no ligament tears
- Normal overlapping of the tibiofibular articulation and of the anterior tubercle over the distal fibula

Medial Anteroposterior Oblique Ankle

Positioning Criteria

- Dorsiflexion of foot remains
- Leg as well as foot should be rotated medially 45 degrees
- Support may be used as needed to hold anatomy in place
- Central ray will remain midway between malleoli

Evaluation Criteria

- The tibiofibular articulation will be open
- The fibula will not superimpose over the talus
- The lateral subtalar joint is open slightly
- Distal tibia, fibula, and talus are demonstrated
- The base of the 5th metatarsal should be within the collimated field because of frequency of fracture in this area

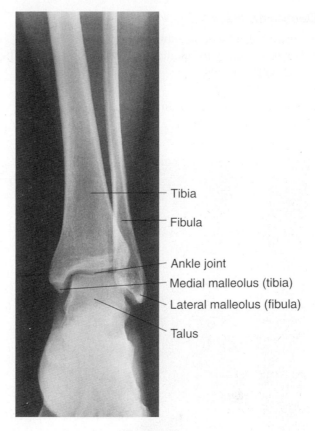

Tibia
Fibula
Ankle joint
Medial malleolus (tibia)
Lateral malleolus (fibula)
Talus

FIGURE 5-30

Demonstrates

- Distal one-third of the lower leg
- Lateral malleolus free of superimposition
- Talus
- Proximal portion of metatarsals
- Distal tibiofibular joint is open

Anteroposterior Mortise Ankle

Positioning Criteria

- Align ankle to midpoint of the IR
- Long axis of distal leg should run parallel with the IR
- Foot should remain in neutral position
- Rotate entire leg, ankle, and foot 15 degrees to 20 degrees internally
- Support may be used as needed to hold anatomy in place
- Central ray should be directed midway between malleoli

Evaluation Criteria

- Ankle joint should be centered to the IR
- The intermalleolar line should be parallel to the IR
- Four-sided collimation, with the distal one-third of tibia and fibula, ankle joint, talus, and proximal metatarsals
- Soft tissue should be included
- Mortise should appear open

Demonstrates

- Entire ankle mortise joint
- Open lateral and medial mortise joints with the malleoli in profile
- Tibial plafond
- Minimal superimposition of distal tibiofibular joint
- Base of 5th metatarsal

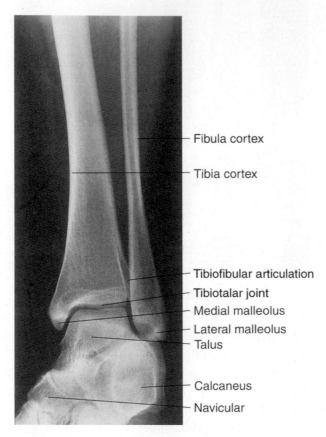

Fibula cortex

Tibia cortex

Tibiofibular articulation

Tibiotalar joint

Medial malleolus

Lateral malleolus

Talus

Calcaneus

Navicular

FIGURE 5-31

Mediolateral Lateral Ankle

Positioning Criteria

- Patient should be in a recumbent lateral position
- Affected lateral side down
- Align ankle and distal leg shaft to long axis of IR
- Dorsiflex foot so the plantar surface is at a right angle to the leg
- Central ray will be directed at medial malleolus

Evaluation Criteria

- Image should be free of motion
- Sharp bony margins should be present
- Lateral malleolus should be seen through distal tibia and talus
- Soft tissue should be demonstrated on the IR
- Four-sided collimation

Demonstrates

- Distal one-third of tibia and fibula with fibula superimposed over the posterior one-third to one-half of tibia
- Talus and calcaneus in profile
- Navicular, cuboid, and base of 5th metatarsal should be included
- Tibiotalar joint will be open

Lateromedial Lateral

Positioning Criteria

- Patient should be in a recumbent lateral position
- Patient's medial aspect of the affected leg should be down
- Align ankle and distal leg shaft to long axis of IR
- Dorsiflex foot so the plantar surface is at a right angle to the leg
- Central ray should be directed to the lateral malleolus

Evaluation Criteria

- Image should be free of motion
- Sharp bony margins should be present
- Lateral malleolus should be seen through distal tibia and talus
- Soft tissue should be demonstrated on the IR
- Four-sided collimation

Demonstrates

- Distal one-third of tibia and fibula with fibula superimposed over the posterior one-third to one-half of tibia
- Talus and calcaneus in profile
- Navicular, cuboid, and base of 5th metatarsal should be included
- Tibiotalar joint will be open
- Truer lateral achieved due to the medial malleolus allowing closer contact with the IR
- This is a difficult position for some patients

Anteroposterior Stress Views

Positioning Criteria

- Ankle joint should be centered to the IR
- The foot should be dorsiflexed
- Plantar surface is turned medially for inversion and laterally for eversion
- Patient must hold position with gauze or another health-care provider may hold the foot in place
- Central ray should be directed midway between malleoli

Evaluation Criteria

- Distal tibia and fibula will be slightly superimposed
- Distal anterior view of tibia, fibula, lateral and medial malleoli, and tibiotalar joint and anterior view of talus should be visualized

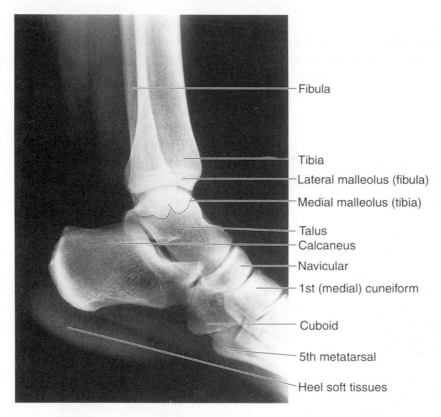

Fibula

Tibia
Lateral malleolus (fibula)
Medial malleolus (tibia)
Talus
Calcaneus
Navicular
1st (medial) cuneiform

Cuboid

5th metatarsal

Heel soft tissues

FIGURE 5-32

- Long axis of distal leg should run parallel with the IR
- Collimation should be four sided, but open enough to include the soft tissue of the ankle

Demonstrates

- Inversion demonstrates the lateral aspect of the joint for lateral ligament tear or rupture
- Eversion demonstrates the medial aspect of the joint for medial ligament tear or rupture

Calcaneus (Os Calcis)
Plantodorsal Axial
Positioning Criteria

- Have a long strip of gauze or a sheet ready
- Patient will be supine
- Angle the tube 40 degrees cephalic from vertical
- Place the patient's 90-degree flexed foot so that the central ray enters the base of the 3rd metatarsal; angle more if the patient can't flex 90 degrees
- Have the patient hold the dorsiflexed position with the gauze or sheet
- Exit through the IR
- Collimate closely to the calcaneus

Evaluation Criteria

- There should be no rotation of the calcaneus
- Calcaneus and subtalar joint should be visualized
- Optimal density and contrast should allow for the visualization of talocalcaneal joint without overexposure to the tuberosity

Demonstrates

- Open talocalcaneal joint, sustentaculum tali, tuberosity, lateral process, and peroneal/trochlear process

Dorsoplantar Axial
Positioning Criteria

- Patient will be prone
- Place sponges or sandbags under the affected side to allow patient to dorsiflex foot
- The long axis of the foot should be perpendicular to the tabletop and the plantar portion of the foot should be directly against the IR
- Angle 40 degrees caudally to the long axis of the foot
- Central ray should enter 2″ (5 cm) superior to the calcaneal tuberosity

Evaluation Criteria

- There should be no rotation of the calcaneus
- Calcaneus and subtalar joint should be visualized
- Optimal density and contrast should allow for the visualization of talocalcaneal joint without overexposure to the calcaneal tuberosity

Demonstrates

- Open talocalcaneal joint, sustentaculum tali, calcaneal tuberosity, lateral process, and peroneal/trochlear process
- Same anatomy as plantodorsal, but exhibits increased recorded detail

Lateral Calcaneus (Os Calcis)

Positioning Criteria

- Patient will be placed in a recumbent lateral
- Affected side closest to the IR
- Adjust the long axis of the plantar surface so that it is parallel with the IR
- Foot should be dorsiflexed
- Central ray should enter at the subtalar joint, which is 1″ (2.5 cm) distal to the medial malleolus

Evaluation Criteria

- The calcaneus should not exhibit rotation
- Distal portion of the tibia and fibula should be present in order to demonstrate the tibiotalar joint
- Sinus tarsi open
- Optimal exposure to demonstrate the calcaneus and soft tissue
- Four-sided collimation including all of the calcaneus and the tibiotalar joint

Demonstrates

- Lateral view of the calcaneus, tibiotalar joint, talus, sinus tarsi, subtalar joint, calcaneal tuberosity, sustentaculum tali, navicular, cuboid, calcaneocuboid joint, and base of 5th metatarsal
- Calcaneal fractures

Tibia and Fibula Projections
Anteroposterior Tibia and Fibula

Positioning Criteria

- Place the lower extremity in the AP position
- Femoral epicondyles parallel to the IR
- Central ray directed perpendicular to midshaft
- Collimate to include both the ankle and knee joints

Evaluation Criteria

- The entire tibia and fibula are included
- Fibula is partially superimposed by tibia at both proximal and distal ends
- If completely superimposed or free from superimposition, extremity is rotated
- Both ankle and knee joints are visible
- The image is properly exposed

Demonstrates

- An AP view of the tibia and fibula
- Medial/lateral displacement

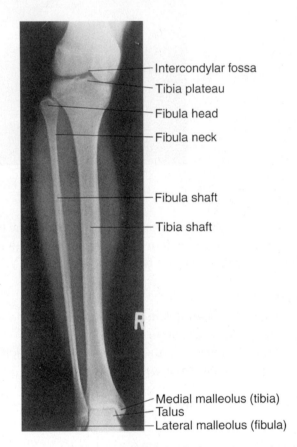

Intercondylar fossa
Tibia plateau
Fibula head
Fibula neck
Fibula shaft
Tibia shaft
Medial malleolus (tibia)
Talus
Lateral malleolus (fibula)

FIGURE 5-33

Lateral Tibia and Fibula

Positioning Criteria

- Rotate the lower extremity laterally
- Patella perpendicular to IR
- Provide support for the ankle and/or foot if necessary to maintain proper position
- Central ray directed perpendicular to midshaft
- Collimate to include both the ankle and knee joints

Evaluation Criteria

- The entire tibia and fibula are included
- Proximal head of fibula superimposed by tibia
- Distal fibula lying over posterior half of tibia
- Both ankle and knee joints are visible
- The image is properly exposed

Demonstrates

- Lateral view of the tibia and fibula
- Tibial tuberosity
- Anterior/posterior displacement

Oblique Tibia and Fibula

Positioning Criteria

- Patient supine with lower extremity extended and rotated 45 degrees (medial or lateral)
- Central ray directed perpendicular to midshaft

Evaluation Criteria

- 45-degree oblique projection
- Entire tibia and fibula visualized
- Optimal exposure

Demonstrates

Medial Rotation Demonstrates

- Proximal and distal tibiofibular articulations
- Interosseous space between tibia and fibula

Lateral Rotation Demonstrates

- Fibula superimposed by lateral portion of tibia

Knee Projections

A grid should be used for all knees measuring more than 4″ (10 cm). For knees measuring less than 4″ (10 cm), it is acceptable to perform imaging without the use of a grid on tabletop.

Anteroposterior Knee

Positioning Criteria

- Patient in AP position
- Lower extremity fully extended
- Femoral epicondyles parallel to the image plane
- Central ray ½″ (1 cm) inferior to apex of patella
- Central ray angled depending on body habitus to open joint space

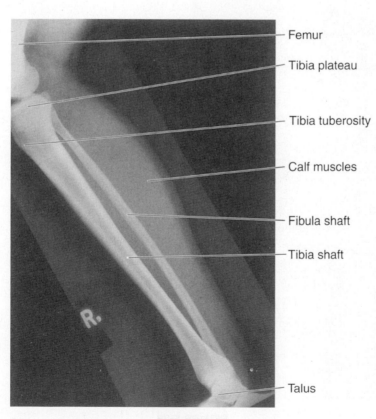

FIGURE 5-34

- Measure tabletop to ASIS and angle as follows:
  Less than 8″ (20 cm): angle 5 degrees caudal
  Between 8″ and 10″ (20 and 25 cm): perpendicular
    central ray
  More than 10″ (25 cm): angle 5 degrees cephalic
- Collimate to include the distal femur, proximal tibia, and
  fibula and medial/lateral to include soft tissue

Evaluation Criteria

- Distal femur and proximal tibia and fibula shown
- Femorotibial joint space is open
- Joint is centered on image
- No rotation of knee
- Image is exposed correctly

Demonstrates

- Femorotibial joint space
- Head of fibula slightly superimposed by tibia
- Medial/lateral fracture displacement

Anteroposterior Medial (Internal) Oblique Knee

Positioning Criteria

- Patient in AP position with lower extremity fully
  extended
- Internally rotated lower extremity 40 degrees to
  45 degrees
- Central ray ½″ (1 cm) inferior to apex of patella
- Central ray angled depending on body habitus to
  open joint space
- Measure tabletop to ASIS and angle as follows:
  Less than 8″ (20 cm): angle 5 degrees caudal
  Between 8″ and 10″ (20 and 25 cm): perpendicular
    central ray
  More than 10″ (25 cm): angle 5 degrees cephalic
- Collimate to include the distal femur, proximal tibia,
  and fibula and medial/lateral to include soft tissue
- Minimum SID: 40″ (100 cm)

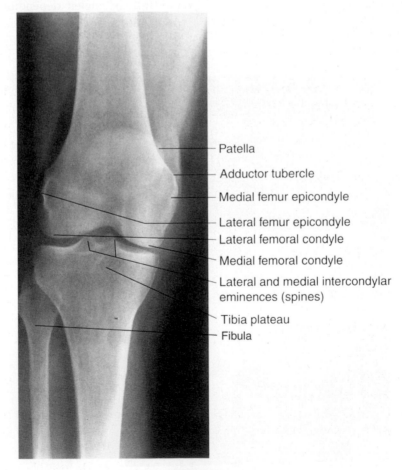

Patella
Adductor tubercle
Medial femur epicondyle
Lateral femur epicondyle
Lateral femoral condyle
Medial femoral condyle
Lateral and medial intercondylar
eminences (spines)
Tibia plateau
Fibula

FIGURE 5-35

Evaluation Criteria

- Distal femur and proximal tibia and fibula shown
- Proximal tibiofibular articulations seen free of super-imposition

Demonstrates

- Head of fibula free of superimposition
- Lateral tibial condyle
- Lateral tibial plateau
- Lateral femoral condyle

Anteroposterior Lateral (External) Oblique Knee

Positioning Criteria

- Patient in AP position
- Lower extremity fully extended
- Lower extremity externally rotated 40 degrees to 45 degrees
- Central ray ½″ (1 cm) inferior to apex of patella
- Central ray angled depending on body habitus to open joint space
- Measure tabletop to ASIS and angle as follows:
  Less than 8″ (20 cm): angle 5 degrees caudal
  Between 8″ and 10″ (20 and 25 cm): perpendicular central ray
  More than 10″ (25 cm): angle 5 degrees cephalic
- Collimate to include the distal femur, proximal tibia, and fibula and medial/lateral to include soft tissue

Evaluation Criteria

- Distal femur and proximal tibia and fibula shown
- Fibula superimposed over midtibia

Demonstrates

- Head of fibula free of superimposition
- Medial tibial condyle
- Medial tibial plateau
- Medial femoral condyle

Lateral Knee (Nontrauma)

Positioning Criteria

- Patient is rotated toward affected side
- Knee flexed 20 degrees to 30 degrees
- Femoral epicondyles perpendicular to IR
- Central ray angled 5 degrees cephalic ½″ (1 cm) inferior to medial condyle
- Four-sided collimation

Evaluation Criteria

- Distal femur and proximal tibia and fibula shown
- Patella is in profile (indicates no rotation)
- Evidence of rotation is seen as follows: underrotated when the abductor tubercle is seen; overrotated when the head of the fibula is seen free of superimposition
- Femoral condyles superimposed

Demonstrates

- Femoropatellar joint space

Lateral Knee (Trauma)

Positioning Criteria

- Patient is supine
- Minimal flexion 5 degrees to 10 degrees
- If transverse fracture of patella is present, no flexion
- Support and elevate the knee
- Femoral epicondyles perpendicular to IR
- Utilize a horizontal central ray
- Central ray directed ½″ (1 cm) inferior to lateral tibial condyle
- Four-sided collimation
- Minimum SID: 40″ (100 cm)

Evaluation Criteria

- Distal femur and proximal tibia and fibula shown
- Patella is in profile (indicates no rotation)
- Evidence of rotation is seen as follows: underrotated when the abductor tubercle is seen; overrotated when the head of the fibula is seen free of superimposition
- Femoral condyles superimposed

Demonstrates

- Femoropatellar joint space
- Femorotibial joint space
- Anterior/posterior fracture displacement
- Presence of joint effusion, indicative of fracture

Anteroposterior Weight-Bearing Knees

Positioning Criteria

- Patient standing AP against upright Bucky
- Typically done bilaterally
- Femoral epicondyles parallel to the image plane
- Central ray perpendicular to joint space
- Central ray ½″ (1 cm) inferior to apex of patella
- 14″ × 17″ (35 × 42.5 cm) IR placed crosswise

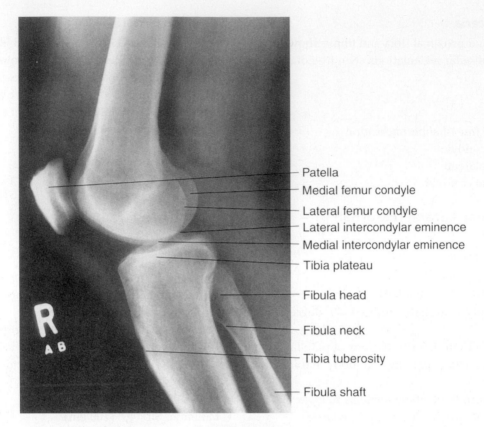

Patella
Medial femur condyle
Lateral femur condyle
Lateral intercondylar eminence
Medial intercondylar eminence
Tibia plateau
Fibula head
Fibula neck
Tibia tuberosity
Fibula shaft

FIGURE 5-36

Evaluation Criteria

- Knee joints centered to collimated area
- No rotation of knees
- Joint spaces are open
- Optimal technique employed

Demonstrates

- More accurate than supine AP image
- Pathology including but not limited to: assessment of degenerative joint disease, joint space narrowing, varus/valgus deformities

Posteroanterior Weight-Bearing Knees (Rosenberg)

Positioning Criteria

- Performed bilaterally
- Patient upright in a PA position
- Flex knees to 45 degrees
- 14″ × 17″ (35 × 42.5 cm) IR placed crosswise aligned with the central ray
- Central ray directed 10 degrees to 15 degrees caudal
- Four-sided collimation

Evaluation Criteria

- Knee joints centered to collimated area
- No rotation of knees
- Joint spaces are open
- Optimal technique employed

Demonstrates

- More accurate than upright AP projection
- Tibial plateaus are superimposed
- Pathology including but not limited to: assessment of degenerative joint disease, joint space narrowing, varus/valgus deformities, assessment of condylar fossa

Knee Axial Projections

Positioning Criteria (Three Methods)
Posteroanterior Axial: Camp-Coventry Method

- Patient prone
- Affected leg flexed 40 degrees and supported
- Central ray angled 40 degrees caudal
- Central ray directed to enter popliteal depression

Posteroanterior Axial Holmblad Method

- Support knee on a chair or other flat surface
- Place patient in kneeling position with lower leg parallel to IR
- Instruct patient to lean forward until femur forms a 70-degree angle to IR
- Central ray perpendicular
- Central ray directed to enter popliteal depression

Anteroposterior Axial Beclere Method

- Utilize a curved IR
- Patient supine with lower extremity extended
- Knee flexed approximately 60 degrees
- Central ray directed ½″ (1 cm) inferior to apex of patella
- Central ray cephalic at an angle perpendicular to tibia

Evaluation Criteria

- Intercondylar fossa centered on image
- Open intercondylar fossa
- Four-sided collimation
- No rotation of knee

Demonstrates

- Intercondylar fossa
- Intercondylar eminence well visualized
- Pathology including but not limited to: avulsion fractures, osteochondritis desiccans, joint space narrowing

Patella Projections
Posteroanterior Patella
Positioning Criteria

- Patient in the prone position with lower extremity extended
- Provide support for ankle and foot
- Femoral condyles should be parallel to IR
- Utilize an 8″ × 10″ (20 × 25 cm) IR aligned with the central ray
- Central ray perpendicular to midpatellar area/popliteal crease
- Increased collimation to anatomy of interest
- Minimum SID: 40″ (100 cm)

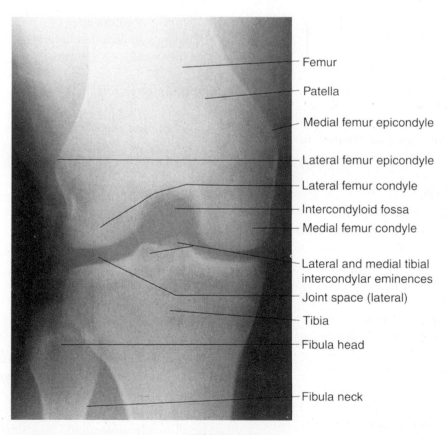

Femur
Patella
Medial femur epicondyle
Lateral femur epicondyle
Lateral femur condyle
Intercondyloid fossa
Medial femur condyle
Lateral and medial tibial intercondylar eminences
Joint space (lateral)
Tibia
Fibula head
Fibula neck

FIGURE 5-37

Evaluation Criteria

- Patella centered in collimated area
- No rotation
- Optimal exposure

Demonstrates

- Patella
- Transverse fracture of patella

Mediolateral Patella

Positioning Criteria

- Patient rotated toward affected side to bring knee into a lateral position
- Flexion of knee should not exceed 5 degrees to 10 degrees
- Utilize an 8″ × 10″ (20 × 25 cm) IR aligned with the central ray
- Central ray perpendicular to distal femoropatellar joint
- Increase collimation to anatomy of interest
- Minimum SID: 40″ (100 cm)

Evaluation Criteria

- Patella centered on image
- Patella in true lateral position
- Optimal exposure

Demonstrates

- Lateral view of patella
- Patellofemoral articulation open
- Pathology including but not limited to: anterior/posterior displacement of fractures

Patella Tangentials

Positioning Criteria (Five Methods)
Orthopedic Physicians Preferred Method

- Requires use of axial viewer
- Viewer aids in creation of 45 degrees of flexion
- Central ray directed 60 degrees caudal to enter base of patella
- Collimate to anatomy of interest
- Minimum SID: 72″ (180 cm) to reduce magnification

Settegast

- Patient positioned prone on the table
- Affected leg slowly flexed approximately 120 degrees until patella is perpendicular to IR
- Have patient hold on to gauze or tape to maintain position

- Place 8″ × 10″ (20 × 25 cm) IR under knee on tabletop
- Central ray is directed 15 degrees to 20 degrees cephalic parallel to patella entering apex of patella
- Increased collimation
- Minimum SID: 40″ (100 cm)

Hughston

- Patient positioned prone on the table
- Affected leg flexed 40 degrees
- Have patient hold on to gauze or tape to maintain position
- Place 8″ × 10″ (20 × 25 cm) IR under knee on tabletop
- Can be performed bilaterally on one larger IR
- Central ray directed 15 degrees to 20 degrees cephalic entering the apex
- Collimate to anatomy of interest
- Minimum SID: 40″ (100 cm)

Inferosuperior Method (Bilateral)

- Patient supine on table
- Knees flexed 40 degrees to 45 degrees and supported
- Place 10″ × 12″ (25 × 30 cm) IR on edge resting on midthighs, tilted to be perpendicular to central ray
- Central ray directed 10 degrees to 15 degrees cephalic
- Central ray enters apex of patella
- Collimate to include bilateral anatomy
- Minimum SID: 40″ (100 cm)

Superoinferior Sitting Method

- Patient seated in chair
- Knees flexed slightly with feet placed under chair
- IR placed on foot stool to reduce OID
- Central ray directed perpendicular to enter base of patella
- Minimum SID: 48″ to 50″ (120 to 125 cm)

Evaluation Criteria

- Intercondylar sulcus and patella visualized
- Patellofemoral joint space is open
- Optimal exposure

Demonstrates

- Patellofemoral joint space
- Pathology including but not limited to: patellar fracture, patellofemoral subluxation syndrome

Femur Projections

For all femur projections, take into consideration the anode heel effect and place the hip of the patient at cathode end of the x-ray beam.

Proximal Femur

Positioning Criteria

- Patient supine and legs fully extended; gonadal region shielded
- Place 10″ × 12″ (25 × 30 cm) IR lengthwise in table Bucky
- Rotate affected leg internally 15 degrees to 20 degrees to provide a true AP projection of the proximal femurs; places femoral heads and necks in profile
- Direct central ray perpendicular to IR, 1″ to 2″ (2.5 to 5 cm) medial and 3″ to 4″ (7.5 to 10 cm) distal to ASIS, or 1″ to 2″ (2.5 to 5 cm) distal to the midfemoral neck for orthopedic devices
- Collimate to four sides to include all pertinent anatomy
- Place appropriate side marker within light field on lateral aspect of image
- Minimum SID: 40″ (100 cm)

Evaluation Criteria

- True AP projection of the proximal one-third of the femur
- Greater trochanter and femoral head and neck in full profile with no evidence of foreshortening
- Femoral neck in the center of IR indicates proper centering of part–IR–central ray
- Lesser trochanters not visible or slightly visible on some patients
- No rotation evident by equidistant ASIS from tabletop
- Optimal exposure factors

Demonstrates

- Proximal one-third of femur; acetabulum and adjacent parts of the pubis, ischium, and ilium
- Medial/lateral displacement of the femoral head
- If patient has an orthopedic device, it should be visualized in its entirety

Anteroposterior Femur: Proximal Femur to Midfemur

Positioning Criteria

- Patient supine and legs fully extended; gonadal region shielded
- Place top of 14″ × 17″ (35 × 42.5 cm) IR at ASIS in table Bucky
- Rotate affected leg 5 degrees internally to bring femoral condyles parallel to IR
- Direct central ray perpendicular and to the midpoint of the IR
- Collimate to four sides to include all pertinent anatomy

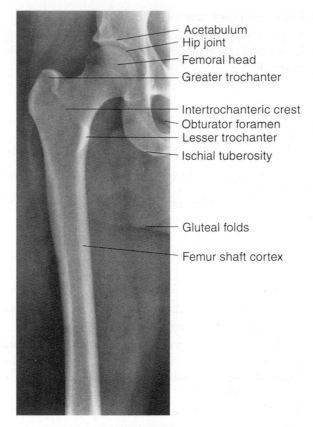

Acetabulum
Hip joint
Femoral head
Greater trochanter

Intertrochanteric crest
Obturator foramen
Lesser trochanter
Ischial tuberosity

Gluteal folds

Femur shaft cortex

FIGURE 5-38

- Place appropriate side marker within light field on lateral aspect of image
- Minimum SID: 40″ (100 cm)

Evaluation Criteria

- Proximal femur to midshaft of femur demonstrated in the AP position
- No rotation evident

Demonstrates

- An AP view of the proximal femur
- Medial/lateral displacement of the proximal femur
- Detection and evaluation of fractures and/or bone lesions

Anteroposterior Femur: Midfemur to Distal Femur

Positioning Criteria

- Patient supine and legs fully extended; gonadal region shielded
- Place 10″ × 12″ (25 × 30 cm) or 14″ × 17″ (35 × 42.5 cm) IR adjacent to the distal aspect of the IR from proximal projection in table Bucky or tabletop depending on part size (moving or stationary grid recommended)

- Ensure internal rotation of the affected leg is maintained at 5 degrees
- Direct central ray perpendicular and to the midpoint of the IR
- Collimate to four sides to include all pertinent anatomy
- Place appropriate side marker within light field on lateral aspect of image
- Minimum SID: 40″ (100 cm)

Evaluation Criteria

- Midfemur to distal shaft of femur demonstrated in the AP position adjacent to the proximal femur image
- Knee joint included
- No rotation evident

Demonstrates

- An AP view of the midfemur to distal femur adjacent to proximal femur image
- Medial/lateral displacement of the midfemur to distal femur
- Detection and evaluation of fractures and/or bone lesions

Lateral Nontrauma Projections: Femur
Lateral Femur: Proximal Femur to Midfemur
Positioning Criteria

- Routine mediolateral
- Patient slightly rotated to affected side with leg bent at 45 degrees with lateral aspect of femur in contact with table and aligned to table midline; gonadal region shielded
- Support foot of affected leg with a sponge; extend and support unaffected leg behind unaffected knee and allow patient to roll posteriorly about 15 degrees to prevent superimposition of proximal femur and hip joint
- Place 10″ × 12″ (25 × 30 cm) or 14″ × 17″ (35 × 42.5 cm) IR in table Bucky with top of IR at ASIS and include hip joint
- Direct central ray perpendicular and to the midpoint of the IR
- Collimate to four sides to include all pertinent anatomy
- Place appropriate side marker within light field on lateral aspect of image
- Minimum SID: 40″ (100 cm)

Evaluation Criteria

- Proximal one-half to two-thirds of proximal femur, including hip joint
- No superimposition by opposite limb
- True lateral of the proximal femur to midfemur

- Superimposition of the greater and lesser trochanters with greater trochanter mostly superimposed by femoral neck
- No evidence of elongation or foreshortening
- Optimal exposure

Demonstrates

- Lateral view of the proximal femur to midshaft of femur
- Anterior/posterior displacement of proximal femur to midfemur
- Detection and evaluation of fractures and/or bone lesions

Lateral Femur: Midfemur to Distal Femur
Positioning Criteria

- Routine mediolateral
- Patient slightly rotated to affected side with leg bent at 45 degrees with lateral aspect of femur in contact with table; gonadal region shielded
- Support foot of affected leg with a sponge; bend unaffected knee and keep behind affected leg to prevent overrotation
- Place top of 10″ × 12″ (25 × 30 cm) or 14″ × 17″ (35 × 42.5 cm) IR adjacent to the distal aspect of the proximal lateral femur image in table Bucky or tabletop depending on part size to include knee joint (lower margin of IR should be 2″ [5 cm] below knee joint)
- Direct central ray perpendicular and to the midpoint of the IR
- Collimate to four sides to include all pertinent anatomy
- Place appropriate side marker within light field on lateral aspect of image
- Minimum SID: 40″ (100 cm)

Evaluation Criteria

- True lateral of distal two-thirds of distal femur, including knee joint
- Knee joint is not open, and distal margins of femoral condyles will not be superimposed due to divergent x-ray beam
- Anterior and posterior margins of medial and lateral femoral condyles superimposed and aligned with open femoropatellar joint space
- Optimal exposure

Demonstrates

- True lateral of distal two-thirds of distal femur, including knee joint
- Anterior/posterior displacement of midfemur to distal femur
- Detection and evaluation of fractures and/or bone lesions

Lateral Trauma Projections: Femur
Lateral Femur: Midfemur to Distal Femur (Trauma)
Positioning Criteria
Mediolateral

- Patient is supine/dorsal decubitus with affected leg elevated with support of radiolucent sponges or pads
- Place 14″ × 17″ (35 × 42.5 cm) IR on the lateral aspect of the affected leg to include midfemur to distal femur and knee joint
- Raise unaffected leg and support with leg lift or step stool to prevent superimposition of soft tissue
- Direct central ray horizontal and perpendicular to midpoint of IR
- Collimate to four sides to include all pertinent anatomy
- Place appropriate side marker within light field on lateral aspect of image
- Minimum SID: 40″ (100 cm)

Lateromedial

- Patient supine/dorsal decubitus with affected leg elevated with the support of radiolucent sponges or pads
- Place 14″ × 17″ (35 × 42.5 cm) IR on the medial aspect (between patient's legs) of the affected leg to include midfemur to distal femur and knee joint
- Direct central ray horizontal and perpendicular to midpoint of IR
- Collimate to four sides to include all pertinent anatomy
- Place appropriate side marker within light field on lateral aspect of image
- Minimum SID: 40″ (100 cm)

Evaluation Criteria

- True lateral of distal two-thirds of distal femur, including knee joint
- Knee joint is not open and distal margins of femoral condyles will not be superimposed due to divergent x-ray beam
- Anterior and posterior margins of medial and lateral femoral condyles superimposed and aligned with open femoropatellar joint space
- Optimal exposure

Demonstrates

- True lateral of distal two-thirds of distal femur, including knee joint
- Anterior/posterior displacement of midfemur to distal femur
- Detection and evaluation of fractures and/or bone lesions

Mediolateral Proximal Femur: Sanderson Method
Positioning Criteria

- Patient supine with support placed under affected hip on stretcher or bed; oblique 20 degrees to 30 degrees from supine
- Align IR so that it is parallel to long axis of foot; place gridded 14″ × 17″ (35 × 42.5 cm) IR against and partially under affected thigh to be near perpendicular to central ray
- Angle central ray mediolaterally to be near perpendicular to long axis of foot
- Employ 10-degree to 20-degree cephalad angle of tube to better visualize the neck and head
- AMOUNT OF CENTRAL RAY CROSS-ANGLE WILL VARY DEPENDING ON EXTERNAL ROTATION OF AFFECTED LEG
- Collimate to four sides to include all pertinent anatomy
- Place appropriate side marker within light field on lateral aspect of image
- Minimum SID: 40″ (100 cm)

Evaluation Criteria

- True lateral view of hip and proximal femur with minimal distortion
- Entire hip prosthesis or pin visualized in its entirety

Demonstrates

- Lateral of proximal femur and hip for patients with limited bilateral lower limb movement due to trauma or arthroplasty
- Alignment of hip prosthesis or pin postoperatively seen with minimal distortion
- Anterior/posterior dislocation or displacement of proximal femur and hip

Posteroanterior Finger
Positioning Criteria

- Patient seated and elbow flexed 90 degrees; full shield
- Place 8″ × 10″ (20 × 25 cm) IR crosswise on table
- Pronate hand and extend fingers
- Direct central ray perpendicular to IR and proximal interphalangeal joint
- Finger of interest should be separated from other fingers and aligned to long axis of IR
- Collimate to four sides to include all pertinent anatomy
- Place appropriate side marker within light field on lateral aspect of image
- Minimum SID: 40″ (100 cm)

Evaluation Criteria

- True PA projection of the digit of interest
- No overlapping of adjacent digits
- Symmetry to soft tissue should be evident
- Interphalangeal joints should be open if hand is truly extended
- Optimal exposure factors, demonstrating short-scale contrast

Demonstrates

- Metacarpal phalangeal joint, proximal phalanx, proximal phalangeal joint, middle phalanx, distal interphalangeal joint, and distal phalanx
- Pathologic conditions of the bone

Posteroanterior Oblique Finger

Positioning Criteria

- Patient seated and elbow flexed 90 degrees; shield
- Place 8″ × 10″ (20 × 25 cm) IR crosswise on table
- Pronate hand and extend fingers along a 45-degree wedge, placing digit of interest in a lateral oblique and parallel to IR
- Collimate from mentum to approximately 1″ (2.5 cm) below the jugular notch and to the soft tissue margins laterally
- Alternate medial oblique may be performed for the 2nd digit only in order to reduce OID
- Direct central ray perpendicular to IR and proximal interphalangeal joint
- Finger of interest should be separated from adjacent fingers and aligned with long axis of IR
- Collimate to four sides
- Place appropriate side marker to lateral aspect of image
- Minimum SID: 40″ (100 cm)

Evaluation Criteria

- 45-degree oblique of finger of interest
- Interphalangeal and metacarpophalangeal joints should appear open
- Optimal exposure factors demonstrating short-scale contrast
- No overlapping of adjacent anatomy

Demonstrates

- 45-degree oblique of metacarpal phalangeal joint, proximal phalangeal joint, proximal phalanx, distal interphalangeal joint, and distal phalanx
- Fractures and dislocations of phalanx of interest
- Pathologic conditions of the bone

Lateral Finger

Positioning Criteria

- Patient seated and elbow flexed 90 degrees; full shield
- Place 8″ × 10″ (20 × 25 cm) IR crosswise on table
- Hand extended in true lateral
- Phalanx of interest parallel with long axis of IR
- Direct central ray perpendicular to IR and proximal interphalangeal joint
- Sponge, pencil eraser, or tape may be necessary to extend phalanx of interest and avoid superimposition of adjacent anatomy
- Collimate to four sides
- Place appropriate side marker
- Minimum SID: 40″ (100 cm)

Evaluation Criteria

- True lateral of entire phalanx of interest
- Interphalangeal and metacarpophalangeal joint spaces should be open
- Concave appearance of anterior aspect of the phalanges
- No superimposition of adjacent digits

Demonstrates

- True lateral of metacarpophalangeal joint, proximal phalanx, proximal interphalangeal joint, middle phalanx, distal interphalangeal joint, and distal phalanx
- Fractures and dislocations to phalanx of interest
- Pathologic conditions of bone

Anteroposterior Thumb

Positioning Criteria

- Patient seated facing the radiographic table
- Place 8″ × 10″ (20 × 25 cm) IR crosswise on table
- Rotate entire arm in order to place the posterior aspect of the thumb against the IR and parallel to long axis of the IR
- A PA thumb allows for easier positioning for the patient at the expense of increased OID and should only be performed if necessary
- Digits 2 to 5 should be pulled back in order to avoid superimposition over the 1st digit
- Direct central ray perpendicular to IR and the 1st metacarpophalangeal joint
- Collimate to four sides
- Place appropriate side marker
- Minimum SID: 40″ (100 cm)

Evaluation Criteria

- AP projection of the thumb
- Interphalangeal and metacarpophalangeal joints should be open

- No superimposition of digits 2 to 5
- No rotation; equal amount of soft tissue present

Demonstrates

- True AP of 1st digit, including the trapezium, entire 1st metacarpal, metacarpophalangeal joint, proximal phalanx, interphalangeal joint, and distal phalanx
- Optimal image demonstrating short-scale contrast

Oblique Thumb

Positioning Criteria

- Patient seated and elbow flexed 90 degrees; full shield
- Place 8″ × 10″ (20 × 25 cm) crosswise on table
- Hand pronated; thumb and hand extended
- Digits 2 to 5 spread apart from the thumb
- Long axis of thumb aligned to long axis of IR
- Central ray perpendicular to IR and directed to the 1st metacarpophalangeal joint
- Collimate to four sides
- Place appropriate side marker
- Minimum SID: 40″ (100 cm)

Evaluation Criteria

- 45-degree oblique projection of the thumb
- Interphalangeal and metacarpophalangeal joints should be open
- No superimposition of digits 2 to 5
- No rotation; equal amount of soft tissue present

Demonstrates

- Oblique of 1st digit, including the trapezium, entire 1st metacarpal, metacarpophalangeal joint, proximal phalanx, interphalangeal joint, and distal phalanx
- Fracture, anterior/posterior dislocation
- Pathologic conditions of the bone
- Optimal image demonstrating short-scale contrast

Lateral Thumb

Positioning Criteria

- Patient seated and elbow flexed 90 degrees; full shield
- Place 8″ × 10″ (20 × 25 cm) IR crosswise on table
- From a PA hand position, internally rotate the thumb slightly in order to place it 90 degrees and parallel to the IR
- Keep digits 2 to 5 away from thumb in order to prevent superimposition
- Direct the central ray perpendicular to the IR and to the 1st metacarpophalangeal joint
- Collimate to four sides
- Place appropriate side marker to lateral aspect of image
- Minimum SID: 40″ (100 cm)

Evaluation Criteria

- True lateral of 1st digit
- Interphalangeal and metacarpophalangeal joints should be open
- No superimposition of anatomy
- Concave appearance of anterior aspect of the phalanges

Demonstrates

- True lateral of 1st digit, including the trapezium, entire 1st metacarpal, metacarpophalangeal joint, proximal phalanx, interphalangeal joint, and distal phalanx
- Anterior/posterior displacement or fracture of the thumb
- Pathologic conditions of the bone
- Optimal image demonstrating short-scale contrast

Posteroanterior Hand

Positioning Criteria

- Patient seated and elbow flexed 90 degrees; full shield
- Place 10″ × 12″ (25 × 30 cm) IR crosswise on table; use half of the IR and cover the other half with lead
- Hand extended and pronated; fingers slightly spread apart
- Long axis of hand and wrist parallel to long axis of IR
- Central ray perpendicular to IR and directed to the 3rd metacarpophalangeal joint
- Collimate to four sides
- Place appropriate side marker on lateral aspect
- Minimum SID: 40″ (100 cm)

Evaluation Criteria

- Digits 2 to 5 in PA projection; thumb is obliqued in this view
- Distal phalanges, distal interphalangeal joints, middle phalanges, proximal interphalangeal joint, proximal phalanges, 5 metacarpals, carpals, and 1″ (2.5 cm) of the distal radius and ulna
- Interphalangeal and metacarpophalangeal joints should be open
- No superimposition of digits
- No rotation; equal amount of soft tissue present

Demonstrates

- Entire hand, including distal phalanges, distal interphalangeal joints, middle phalanges, proximal interphalangeal joints, proximal phalanges, 5 metacarpals, carpals, and 1″ (2.5 cm) of the distal radius and ulna
- The base of the 3rd to 5th metacarpals are free of superimposition
- Fracture, anterior/posterior dislocation
- Pathologic conditions of the bone
- Optimal image demonstrating short-scale contrast

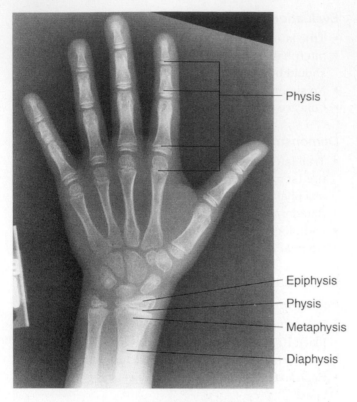

- Physis
- Epiphysis
- Physis
- Metaphysis
- Diaphysis

FIGURE 5-39

- Rotate hand laterally 45 degrees using a sponge to hold hand in place
- All digits should be separated and parallel to IR unless only the metacarpals are of interest, in which case the digits may be slightly bent
- Central ray perpendicular to IR and directed to the 3rd metacarpophalangeal joint
- Collimate to four sides
- Place appropriate side marker on lateral aspect
- Minimum SID: 40″ (100 cm)

Evaluation Criteria

- True 45-degree oblique of hand
- Interphalangeal and metacarpophalangeal joints should be open unless the digits are not parallel to IR
- No superimposition of digits
- The bases of metacarpals 1 and 2 are free of superimposition, and the bases of metacarpals 3 to 5 are superimposed
- Equal amount of soft tissue present

Demonstrates

- Entire hand, including distal phalanges, distal interphalangeal joints, middle phalanges, proximal interphalangeal joints, proximal phalanges, 5 metacarpals, carpals, and 1″ (2.5 cm) of the distal radius and ulna
- Fracture, anterior/posterior dislocation
- Pathologic conditions of the bone
- Optimal image demonstrating short-scale contrast

Posteroanterior Oblique Hand

Positioning Criteria

- Patient seated and elbow flexed 90 degrees; full shield
- Place 10″ × 12″ (25 × 30 cm) IR crosswise on table; use half of the IR and cover the other half with lead

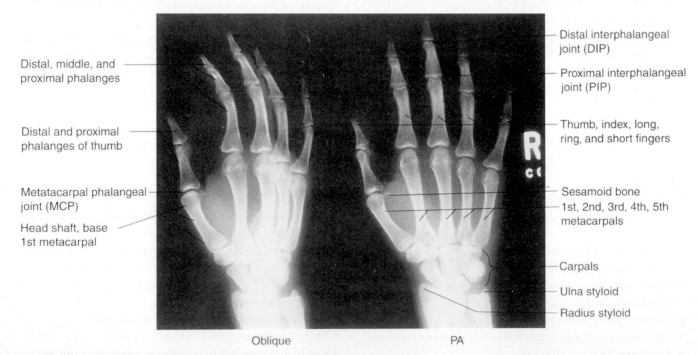

- Distal, middle, and proximal phalanges
- Distal and proximal phalanges of thumb
- Metatacarpal phalangeal joint (MCP)
- Head shaft, base 1st metacarpal

- Distal interphalangeal joint (DIP)
- Proximal interphalangeal joint (PIP)
- Thumb, index, long, ring, and short fingers
- Sesamoid bone
- 1st, 2nd, 3rd, 4th, 5th metacarpals
- Carpals
- Ulna styloid
- Radius styloid

Oblique   PA

FIGURE 5-40

Fan Lateral, Extended Lateral, and Lateral in Partial Flexion

Positioning Criteria

- Patient seated and elbow flexed 90 degrees; full shield
- Place 8″ × 10″ (20 × 25 cm) IR lengthwise on table
- Patient's hand and wrist should be placed in a true lateral, 5th digit down
- Fingers should then be fanned out in order to avoid superimposition of the digits and placed on step wedge sponge
- Digits should be parallel to the IR; metacarpals are in a true lateral
- The central ray is perpendicular to the IR and directed to the 2nd metacarpophalangeal joint
- Collimate to four sides
- Place appropriate side marker on lateral aspect
- Minimum SID: 40″ (100 cm)

Evaluation Criteria

- Fan lateral of hand
- Interphalangeal joints should be free of superimposition; however, metacarpals should be superimposed
- Distal 1″ (2.5 cm) of radius and ulna should be superimposed
- Digits should have equal amount of distance between them
- Equal amount of soft tissue present

Demonstrates

- Lateral of entire hand, including distal phalanges, distal interphalangeal joints, middle phalanges, proximal interphalangeal joints, proximal phalanges, 5 metacarpals, carpals, the thumb in a slight oblique, and 1″ (2.5 cm) of the distal radius and ulna
- Fracture and dislocations of the phalanges
- Anterior/posterior dislocation of the metacarpals
- Pathologic conditions of the bone
- Optimal image demonstrating short-scale contrast

Extension Lateral/Partial Flexion Lateral

Positioning Criteria

- Patient seated and elbow flexed 90 degrees; full shield
- Place 8″ × 10″ (20 × 25 cm) IR lengthwise on table
- Patient's hand and wrist should be placed in a true lateral, 5th digit down
- Fingers and metacarpals should be superimposed and extended, directed parallel to the long axis of the IR
- The partial flexion lateral is used for patients unable to extend hand because of pain, fracture, or surgery
- The central ray is perpendicular to the IR and directed to the 2nd metacarpophalangeal joint

- Collimate to four sides
- Place appropriate side marker on lateral aspect
- Minimum SID: 40″ (100 cm)

Evaluation Criteria for Extension Lateral of Hand

- Superimposition of entire hand and wrist, including phalanges, metacarpals, and carpals
- Distal 1″ (2.5 cm) of radius and ulna should be superimposed

Demonstrates

- Foreign bodies to hand
- Anterior/posterior dislocation of the metacarpals

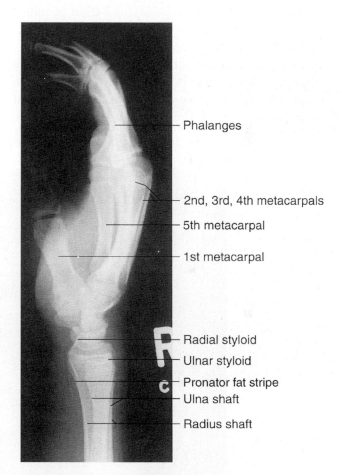

Phalanges

2nd, 3rd, 4th metacarpals

5th metacarpal

1st metacarpal

Radial styloid

Ulnar styloid

Pronator fat stripe

Ulna shaft

Radius shaft

FIGURE 5-41

- Pathologic conditions of the bone
- Optimal image demonstrating short-scale contrast

Posteroanterior Wrist

Positioning Criteria

- Patient seated and elbow flexed 90 degrees; full shield
- Place 10″ × 12″ (25 × 30 cm) IR crosswise on table; use half of the IR and cover the other half with lead

- Hand pronated and fingers clenched, making a fist and bringing the carpals closer to the IR
- The central ray is perpendicular to the IR and directed to the midcarpal area
- Collimate to four sides
- Place appropriate side marker on lateral aspect
- Minimum SID: 40″ (100 cm)

Evaluation Criteria

- True PA of the wrist
- Equal distance evident between the carpals
- Separation of the radius and ulna

Demonstrates

- Metacarpals, carpals, and distal one-third of radius and ulna
- Scaphoid, capitate, hamate free of superimposition
- An AP wrist with a slight arch may be done to place carpals in close contact with the IR to better demonstrate intercarpal spaces and rule out ligament disruption

- Fractures of the carpals, distal radius, ulna, and radial or ulna styloid
- Pathologic conditions of the bone

Posteroanterior Oblique Wrist

Positioning Criteria

- Patient seated and elbow flexed 90 degrees; full shield
- Place 10″ × 12″ (25 × 30 cm) IR crosswise on table; use half of the IR and cover the other half with lead
- Hand pronated, fingers extended and rotated 45 degrees externally, parallel with the long axis of the IR
- The central ray is perpendicular to the IR and directed to the midcarpal area
- Collimate to four sides
- Place appropriate side marker on lateral aspect
- Minimum SID: 40″ (100 cm)

Evaluation Criteria

- 45-degree oblique of the wrist
- Separation of the radius and ulna

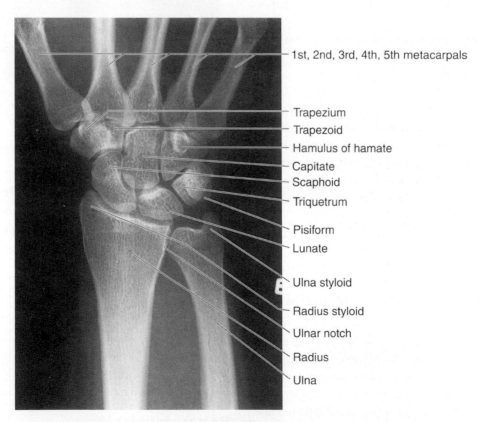

1st, 2nd, 3rd, 4th, 5th metacarpals

Trapezium
Trapezoid
Hamulus of hamate
Capitate
Scaphoid
Triquetrum

Pisiform
Lunate

Ulna styloid

Radius styloid
Ulnar notch
Radius
Ulna

FIGURE 5-42

Demonstrates

- Metacarpals, carpals, and distal one-third of radius and ulna
- Trapezium, scaphoid, and trapezoid are best demonstrated
- Ulnar head is superimposed over the distal radius
- Fractures of the carpals, distal radius, ulna, and radial or ulna styloid
- Pathologic conditions of the bone

Anteroposterior Oblique Wrist

Positioning Criteria

- Patient seated and elbow flexed 90 degrees; full shield
- Place 10″ × 12″ (25 × 30 cm) IR crosswise on table; use half of the IR and cover the other half with lead
- Hand supinated, fingers extended and rotated 45 degrees medially, parallel with the long axis of the IR
- The central ray is perpendicular to the IR and directed to the midcarpal area
- Collimate to four sides
- Place appropriate side marker on lateral aspect
- Minimum SID: 40″ (100 cm)

Evaluation Criteria

- 45-degree oblique of the wrist
- Separation of the radius and ulna

Demonstrates

- Metacarpals, carpals, and distal one-third of radius and ulna
- Triquetrum and pisiform are best demonstrated, free of superimposition
- Ulnar head is superimposed over the distal radius
- Fractures of the carpals, distal radius, ulna, and radial or ulna styloid
- Pathologic conditions of the bone

Lateral Wrist

Positioning Criteria

- Patient seated and elbow flexed 90 degrees; full shield
- Place 8″ × 10″ (20 × 25 cm) IR lengthwise on table
- Hand and wrist extended in a true lateral, ulnar side down
- Hand and wrist parallel with the long axis of the IR
- The central ray is perpendicular to the IR and directed to the midcarpal area
- Collimate to four sides
- Place appropriate side marker
- Minimum SID: 40″ (100 cm)

Evaluation Criteria

- True lateral of wrist
- Centered to IR
- Four-sided collimation

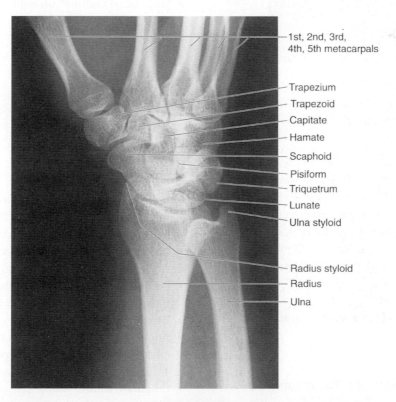

1st, 2nd, 3rd, 4th, 5th metacarpals
Trapezium
Trapezoid
Capitate
Hamate
Scaphoid
Pisiform
Triquetrum
Lunate
Ulna styloid
Radius styloid
Radius
Ulna

FIGURE 5-43

Demonstrates

- Metacarpals, carpals, and distal one-third of radius and ulna superimposed
- Pronator fat pad demonstrated ½″ (1 cm) anteriorly to radius
- Barton, Colles, and Smith fractures
- Anterior/posterior displacement and fractures of the carpals, distal radius, and ulna
- Pathologic conditions of the bone

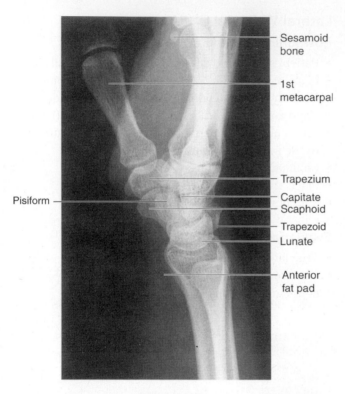

Sesamoid bone

1st metacarpal

Trapezium

Capitate
Scaphoid

Trapezoid

Lunate

Anterior fat pad

Pisiform

FIGURE 5-44

Posteroanterior Scaphoid

Positioning Criteria

- Patient seated and elbow flexed 90 degrees; full shield
- Place 8″ × 10″ (20 × 25 cm) IR lengthwise on table
- Hand and wrist placed PA and deviated toward ulna
- Lateral hand and wrist elevated 20 degrees on a sponge
- Central ray is perpendicular to the IR and directed to the scaphoid, or snuff box, located (2 cm, or ¾ inch, proximal and 2 cm, or ¾ inch lateral to first carpometacarpal joint)[1]
- Collimate to four sides
- Place appropriate side marker on lateral aspect
- Minimum SID: 40″ (100 cm)

Evaluation Criteria

- PA scaphoid demonstrated without superimposition of adjacent carpals

- Scaphoid centered to IR
- Four-sided collimation evident

Demonstrates

- Scaphoid is best demonstrated without superimposition or foreshortening
- Distal radius and ulna
- Lateral carpals and interspaces open
- Best demonstrates fracture of the scaphoid

Posteroanterior Stecher

Positioning Criteria

- Patient seated and elbow flexed 90 degrees; full shield
- Place 8″ × 10″ (20 × 25 cm) IR lengthwise on table
- Hand and wrist placed PA and deviated toward ulna
- Central ray is angled 15 degrees to 20 degrees proximally and directed to the scaphoid, or snuff box, located (2 cm, or ¾ inch, proximal and 2 cm, or ¾ inch lateral to first carpometacarpal joint)[1]
- Collimate to four sides
- Place appropriate side marker on lateral aspect
- Minimum SID: 40″ (100 cm)

Evaluation Criteria

- PA scaphoid demonstrated without superimposition of adjacent carpals
- Scaphoid centered to IR
- Four-sided collimation evident

Demonstrates

- Scaphoid is best demonstrated without superimposition or foreshortening
- Distal radius and ulna
- Lateral carpals and interspaces open
- Best demonstrates fracture of the scaphoid

Carpal Canal

Positioning Criteria

- Patient seated facing the radiographic table; full shield
- Place 8″ × 10″ (20 × 25 cm) IR crosswise on table
- Instruct patient to hyperextend fingers in order to bring metacarpals and digits as vertical as possible, while leaving the carpals and forearm on IR
- Patient may use opposite hand to hold the dorsiflexed fingers of the affected hand in position
- Rotate hand and wrist 10 degrees toward thumb
- Angle central ray 25 degrees to 30 degrees to the long axis of the hand, more if dorsiflexion is minimal, and 1″ (2.5 cm) distal to the base of the 3rd metacarpal
- Collimate to four sides
- Place appropriate side marker on lateral aspect

Evaluation Criteria

- Carpals appear arched
- Collimation visible on four sides
- 10-degree internal rotation evident by hamulus and pisiform free of superimposition

Demonstrates

- Pisiform and hamulus demonstrated in profile
- Demonstrates abnormal calcifications and bony changes in carpal sulcus, causing impingement on median nerve
- Capitate, scaphoid, and trapezium also well demonstrated

Forearm

FOR FOREARM PROJECTIONS, TAKE INTO CONSIDERATION ANODE HEEL EFFECT AND PLACE WRIST UNDER ANODE ASPECT OF X-RAY BEAM.

Positioning Criteria

- Patient seated facing the table and elbow extended; full shield
- Place 14″ × 17″ (35 × 42.5 cm) IR
- Entire forearm to humerus parallel to IR
- Central ray perpendicular to IR and midway between elbow and wrist
- Collimate to lateral margins of forearm and vertically if possible
- Place appropriate side marker on lateral aspect
- Minimum SID: 40″ (100 cm)

Evaluation Criteria

- True AP of forearm
- No superimposition of distal radius and ulna
- Collimation evident

Demonstrates

- AP of radius and ulna
- The distal row of carpal bones
- Superimposition of radial tuberosity over proximal ulna
- Pathology of radius and ulna
- Fractures

Lateral Forearm

Positioning Criteria

- Patient seated and elbow flexed 90 degrees; full shield
- Hand in extension lateral
- Place 10″ × 12″ (25 × 30 cm) IR
- The central ray is perpendicular to the IR and directed to the midshaft of radius and ulna

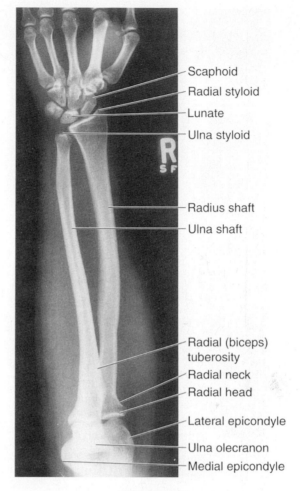

FIGURE 5-45

- Collimate to four sides
- Place appropriate side marker on lateral aspect
- Minimum SID: 40″ (100 cm)

Evaluation Criteria

- True lateral of forearm
- Collimation evident

Demonstrates

- Superimposition of carpals, distal radius, and ulna
- Epicondyles of the humerus should be superimposed and perpendicular to the table
- The radial head will slightly superimpose over the ulna
- Pathologies of the forearm

Elbow

FOR ELBOW PROJECTIONS, TAKE INTO CONSIDERATION ANODE HEEL EFFECT AND PLACE WRIST UNDER ANODE ASPECT OF X-RAY BEAM.

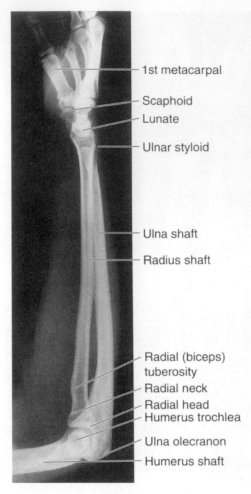

1st metacarpal
Scaphoid
Lunate
Ulnar styloid

Ulna shaft
Radius shaft

Radial (biceps) tuberosity
Radial neck
Radial head
Humerus trochlea
Ulna olecranon
Humerus shaft

FIGURE 5-46

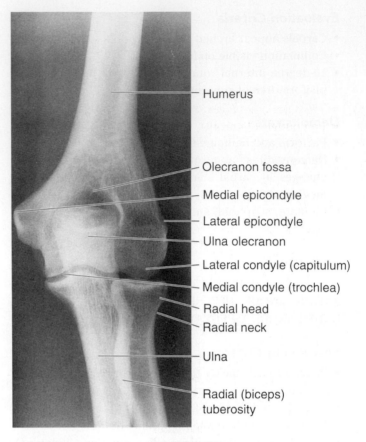

Humerus

Olecranon fossa
Medial epicondyle
Lateral epicondyle
Ulna olecranon
Lateral condyle (capitulum)
Medial condyle (trochlea)
Radial head
Radial neck
Ulna
Radial (biceps) tuberosity

FIGURE 5-47

Positioning Criteria

- Patient seated facing the table and elbow extended; full shield
- Place 10″ × 12″ (25 × 30 cm) IR
- Entire forearm to proximal humerus parallel to IR
- Central ray perpendicular to IR, midway between humeral epicondyles, and ¾″ to 1″ (2 to 2.5 cm) distal to the epicondyles
- Collimate to lateral margins of elbow
- Place appropriate side marker on lateral aspect
- Minimum SID: 40″ (100 cm)

Evaluation Criteria

- True AP of elbow
- Four-sided collimation evident

Demonstrates

- AP of elbow
- Radial tuberosity superimposed over ulna
- Pathology

- Fractures
- Dislocations

Anteroposterior Partial Flexion Elbow

This view is necessary in a trauma situation in which the patient is unable to fully extend the elbow. The patient would be instructed to extend the elbow as much as possible. The first view would be with the forearm parallel or against the IR, and the second view would be with the humerus parallel to the IR.

Positioning Criteria

- Patient seated facing the table and elbow extended in this case as much as possible; full shield
- Place 10″ × 12″ (25 × 30 cm) IR
- First image: entire forearm parallel to the IR
- Second image: humerus parallel to IR
- Central ray perpendicular to IR, midway between humeral epicondyles, and ¾″ to 1″ (2 to 2.5 cm) distal to the epicondyles
- Collimate to lateral margins of elbow
- Place appropriate side marker on lateral aspect
- Minimum SID: 40″ (100 cm)

Evaluation Criteria

- AP of elbow
- Four-sided collimation evident

Demonstrates

- AP of proximal forearm and distal humerus
- Epicondyles in profile
- Radial tuberosity superimposed over ulna
- Pathology
- Fracture
- Dislocations

Internal Oblique Elbow

Positioning Criteria

- Patient seated facing the table and elbow extended; full shield
- Place 10″ × 12″ (25 × 30 cm) IR
- From the true AP elbow position, roll forearm internally and pronate hand
- Central ray perpendicular to IR, midway between humeral epicondyles, and ¾″ to 1″ (2 to 2.5 cm) distal to the epicondyles
- Collimate to lateral margins of elbow
- Place appropriate side marker on lateral aspect
- Minimum SID: 40″ (100 cm)

Evaluation Criteria

- 45-degree internal oblique of elbow
- Four-sided collimation evident
- Long axis of forearm and humerus parallel to IR

Demonstrates

- Coronoid process best demonstrated
- Radial head and neck superimposed over ulna
- Medial epicondyle and trochlea partially in profile
- Trochlea notch partially open
- Olecranon situated in olecranon fossa
- Pathology
- Fractures

External Oblique Elbow

Positioning Criteria

- Patient seated facing the table and elbow extended; full shield
- Place 10″ × 12″ (25 × 30 cm) IR
- From the true AP elbow position, roll forearm externally 45 degrees
- Central ray perpendicular to IR, midway between humeral epicondyles, and ¾″ to 1″ (2 to 2.5 cm) distal to the epicondyles

- Collimate to lateral margins of elbow
- Place appropriate side marker on lateral aspect
- Minimum SID: 40″ (100 cm)

Evaluation Criteria

- 45-degree external oblique of elbow
- Four-sided collimation evident
- Long axis of forearm and humerus parallel to IR

Demonstrates

- Radial head, neck, and tuberosity free of superimposition
- Lateral epicondyle and capitulum in profile
- Pathology
- Fractures

Lateral Elbow

Positioning Criteria

- Patient seated and elbow flexed 90 degrees; full shield
- Hand in extension lateral
- Place 10″ × 12″ (25 × 30 cm) IR
- The central ray is perpendicular to the IR and directed approximately ½″ (1 cm) medial to olecranon
- Collimate to four sides
- Place appropriate side marker on lateral aspect
- Minimum SID: 40″ (100 cm)

Evaluation Criteria

- True lateral of elbow
- Four-sided collimation evident
- Include approximately 2″ (5 cm) of distal humerus and proximal radius/ulna

Demonstrates

- Three arcs of elbow: arc of capitulum/trochlea, trochlear notch, and trochlear sulcus
- Anterior fat pad
- Visibility of posterior fat pad on true lateral indicates pathology to elbow joint
- Supinator fat pad indicator of radial head fractures
- Superimposition of carpals, distal radius, and ulna
- Epicondyles of the humerus should be superimposed and perpendicular to the table
- The radial head will slightly superimpose over the ulna
- Pathologies of the forearm
- Anterior/posterior dislocations

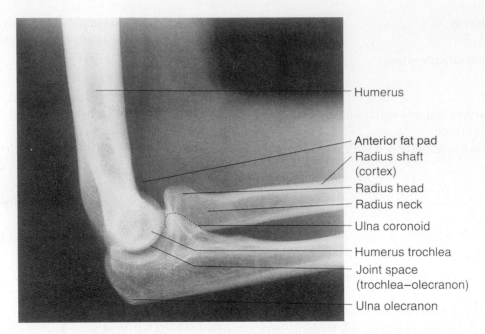

Humerus

Anterior fat pad
Radius shaft
(cortex)
Radius head
Radius neck
Ulna coronoid
Humerus trochlea
Joint space
(trochlea–olecranon)
Ulna olecranon

FIGURE 5-48

Axial Trauma (Coyle of Elbow)

IN A TRAUMA SITUATION IN WHICH A PATIENT IS UNABLE TO OBLIQUE THE ARM, TWO AXIAL VIEWS MAY BE PERFORMED WITH THE PATIENT MAINTAINING THE COMMON TRAUMA POSITIONING OF FLEXION AT THE ELBOW.

Positioning Criteria

- Patient seated and elbow flexed 90 degrees; full shield
- Hand pronated
- Place 10″ × 12″ (25 × 30 cm) IR
- First image: central ray angled 45 degrees proximally or toward the shoulder
- Second image: central ray directed to radial head, or approximately ½″ (1 cm) medial and distal to olecranon
- Collimate to four sides
- Place appropriate side marker on lateral aspect
- Minimum SID: 40″ (100 cm)

Evaluation Criteria

- Axial lateral of elbow
- Four-sided collimation evident
- Include approximately 2″ (5 cm) of distal humerus and proximal radius/ulna

Demonstrates

- Radial neck and tuberosity free of superimposition from ulna and in profile
- Majority of radial head free from superimposition except for slight coronoid superimposition

- Radial head and capitulum joint space open
- Distortion to epicondyles due to angle on tube
- Pathologies and fractures of the elbow, especially to radial head, neck, and tuberosity

Coyle for Coronoid

Positioning Criteria

- Patient seated and elbow flexed 80 degrees; full shield
- Hand pronated
- Place 10″ × 12″ (25 × 30 cm) IR
- Central ray angled 45 degrees distally or away from shoulder
- Central ray directed approximately ½″ (1 cm) medial and proximal to olecranon
- Collimate to four sides
- Place appropriate side marker on lateral aspect
- Minimum SID: 40″ (100 cm)

Evaluation Criteria

- Axial lateral of elbow
- 80 degrees flexion of elbow in order for coronoid to be demonstrated
- Four-sided collimation evident
- Include approximately 2″ (5 cm) of distal humerus and proximal radius/ulna

Demonstrates

- Distal coronoid elongated and in profile
- Coronoid and trochlea joint space open
- Radial head and neck superimposed over ulna
- Fractures and pathology especially to coronoid process

Humerus (Nontrauma)
Anteroposterior
Positioning Criteria

- Patient supine or erect AP
- 14″ × 17″ (35 × 42.5 cm) IR lengthwise
- Central ray to midpoint of humerus
- Hand supinated
- Collimate to four sides, including pertinent anatomy
- Correct marker on lateral aspect of anatomy
- Minimum SID: 40″ (100 cm)

Evaluation Criteria

- True AP of humerus
- Shoulder to elbow joint visible
- Optimal exposure factors

Demonstrates

- Greater tuberosity in profile laterally
- Shoulder down to elbow
- Medial aspect of humeral head in profile partially
- Medial aspect of humeral head slightly superimposed by glenoid cavity
- Epicondyles of distal humerus parallel to IR and in profile
- Fractures and pathology of humerus

Lateral Humerus (Nontrauma)
Positioning Criteria

- Patient supine or erect AP; gonad region shielded
- 14″ × 17″ (35 × 42.5 cm) IR lengthwise
- Internally rotate (mediolateral) arm and pronate hand
- Central ray to midpoint of humerus
- Second option (lateromedial) will decrease gonadal dose: patient PA, elbow flexed 90 degrees
- Oblique patient enough to bring humerus against IR
- Collimate to four sides, including pertinent anatomy
- Correct marker on lateral aspect of anatomy
- Minimum SID: 40″ (100 cm)

Evaluation Criteria

- True lateral of humerus
- Shoulder to elbow joint visible
- Optimal exposure factors

Demonstrates

- Lesser tuberosity in profile medially
- Slight superimposition of glenoid cavity over lesser tuberosity
- Epicondyles of distal humerus perpendicular to IR
- Fractures and pathology of humerus

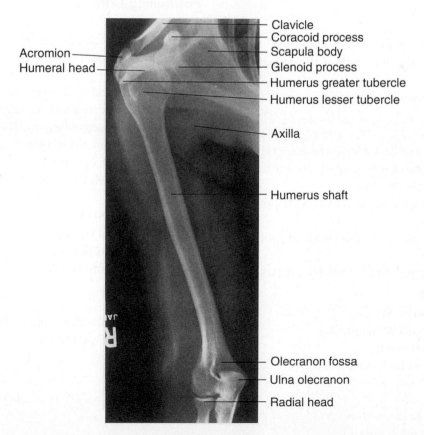

Acromion
Humeral head

Clavicle
Coracoid process
Scapula body
Glenoid process
Humerus greater tubercle
Humerus lesser tubercle

Axilla

Humerus shaft

Olecranon fossa
Ulna olecranon
Radial head

FIGURE 5-49

Anteroposterior Neutral Trauma Humerus

The AP neutral trauma may be performed when the patient is unable to supinate hand and rotate humerus in order to get true AP projection. Patient may be supine, with IR placed carefully under the humerus. Adjust the patient's humerus in order to get the truest AP possible. All other instructions remain the same as the nontrauma AP humerus.

Scapula Y Trauma Proximal Humerus (Anteroposterior and Posteroanterior)

Positioning Criteria

- Patient supine or erect, AP or PA, with a gonad shield
- 10″ × 12″ (25 × 30 cm) IR lengthwise
- AP: patient obliqued approximately 60 degrees away from affected shoulder
- PA: patient obliqued toward affected humerus, approximately 30 degrees to 40 degrees
- Palpating the acromial tip and superior border of scapula will help determine the proper amount of obliquity necessary for each patient
- Central ray directed to midscapula
- Collimate to four sides, including pertinent anatomy
- Correct marker on lateral aspect of anatomy
- Minimum SID: 40″ (100 cm)

Evaluation Criteria

- Lateral of proximal humerus
- Shoulder joint down to as much of the humerus as possible
- Optimal exposure factors

Demonstrates

- Done for fractures and dislocations of humeral head
- Humeral head will be demonstrated inferior to coracoid with anterior dislocation
- Humeral head superior to acromion with posterior dislocations
- Demonstrates scapula spine and coracoid process

Transthoracic Lateral Proximal Humerus

Positioning Criteria

- Patient supine or erect AP
- 10″ × 12″ (25 × 30 cm) IR lengthwise
- Affected side against the IR
- Raise unaffected arm up toward head

- A 10-degree to 15-degree cephalic angle may be used if patient is unable to extend unaffected arm up
- Central ray directed to surgical neck and through midaxillary
- Collimate to four sides, including pertinent anatomy
- Correct marker on lateral aspect of anatomy
- Autotomography to blur out lung and vascular markings
- Minimum SID: 40″ (100 cm)

Evaluation Criteria

- Lateral of proximal humerus and glenohumeral joint
- Shoulder joint down to as much of the humerus as possible
- Optimal exposure factors

Demonstrates

- Proximal humerus and glenohumeral joint free of superimposition from opposite shoulder
- Done for fractures and dislocations of humeral head
- Humerus visualized anterior to thoracic cavity and free from vascular markings

Lateral Trauma Midhumerus to Distal Humerus

Positioning Criteria

- Patient supine
- 10″ × 12″ (25 × 30 cm) or 14″ × 17″ (35 × 42.5 cm) IR lengthwise, patient shielded
- Build up humerus slightly, and place the IR between the patient's body and humerus
- Central ray directed horizontally and to the midpoint of distal two-thirds of the humerus
- Collimate to four sides, including pertinent anatomy
- Correct marker on lateral aspect of anatomy
- Minimum SID: 40″ (100 cm)

Evaluation Criteria

- Lateral of distal humerus
- Elbow joint to as much of the humerus as possible
- Optimal exposure factors

Demonstrates

- Fractures and dislocations of distal humerus
- Epicondyles perpendicular to IR
- Pathology

SHOULDER

Anteroposterior Neutral Shoulder

Positioning Criteria

- Patient supine or erect, AP, and shielded
- 10″ × 12″ (25 × 30 cm) IR crosswise
- Patient's arm in neutral position
- Central ray directed 1″ (2.5 cm) inferior to coracoid, or approximately 1½″ (4 cm) inferior to clavicle and midway between the humerus and sternum
- Hand neutral
- Collimate to four sides, including pertinent anatomy
- Correct marker on lateral aspect of anatomy
- Minimum SID: 40″ (100 cm)

Evaluation Criteria

- Oblique of humerus
- Sternoclavicular joint to humerus
- Clavicle to upper scapula
- Scapulohumeral joint centered
- Optimal exposure factors

Demonstrates

- Greater and lesser tubercles superimposed by humeral head
- Oblique of humerus
- Epicondyles 45 degrees to IR
- Calcium deposits
- Bony pathologies
- Fractures and dislocations of proximal humerus

Internal Shoulder

Positioning Criteria

- Patient supine or erect, AP, and shielded
- 10″ × 12″ (25 × 30 cm) IR crosswise
- Instruct patient to rotate entire arm internally
- Central ray directed 1″ (2.5 cm) inferior to coracoid, or approximately 1½″ (4 cm) inferior to clavicle and midway between the humerus and sternum
- Hand supinated
- Collimate to four sides, including pertinent anatomy
- Correct marker on lateral aspect of anatomy
- Minimum SID: 40″ (100 cm)

Evaluation Criteria

- True lateral of humerus
- Sternoclavicular joint to humerus
- Clavicle to upper scapula
- Scapulohumeral joint centered
- Optimal exposure factors

Demonstrates

- Lesser tubercle moves inferomedial and into profile
- Brings the humerus into a true lateral
- Epicondyles perpendicular to IR
- Bursitis, tendonitis, and Hill-Sachs defect
- Fractures and dislocations of proximal humerus

External Shoulder

Positioning Criteria

- Patient supine or erect, AP, and shielded
- 10″ × 12″ (25 × 30 cm) IR crosswise
- Instruct patient to rotate entire arm externally
- Central ray directed 1″ (2.5 cm) inferior to coracoid, or approximately 1½″ (4 cm) inferior to clavicle and midway between the humerus and sternum
- Hand pronated
- Collimate to four sides, including pertinent anatomy
- Correct marker on lateral aspect of anatomy
- Minimum SID: 40″ (100 cm)

Evaluation Criteria

- True AP of humerus
- Sternoclavicular joint to humerus
- Clavicle to upper scapula
- Scapulohumeral joint centered
- Optimal exposure factors

Demonstrates

- Moves greater tubercle superolateral and into profile
- True AP of humerus
- Epicondyles parallel to IR
- Bankart lesions
- Fractures and dislocations of proximal humerus

Inferosuperior Axial, Nontrauma Shoulder

Positioning Criteria

- Patient supine and shoulder propped up on a sponge
- Instruct patient to turn head toward unaffected aspect of body; shield patient
- 10″ × 12″ (25 × 30 cm) IR crosswise, placed posterior to affected shoulder and as close to neck as possible
- Arm abducted 90 degrees and externally rotated
- Central ray directed medially 15 degrees to 20 degrees and centered horizontally to axilla and humeral head
- Collimate to four sides, including pertinent anatomy
- Correct marker on lateral aspect of anatomy
- Minimum SID: 40″ (100 cm)

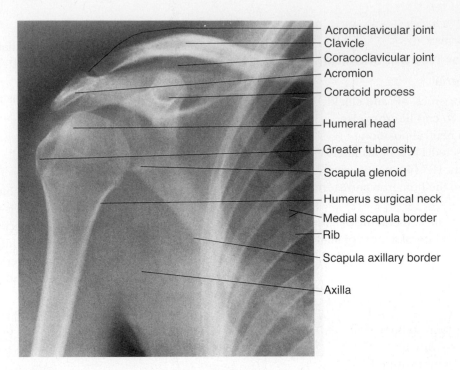

Acromiclavicular joint
Clavicle
Coracoclavicular joint
Acromion
Coracoid process
Humeral head
Greater tuberosity
Scapula glenoid
Humerus surgical neck
Medial scapula border
Rib
Scapula axillary border
Axilla

FIGURE 5-50

Evaluation Criteria

- Arm abducted 90 degrees
- Lateral view of proximal humerus
- Superior and inferior glenoid cavity borders superimposed
- Clavicle to humerus included

Demonstrates

- Orthopedic physicians preferred method for lateral view of head and neck of humerus
- Demonstrates scapulohumeral joint
- Coracoid and lesser tuberosity in profile
- Scapula spine below scapulohumeral joint
- Osteoporosis, osteoarthritis, and, with exaggerated external rotation, Hill-Sachs defect
- Fractures and dislocations

Posterior Oblique, Grashey

Positioning Criteria

- Patient supine or erect and shielded
- 10″ × 12″ (25 × 30 cm) IR crosswise
- Patient AP and obliqued toward affected side 35 degrees to 45 degrees
- Central ray perpendicular to glenohumeral joint, 2″ (5 cm) medial and inferior to superior and lateral shoulder border
- Arm neutral
- Collimate to four sides, including pertinent anatomy
- Minimum SID: 40″ (100 cm)

Evaluation Criteria

- Scapulohumeral (glenohumeral) joint open and centered to the image

Demonstrates

- Shows glenoid in profile and glenohumeral interspace open
- Orthopedic physicians preferred method for lateral view of head and neck of humerus
- Fracture of proximal humerus and glenoid labrum
- Bankart lesions
- Erosion to rim of glenohumeral joint
- Pathology to scapulohumeral joint

Tangential Nontrauma

Positioning Criteria

- Method one: patient supine
  Instruct patient to turn head toward unaffected aspect of body
  10″ × 12″ (25 × 30 cm) IR crosswise, placed posterior to affected shoulder and as close to neck as possible
  Arm extended and close to body
  Central ray 10 degrees to 15 degrees posterior from horizontal and directed to intertubercular groove
- Method two: patient erect, leaning over IR
  IR placed over forearm and held in place by patient's supinated hand

Instruct patient to lean shoulder forward so humerus is 10 degrees to 15 degrees from vertical

Central ray perpendicular to IR and directed to bicipital (intertubercular) groove

- Collimate to four sides, including pertinent anatomy
- Correct marker on lateral aspect of anatomy
- Shield patient
- Minimum SID: 40″ (100 cm)
- Respiration suspended

Evaluation Criteria

- Humeral head, bicipital groove, and tuberosities visualized
- Close collimation

Demonstrates

- Humeral head, bicipital groove, greater and lesser tuberosity in profile
- No superimposition of the acromion
- Pathology within bicipital groove

Scapula Y Shoulder

Positioning Criteria

- Patient supine or erect, AP or PA
- 10″ × 12″ (25 × 30 cm) IR lengthwise
- AP: patient obliqued approximately 60 degrees away from affected shoulder
- PA: patient obliqued toward affected humerus, approximately 30 degrees to 40 degrees
- Palpating the acromial tip and superior border of scapula will help determine the proper amount of obliquity necessary for each patient
- Central ray directed to midscapula
- Collimate to four sides, including pertinent anatomy
- Correct marker on lateral aspect of anatomy
- Shield patient
- Minimum SID: 40″ (100 cm)

Evaluation Criteria

- Lateral of proximal humerus and scapula
- Scapulohumeral joint
- Shoulder joint down to as much of the humerus as possible
- Optimal exposure factors

Demonstrates

- True lateral of scapula and humerus
- Done for fractures and dislocations
- Scapula body on end, without rib superimposition
- Acromion and coracoid
- Humeral head superimposed over body of scapula

- Humeral head will be demonstrated inferior to coracoid with anterior dislocation
- Humeral head superior to acromion with posterior dislocations

Transthoracic Lateral Shoulder Trauma

Positioning Criteria

- Patient supine or erect, AP, and shielded
- 10″ × 12″ (25 × 30 cm) IR lengthwise
- Affected side against the IR
- Raise unaffected arm up toward head
- A 10-degree to 15-degree cephalic angle may be used if patient is unable to extend unaffected arm up
- Central ray directed to surgical neck and through midaxillary
- Collimate to four sides, including pertinent anatomy
- Correct marker on lateral aspect of anatomy
- Autotomography to blur out lung and vascular markings
- Minimum SID: 40″ (100 cm)

Evaluation Criteria

- Lateral of proximal humerus and glenohumeral joint
- Shoulder joint down to as much of the humerus as possible
- Optimal exposure factors

Demonstrates

- Proximal humerus and glenohumeral joint free of superimposition from opposite shoulder
- Done for fractures and dislocations of humeral head
- Humerus visualized anterior to thoracic cavity and free from vascular markings

Anteroposterior Scapula

Positioning Criteria

- Patient supine or erect, AP, and shielded
- 10″ × 12″ (25 × 30 cm) IR lengthwise
- Affected arm is abducted 90 degrees with hand in supination
- Central ray directed perpendicular to IR, 2″ (5 cm) medial to axilla, and 2″ (5 cm) inferior to coracoid
- Use autotomography or full exhalation to improve visibility of scapula
- Collimate to four sides, including pertinent anatomy
- Correct marker on lateral aspect of anatomy
- Minimum SID: 40″ (100 cm)

Evaluation Criteria

- AP of scapula
- Superior to inferior border of scapula visualized
- Optimal exposure factors

Demonstrates

- Entire scapula demonstrated
- Lateral border of scapula free of ribs and lungs
- Medial aspect through thoracic structures
- Fractures of scapula

Lateral Scapula Anterior/Posterior Oblique

Positioning Criteria

- Patient supine or erect, AP or PA, and shielded
- 10″ × 12″ (25 × 30 cm) IR lengthwise
- AP: patient obliqued approximately 60 degrees away from affected shoulder
- PA: patient obliqued toward affected humerus, approximately 30 degrees to 45 degrees from lateral position
- Palpate medial and lateral border of scapula and rotate patient until scapular body is perpendicular to the IR
- Central ray directed to midscapula lateral border
- Affected arm brought across chest with hand resting on unaffected shoulder
- Alternative method: Bend elbow of affected side and rest forearm across lower back
- Collimate to four sides, including pertinent anatomy
- Correct marker on lateral aspect of anatomy
- Suspend respiration

Evaluation Criteria

- Lateral of scapula
- Ribs should not superimpose over the scapula
- Optimal exposure factors

Demonstrates

- True lateral of scapula evident by superimposition of vertebral and lateral borders
- Scapular body in profile
- When affected arm brought over chest, the scapular body is best demonstrated
- When affected arm is bent behind back, the acromion and coracoid are demonstrated
- Fractures and dislocations
- Scapula body on end, without rib superimposition
- Humeral head will be demonstrated inferior to coracoid with anterior dislocation
- Humeral head superior to acromion, with posterior dislocations
- Done for fractures and anterior/posterior dislocations

Clavicle Anteroposterior/Posteroanterior

Positioning Criteria

- Patient AP, arm in neutral position; shield patient
- 10″ × 12″ (25 × 30 cm) IR crosswise

- Central ray perpendicular to midclavicle
- PA: Everything remains the same; however, finding the midshaft of the clavicle is difficult PA
- Palpate the vertebral prominence and center 2″ (5 cm) inferior, midway between the vertebrae and humerus
- Collimate to four sides, including pertinent anatomy
- Correct marker on lateral aspect of anatomy
- Autotomography to blur out lung and vascular markings
- Minimum SID: 40″ (100 cm)
- Respiration: inhalation elevates clavicles

Evaluation Criteria

- Optimal exposure

Demonstrates

- Visualization of clavicle, sternoclavicular joint, and acromioclavicular joint
- Clavicle will be superimposed over superior ribs
- PA brings clavicle closer to IR and reduces gonadal dose
- Fracture

Anteroposterior Axial

Positioning Criteria

- Patient AP, arm in neutral position, and shielded
- 10″ × 12″ (25 × 30 cm) IR crosswise
- Central ray angled 15 degrees to 30 degrees cephalic to midclavicle and slightly inferior to clavicle
- Collimate to four sides, including pertinent anatomy
- Correct marker on lateral aspect of anatomy
- Autotomography to blur out lung and vascular markings
- Minimum SID: 40″ (100 cm)
- Respiration: inhalation elevates clavicles

Evaluation Criteria

- Optimal exposure

Demonstrates

- Visualization of clavicle, sternoclavicular joint, and acromioclavicular joint
- Clavicle will not be superimposed over ribs
- Fracture/pathology

Posteroanterior Axial

Positioning Criteria

- Patient PA, arm in neutral position, and shielded
- 10″ × 12″ (25 × 30 cm) IR crosswise
- Central ray directed to midclavicle, angled 15 degrees to 30 degrees caudal and slightly superior from PA clavicle
- Collimate to four sides, including pertinent anatomy

- Correct marker on lateral aspect of anatomy
- Minimum SID: 40″ (100 cm)
- Respiration: inhalation elevates clavicles

Evaluation Criteria

- Optimal exposure

Demonstrates

- Visualization of clavicle, sternoclavicular joint, and acromioclavicular joint
- Clavicle free of superimposition from scapula and ribs
- PA will reduce patient dose
- Fractures/pathology

Acromioclavicular Joints

Positioning Criteria

- Patient PA, arm in neutral position, and shielded
- 14″ × 17″ (35 × 42.5 cm) IR crosswise
- Central ray perpendicular to sternum at the level of the acromioclavicular joint
- Collimate to four sides, including pertinent anatomy
- Correct markers on lateral aspects of anatomy
- Minimum SID: 72″ (180 cm)
- Suspend respiration

Evaluation Criteria

- Optimal exposure
- Marker indicating without weights

Demonstrates

- Visualization of clavicle, sternoclavicular joint, and acromioclavicular joint
- PA brings clavicle closer to IR and reduces gonadal dose
- Done to demonstrate separation/dislocation of the acromioclavicular joint
- Evidenced by widening of the joint of one side versus the other

Acromioclavicular Joints with Weights

Everything remains the same except the patient is instructed to hold a set of 8- to 10-pound weights around the wrists.

Student should note, hypersthenic patients may not allow imaging of both acromioclavicular joints on one 14″ × 17″ (35 × 42.5 cm) IR, so a 10″ × 12″ (25 × 30 cm) IR on each acromioclavicular joint may be necessary.

Bone Survey

Bone surveys are performed in order to demonstrate fractures and metastasis. They are usually performed in conjunction with nuclear medicine. The following images are performed in a bone survey study, and all criteria listed previously in this review apply to the list of positions below:

AP and lateral images of: skull, humerus, forearm, T-spine, lateral spine, proximal and distal femur, tibia, and fibula.

Imaging of the ribs is also frequently included.

Long Bone Measurement (Orthoroentgenography)

Positioning Criteria

- The central ray is placed directly over the joint rather than allowing a divergent when trying to fit the entire length of a femur, for example

Lower Limb Measurement

- A Bell-Thompson ruler is used to measure limb length
- AP hip: central ray directed to femoral neck; collimate in close; ruler placed high enough to incorporate calibrated readings throughout the exposures
- AP knee: central ray directed to knee joint; close collimation and ruler measurement evident on image
- AP ankle: central ray midway between malleoli; close collimation and ruler measurement evident on image

Upper Limb Measurements

- AP shoulder: central ray to midshoulder; tight collimation; ruler measurement evident on image
- AP elbow: central ray to midelbow joint
- AP wrist: central ray to midrise

Evaluation Criteria

- All images must include close collimation and the calibrated ruler measurement

Demonstrates

- Limb length discrepancies

Bone Age

Bone age studies are performed to measure the epiphysis of a pediatric patient's hand in order to determine growth and development·

Soft Tissue/Foreign Body

Soft tissue/foreign body techniques with analogue imaging are performed by halving the milliamperes per second (mA/s), allowing better visualization of the soft tissue, rather than bone.

Computed and digital radiography allow the manipulation of window width in order to demonstrate soft tissue techniques.

Arthrography

Arthrography is imaging of synovial joints and soft tissue structures. Contrast media are injected into the joint space with the use of fluoroscopy or computed tomography, and then overhead images are taken, or cross-sectional images with magnetic resonance. The knee and shoulder are the most frequent arthrograms performed.

- A sterile tray will be set for the radiologist or radiology assistant
- A scout image is normally necessary
- The area will be treated with lidocaine in order to help numb the area
- The radiologist will locate the joint space under fluoroscopy or computed tomography
- Once the joint space is located, contrast media will be injected
- The doctor will manipulate the joint and take overheads or will send the patient to MRI

- The technologist should be available to assist the radiologist as well as to comfort the patient

Myelography

Myelography is the study of the spinal canal through injection of contract media into the subarachnoid space.

Pathologic Conditions

- Lesions
- Cancer
- Herniated nucleus pulposus (HNP)
- Benign tumors and cysts

Contraindications

- Blood in the cerebrospinal fluid
- Inflammation of the arachnoid membrane (arachnoiditis)
- Increased intracranial pressure
- Recent lumbar puncture, within 2 weeks

REVIEW QUESTIONS

1. The PA projection of the chest is preferred to an AP because:

    a. The heart shadow is magnified
    b. Maximum engorgement of the aorta is obtained
    c. Maximum aeration of the lungs is obtained
    d. There is minimal cardiac magnification

2. A requisition is received for a three-way abdomen series. The patient arrives in a wheelchair and is able to stand. In what order should the procedure be performed?

    a. Chest—upright abdomen—supine abdomen
    b. Upright abdomen—supine abdomen—chest
    c. Supine abdomen—chest—upright abdomen
    d. Left lateral decubitus—chest—supine abdomen

3. The trochlear process of the elbow would be best demonstrated in which projection?

    a. Lateral
    b. Lateral oblique
    c. Medial oblique
    d. AP

4. Which oblique is appropriate in order to demonstrate the entire mortise joint open?

    a. 30-degree internal oblique
    b. 45-degree internal oblique
    c. 15-degree to 20-degree internal rotation
    d. 5-degree internal oblique

5. Would the neck-shaft angle (femur) increase or decrease on a short adult?

    a. Decrease
    b. Increase
    c. The height of a patient will not matter
    d. All of the answers are correct

6. What should be done to place the femoral neck parallel for a true AP hip?
    a. Externally rotate the leg
    b. Internally rotate the entire leg
    c. The neck is naturally parallel
    d. Rotate the leg and angle to tube

7. What is the significance of a 45-degree oblique position for a cervical spine examination?

    a. The 45-degree oblique opens the pedicle
    b. There is no significance to a 45-degree oblique
    c. The 45-degree oblique demonstrates the zygapophyseal joints
    d. The 45-degree oblique allows the intervertebral foramina to open

8. When performing an oblique of the T-spine, what anatomy is best demonstrated?

    a. Zygapophyseal joints
    b. Intervertebral foramina
    c. Pars
    d. Pedicles

9. What images would assess the mobility of the lumbar spine?

   a. AP
   b. Axial
   c. Flexion/extension laterals
   d. Obliques

10. When performing a PA Caldwell view, what would be the correct central ray orientation, in order to demonstrate the petrous ridges below the orbital floor?

    a. 25-degree cephalic angle
    b. 15-degree cephalic angle
    c. No angle is necessary
    d. 30-degree caudal angle exiting the nasion

11. What position would demonstrate the stomach free of superimposition from the spine and the body air filled?

    a. RAO
    b. LPO
    c. AP
    d. LAO

12. What position would best demonstrate the splenic flexure?

    a. LPO
    b. RPO
    c. AP axial
    d. PA axial

13. An RPO position would best demonstrate what anatomy?

    a. Left kidney and right ureter
    b. Right kidney and left ureter
    c. Right kidney only
    d. Left kidney only

14. How would a technologist know when an SBS is complete?

    a. Barium fills the duodenum
    b. Barium fills the jejunum
    c. Barium fills the ileocecal valve
    d. Barium fills the ileum

15. What position would best demonstrate the esophagus between the heart and spine?

    a. PA
    b. LPO
    c. AP
    d. RAO

REFERENCE

1. Bontrager KL, Lampignano JP. *Textbook of Radiographic Positioning and Related Anatomy.* 7th ed. St. Louis, MO: Mosby; 2010.

CHAPTER 6

Patient Care and Education

The Patient Care and Education portion of the ARRT Examination in Radiography comprises 15% or 30 total questions on the examination. The content specifications for this examination category include seven sections:

1. Ethical and Legal Aspects
2. Interpersonal Communication
3. Infection Control
4. Physical Assistance and Transfer
5. Medical Emergencies
6. Pharmacology
7. Contrast Media

ETHICAL AND LEGAL ASPECTS

This section of the Patient Care and Education portion of the ARRT examination consists of four total questions.

Patient's Rights

Informed Consent

Informed consent is required for any procedure that is either experimental or has substantial risk involved. Consent to perform a medical procedure can be granted by one of the following methods: written consent, oral consent, or implied consent. Oral consent is also termed *verbal consent*; this is the most difficult method for which to prove consent was granted. Implied consent is given during emergent situations when the patient is unable to provide consent. Written consent is the preferred method of providing consent. For a consent form to be legal, the following elements must be included[1]:

- Full explanation of the procedure
- Risks of the procedure
- Benefits of the procedure
- Alternates to the procedure
- Date of the procedure
- Facility name

- Physician performing the procedure
- Witness signature
- Physician signature, patient signature (patient's guardian's signature)

Any patient over the age of 18 years and competent to make decisions must sign the form. A minor or a patient not legally competent can have a parent, legal guardian, or health-care proxy sign the form. A patient who does not speak or understand English must be provided with a medically trained interpreter.[2] Consent for the performance of a procedure is not transferrable; the procedure can be performed only by the physician stated. All conditions of the consent form must be met at the time of the procedure.

Confidentiality

The Health Insurance Portability and Accountability Act (HIPAA) protects the release of protected health information (PHI) without the patient's written consent. HIPAA also standardizes how electronic data is shared. HIPAA requires that all of the following be met[1,3]:

- Written explanation of how provider uses PHI
- Patients must be permitted to see, copy, and request amendments to their medical records
- Provider must provide history of routine disclosures of PHI upon request
- Patient must give consent before PHI related to treatment, payment, or health-care operations is shared
- Documents with patient names cannot be in public areas
- Access to PHI is restricted to trained HIPAA compliance officer for the facility
- All computer files must be encrypted and computer access secured

Patients have the right to place restrictions on how PHI is disclosed by the provider and may file complaints with the provider or with the U.S. Department of Health and Human Services.

Additional Rights

The Patient's Bill of Rights was created to accomplish three major goals:

1. Ensure all patients receive fair and adequate medical care
2. Provide a resource for patients to address concerns regarding care
3. Encourage patients to be active participants in their health

The bill includes 12 rights for all patients[1]:

1. Right to considerate and respectful care
2. Right to current and understandable information pertaining to their medical condition when applicable (exclusions, e.g., in emergent situations)
3. Right to be active participants in decisions related to care including the right to refuse care
4. Right to advanced directives
5. Right to privacy (respect for modesty, maintain dignity)
6. Right to confidentiality
7. Right to review medical records except when restricted by law
8. Right to receive medical services from a facility when capable or be transferred to an appropriate facility
9. Right to be informed of business relationships that may influence care
10. Right to consent or decline participation in research studies
11. Right to continuity of care
12. Right to information regarding policies related to complaints, grievances, billing practices, and payment methods

Patients who refuse to participate in research studies must continue to receive the highest level of care and treatment available by the medical facility. Patients who opt to participate in research studies must be provided a full, understandable explanation of the study prior to providing consent.

As stated in the Patient's Bill of Rights, patients have the right to advanced directives. An advanced directive (living will) is a legal document that states the specific wishes of a patient related to medical treatment once that patient cannot communicate his or her wishes. Advanced directives are part of the patient's permanent medical record. Often, part of an advanced directive is the appointment of a durable power of attorney or health-care proxy. This person, designated by the patient, acts on behalf of the patient and is empowered to make medical decisions and provide consent. Also,

patients have the right to choose a do-not-resuscitate (DNR) order. A DNR order means that no efforts will be made to save the patient's life if death is imminent.[1,2,4,5]

Hospice care is provided to patients who have a terminal illness. Patients under hospice care, whether at home or in a hospice facility, receive palliative care. Palliative care is meant to provide care and management of the pain and symptoms of serious illness. Palliative care can occur at any stage of an illness; it is not only provided by hospice.

Legal Issues

Examination Documentation

The patient's medical record is a legal document that includes all information pertaining to the patient's care and treatment. Often referred to as the patient's *chart*, this document is an extensive compilation of all information related to the patient. The chart must be accurate, be legible, and contain all pertinent information. Such information includes, but is not limited to, patient diagnosis, medications, treatments, laboratory results, and radiographs.

Part of the responsibility of a radiologic technologist is to take a patient's clinical history. The clinical history is a valuable tool used to assist the radiologist when making a diagnosis. A clinical history may contain both objective and subjective data.[4] Objective data is data that can be observed or evaluated by the senses (heard, seen, felt) or that can be reported (such as laboratory results). Subjective data is what the patient perceives or experiences (such as pain). Subjective data cannot be observed or evaluated by the radiologic technologist's senses.

To obtain an accurate clinical history, radiologic technologists can use the following tools[1,2,4]:

- Open-ended questions that are nonleading and require no specific or correct response
- Facilitation, which includes affirmation of what is said and encouragement of elaboration by the patient
- Silence to allow the patient time to gather thoughts
- Probing questions to acquire additional detail from the patient
- Rewording (repetition) of information to ensure clarity
- Summarizing the information to ensure accuracy

Another guide to use when taking a clinical history is to follow the SACRED SEVEN[4]:

1. Localization—precise area involved
2. Chronology—onset, duration, frequency, and progression of symptoms
3. Quality—description of the character of the symptoms (e.g., dull, sharp, color, and size)

4. Severity—intensity of the condition
5. Onset—explanation by the patient of what the patient was doing when condition began
6. Aggravating or alleviating factors—things that either intensify, relieve, or modify symptoms
7. Associated manifestations—additional symptoms that occur at time of primary complaint

Common Terminology[1,2,4,5]

- Criminal offense—crime that violates a state or federal law and is punishable by fine or imprisonment
- Civil offense—violation of the rights or duties of an individual or society that is not punishable by imprisonment
- Felony—punishable by imprisonment
- Misdemeanor—less significant crime; punishable by fine and/or less than 1 year in prison
- Tort—civil wrongdoing against another person or property; can be intentional (e.g., assault, battery, false imprisonment, libel, slander) or unintentional (negligence)
- False imprisonment—unjustified detention of a person against his or her will (e.g., use of restraints without a physician order)
- Libel or slander—defamation of a person's character; libel is written and slander is verbal
- Assault—threat of touching a person to inflict injury
- Battery—touching of another person without consent
- Fraud—willful attempt to misrepresent information that may cause harm or loss to another person

Negligence is an unintentional tort and is defined as the omission of reasonable care or caution.[1] *Reasonable care or caution* is defined as what a reasonable person would do in the same situation. When negligence is between a patient and a health-care provider, it is termed *malpractice*. There are three different types of malpractice[1,2,4]:

1. Gross malpractice—reckless disregard for a person
2. Contributory malpractice—person's behavior directly contributed to the injury
3. Corporate malpractice—facility is responsible as a whole

For a health-care provider to be found guilty of malpractice or negligence, all four of the following conditions must be met[1,2,4]:

1. There was an established standard of care.
2. There was a breach of accepted standard of care.
3. The patient suffered a loss or injury.
4. The defendant is partly responsible for the loss or injury.

Legal Doctrines[1]

- Res ipsa loquitur—"the thing speaks for itself"; injury was caused by negligent act because the accident would not have occurred unless person was negligent (e.g., surgical instrument left in a patient)
- Respondeat superior—"the boss answers for what the employee does"; employer is liable for the actions of the employee
- Borrowed servant—physician liable for those acting under his or her orders
- Vicarious liability—responsibility of a superior for the acts of his or her subordinate
- Rule of personal liability—each person responsible is liable for himself or herself
- Duty of care—individuals must adhere to reasonable standard of care

Restraints versus Immobilization[1,2,4,5]

Immobilization devices are not the same as physical restraints. Immobilization devices are used to keep patients from moving during radiographic procedures and do not require a physician order to be applied. Restraints are devices used to prevent people from harming themselves or others and require a physician order to be applied.

Examples of immobilization devices include sponges, tape, and a Pigg-O-Stat. Examples of restraints include wrist and ankle restraints, vest restraints, and hand mitts.

ARRT Standard of Ethics

The ARRT Standard of Ethics contains two components: the Code of Ethics and the Rules of Ethics. The Code of Ethics is a list of broad principles that outline professional code of conduct. The Rules of Ethics are mandatory, specific standards that are enforceable.

INTERPERSONAL COMMUNICATION

Modes of Communication

Verbal/Written

Verbal communication is the primary method radiographers use to communicate with patients. Verbal communication refers to how a radiographer speaks to the patient prior to, during, and after an examination. Speech should be clear, use terminology appropriate for the patient, and use proper grammar and sentence structure. Verbal communication should be performed face to face when possible. Part of verbal communication may be the use of humor. Humor can help to ease a patient's anxiety and connect with the patient. Radiographers must use humor in an appropriate manner: no references to sex, gender, diseases, physical or mental disabilities, or sensitive subjects such as religion and politics.[4] In addition, radiographers should not engage in self-deprecating humor even if the patient does so first.[4]

Nonverbal

Nonverbal communication is influenced by a patient's culture. Radiographers must be aware that various cultures interpret nonverbal communication differently. A primary example is eye contact; in the United States, eye contact while speaking is considered a positive nonverbal method of communication demonstrating interest, concern, and honesty. However, in other cultures, such as Asian, eye contact while speaking is considered disrespectful.[1,4] The following is a list of types of nonverbal communication techniques[1,2,4]:

1. Touch can be either positive or negative depending on the type. Touch that is abrupt or tentative in nature can be perceived by the patient as anger, frustration, dominance, or reluctance to be of assistance. Positive touch should be done using light pressure (termed *palpation*) and demonstrate to the patient support, encouragement, and reassurance. Positive touch can help form a connection with the patient, place emphasis on important aspects of the exam, and provide emotional support when needed. It is important to explain to the patient what you are going to do prior to touching the patient.
2. Appearance is a vital component to the professionalism of a radiographer. Radiographers should maintain good hygiene, have a neat and clean uniform, and not wear any perfumes or colognes in the clinical environment. Appearance also applies to the clinical environment. Radiography rooms and other patient areas should be clean and organized.
3. Paralanguage refers to the manner in which a person speaks. Although speech is verbal communication, paralanguage is not what the radiographer says but how the patient interprets the manner in which it is said. The tone, pitch, volume, rate, and quality of the spoken word can alter the perceived intentions of the radiographer's spoken words.
4. Body language is often more important in how a patient responds to a radiographer than the spoken word. Radiographers need to maintain an appropriate distance from the patient when speaking, approximately 3 feet (ft); avoid standing with arms crossed over chest;

and be aware of facial expressions when speaking or reacting to others and their physical presence.

Challenges to Communication/Patient Characteristics

Communication with a patient is vital to achieving a quality diagnostic examination; however, there are numerous challenges for radiographers when communicating with patients. One of the main challenges is age; the list below provides techniques for communication with patients of different age ranges (ranges vary by reference; those provided are averages).[1,2,4]

- Neonate/infant (birth to 1 year): Use a calm voice, talk to the neonate/infant, smile, and employ gentle touch during the examination. Involve the parent/guardian if needed.
- Toddler (1–2 years): Call the child by the name used at home, use familiar words and phrases, involve play in the examination, and use demonstration and short directions. Involve the parent/guardian if needed.
- Preschool (3–5 years): This age group has increasing independence and appreciates options. Use simple explanations, clear instructions, demonstration, and praise or rewards to facilitate the examination.
- School-aged (5–10 years): Be specific with instructions, use demonstration, and ask the patient to assist with the examination.
- Adolescents (10–25 years): Maintain modesty at all times during examinations, engage the patient in conversation about interests, show empathy, involve the patient in the examination, and be thorough in your explanations.
- Young adult (25–45 years): Provide thorough explanations of the examination to the patient and use correct terminology.
- Middle adult (46–64 years): Be mindful of changes to both physical and mental health when communicating with the patient. Adjust communication based on these changes; for example, patients with hearing loss may need volume of speech to be higher.
- Late adult (65–79 years) and old adult (80+ years): It is important not to stereotype patients; assess each individually for mental and physical changes and adjust communication technique based on these changes. For patients with mental changes, speak slowly, provide one explanation at a time, and use concrete wording for explanations.

In addition to age, other challenges to communication can include[1,2,4]:

- Non–English-speaking patients: Use of trained interpreters, either in person or through a telephone service, is preferred over family or friends when discussing medical examinations. When using an interpreter, talk to the patient, not the interpreter, and use nonverbal communication including touch, facial expressions, and pantomime (gestures) to emphasize important aspects of the examinations.

- Speech- and hearing-impaired patients: Hearing loss and deafness are not the same; hearing loss is gradual loss of hearing, whereas deafness is apparent at birth. Prior to addressing a patient with hearing loss, get the patient's attention, talk directly to the patient (face patient), speak in a lower volume as that range is easier for the patient to hear, use a moderate pace with clearly spoken words, communicate in a quiet environment, rephrase if the patient seems to be confused, and most importantly, have patience. Deaf patients often use lip reading as a way to understand speech so it is important to look at the patient when talking. In addition, it may be necessary to use an interpreter who uses sign language to facilitate the examination. Last, if an interpreter is not available, a pen and paper may be provided to assist. For patients with aphasia (inability to speak or difficulty speaking), it is best to ask how they best communicate and follow the patient's lead.
- Vision-impaired patients: Patients with limited or complete loss of vision often use hearing, touch, and memory to navigate their environments. Radiographers should ask the patient how best to communicate with the patient and how best they can be of assistance to the patient. When providing instructions, be very descriptive and clear about what is needed.
- Mentally impaired patients: Mental impairment can be either congenital (e.g., Down syndrome), due to an illness of the brain (e.g., brain tumor), or caused by emotional disorders (e.g., schizophrenia). The radiographer should assess the patient's level of understanding, give clear and simple instructions, and communicate appropriately for the patient's age.
- Substance abusers: Patients under the influence of either drugs or alcohol should be assessed for level of comprehension. Patients may not be able to understand directions and also may not be in control of their actions.
- Mobile and surgical patients: Patients may be nonresponsive to verbal commands but still may hear when spoken to. Introduce yourself prior to beginning the examination and explain what is occurring during the examination; in addition, use a gentle, nonaggressive touch.

Explanation of Medical Terms

When speaking to a patient, it is important to use appropriate levels of vocabulary and medical terminology. The explanation of medical terms should be done using easily understood wording and, if appropriate, examples.

Strategies to Improve Understanding

Use open-ended questions to determine patient understanding, allow for silence to give patient time to process information, attempt different approaches to explaining the terminology if needed, and encourage questions from the patient. It is important to determine the type of learner (learning style) and modify explanations accordingly. Types of learning styles include[1,2]:

- Global learner—can look at entire picture at once to learn information
- Linear learner—needs to learn information in sequential steps/order
- Visual learner—material is best presented in picture or graphic format
- Auditory learner—learns best through verbal explanations
- Kinesthetic learner—learns through demonstration and return demonstration

Cultural Diversity

Culture can be defined in numerous ways. These ways include, but are not limited to[4]:

- Gender
- Race
- Generational
- Geographic
- Sexual orientation
- Religion
- Nonrace characteristics (e.g., deaf, blind)
- Socioeconomic
- Family structure (e.g., single parent)

Radiographers need to be sensitive to areas of concern for individuals of different cultures including modesty, physical contact, familial hierarchy, male/female interactions, economics, and previous experience with health-care providers.

Cultural competency is important for radiographers as the patient population being treated becomes increasingly diverse. The five elements for becoming culturally competent include[4]:

1. Value diversity
2. Capacity for self-assessment
3. Understand cross-cultural interactions
4. Applying cultural knowledge to medical care
5. Adapting patient services that reflect cultural understanding

Patient Education/Explanation of Procedure

It is part of the radiographer's job responsibility to educate patients regarding medical procedures and to provide appropriate preexamination preparation and postexamination instructions. Opportunities for the radiographer to educate the patient include the following:

1. Providing preparation instruction for the examination by detailing the specific steps of the preparation
2. During the procedure, explain the purpose, how it is performed including equipment used, average time of the procedure, and what is expected of the patient during the procedure
3. Responding to patient's questions and concerns regarding the examination
4. Providing postexamination instructions and follow-up care

When providing instructions to patients, it is important to not use technical terms, focus on the level of understanding of the patient, and be attentive to the concerns of and questions from the patient. To provide the most information to the patient, avoid standardized responses to questions; give focused responses specific to the patient's circumstances.

During the process of educating the patient, it may be beneficial to include the following techniques:

- Use written materials to support information
- Review each step with the patient throughout the discussion
- Validate the patient's understanding with open-ended questions
- Use the best communication skills for the patient's learning style

Respond to Inquiries about Other Imaging Modalities

Radiographers often have to provide information to patients.

INFECTION CONTROL

Terminology and Basic Concepts

Medical Asepsis

Medical asepsis (microbial dilution) is meant to reduce the probability of pathogens being present and able to cause infection; the risk of infection is never completely zero. The primary method to perform medical asepsis is hand-washing; it reduces the number of infectious agents. Medical asepsis alters the environment of the pathogen and makes it not conducive for growth and replication.

The process of reducing the number of pathogens can be achieved through proper hand-washing (soap, water, and friction) and the use of disinfectants. The technique for proper hand-washing is as follows[1]:

1. Turn on the water using either a foot pedal or paper towel
2. Wet hands thoroughly, keeping hands lower than elbows
3. Apply soap and lather hands well
4. Wash all hand surfaces including fingers for at least 20 seconds
5. Rinse hands thoroughly
6. Dry hands
7. Turn off water with foot pedal or using a paper towel

Surgical Asepsis

Surgical asepsis (sterilization) is the complete destruction of pathogens and spores from equipment.[1,2,4] There are numerous methods to perform surgical asepsis; these methods include the following:

- Chemical: use of a germicidal solution with a sterile rinse; instructions vary by manufacturer. Effectiveness is dependent on the strength of the sterilization solution, temperature of the solution, and the immersion time. Chemical sterilization is not a highly effective method.
- Dry heat: use of an oven at temperatures between 329° and 338°F (165° and 170°C). Items are sterilized for 1 to 6 hours. Dry heat is used for some sharp instruments, powders, and greasy items. The use of dry heat is not a preferred method of sterilization and cannot be used for items that cannot withstand extremely high temperatures.
- Conventional gas: uses a mix of gases heated to approximately 135°F (57°C). Conventional gas is used for items that cannot withstand high temperatures, such as electrical devices, plastics, and optical devices. Conventional gas is an effective method of sterilization, but the gas is poisonous to people when used in the sterilization process.
- Gas plasma: uses low-temperature and low-moisture hydrogen peroxide plasma for sterilization. Process is nontoxic and can be used for most items except long lumens, powders, liquids, and cellulose.
- Autoclave: uses steam under pressure to sterilize equipment. Process is quick, convenient, and effective.

Sterile Technique/Sterile Fields

Items and people are either sterile or not sterile. If something is questionable, it is considered not sterile. Only sterile persons can touch sterile items; all persons must wear sterile gowns and gloves. When passing, persons need to pass back-to-back. A person is only considered sterile from the level of the tabletop up or the waist of the person and up. Below this level is not considered sterile. In addition, the arm is considered sterile 2 inches above the elbow to the cuff of the sterile gown. The cuff is not considered sterile because is made of an absorbent material.[1,2,4,5]

Sterile fields are areas that are free of microorganisms for the placement of supplies and equipment. Any item placed in a sterile field must be sterile: clean, dry, unopened, and not expired. Sterile packages are opened in the following manner[1]:

1. Place the sterile pack on the tray
2. Open the corner farthest away from you
3. Open sides of the pack by grasping the tips of the packaging
4. Pull remaining side toward you

All sterile items must be covered prior to use. Once an item is removed from the sterile field, it should not be returned, and contaminated items should be discarded immediately to avoid cross-contamination. The edges of all packaging are considered unsterile, and all handles of equipment must be kept out of the sterile field. When pouring a liquid into a sterile field, the bottle should not come in contact with the sterile field; a small amount of liquid should be poured off and discarded before the required amount is poured into the sterile field. Finally, no person is permitted to reach across a sterile field.[1,2,4,5]

When adding items to a sterile field, it is important to maintain the field and not contaminate the area. For sterilized items being added, hold the package in the nondominant hand and open the outer wrapping by opening the first fold away from you. Next, grasp the corners of the package and drop onto the sterile tray. When adding disposable items to the tray, open the packaging (partially as not to let the item fall out) per manufacturer instructions, invert the package, and drop the item onto the sterile field.[1]

A sterile scrub is required when a person is entering a sterile environment and will be touching the sterile field. The procedure for a sterile (surgical) scrub is as follows[1]:

1. Put on hood/cap, mask, and goggles (if necessary)
2. Using the foot pedal or lever, turn on the water and adjust flow to prevent splashing
3. With hands above the level of the elbows, wet hands and forearms
4. Add soap and use friction to form lather
5. Wash all surfaces of hands, fingers, and forearms for at least 1 minute and clean under nails
6. Rinse, maintaining hands above elbows

7. Using a second brush, scrub nails for 30 strokes; 20 strokes for each skin surface including all sides of fingers, forearms, and elbows
8. Rinse
9. Dry using a sterile towel starting with fingers and working toward elbows
10. Do not touch any nonsterile surface once finished

Once a sterile scrub is complete, the radiographer may begin the process of sterile gowning and gloving[1]:

1. Lift sterile gown and allow to unfold
2. Insert arms into sleeves, keeping hands inside cuffs
3. Using dominant hand inside sleeve, pick up sterile glove
4. Insert nondominant hand into sterile glove
5. Using dominant hand inside sleeve, stretch cuff over glove
6. With gloved hand, pick up other glove and insert hand
7. Stretch cuff over glove
8. Separate waist tie from gown
9. Give protective tab to another person then turn around to wrap tie around waist
10. Using a sharp tug, separate tab from tie; secure tie

Pathogens

Pathogens are microorganisms that have the ability to cause infection and disease. Pathogens can multiply by large numbers and cause tissue damage. They have the ability to secrete exotoxins, which are substances that increase temperature and cause nausea, vomiting, and other disease symptoms. There are four different types of pathogens of primary concern to radiologic technologists: bacteria, viruses, fungi, and protozoans (parasites).[1,2,4,5]

1. Bacteria are single-celled microorganisms that can replicate without a host cell and are prokaryotes (lack nuclei but have DNA/RNA). Bacteria are classified by their shape or morphology: spherical (cocci), rod (bacilli), and spiral (spirilla or spirochetes). In addition, bacteria are classified as either gram-positive or gram-negative. Finally, bacteria can be obligate aerobes (require oxygen), anaerobes (do not need oxygen), or facultative (can survive with or without oxygen). Bacteria produce endospores, which are a resistance form of the bacteria that can remain dormant for years and germinate once conditions are ideal. Endospores can be found in such places as soil, air, and dust particles. Examples of bacteria include *Mycobacterium tuberculosis* and *Escherichia coli*.
2. Viruses are the smallest disease-causing microorganism and are called *obligate intracellular parasites*. This

means that viruses need a host cell to survive and replicate. A virus has either DNA or RNA protected by a capsid and sometimes lipoproteins in the shape of spikes. Either the capsid or spikes helps the virus attach to the host cell. When the virus is fully developed, it is termed a *virion*.

3. Fungi are either single-celled yeasts or long-branched structures called *molds*. Some fungi are dimorphic, meaning they can exist as either a mold or yeast. The replication process for molds and yeasts are different: Molds replicate through spore formation (conidia) and yeasts replicate through bud formation. Fungi are eukaryotic, meaning they have a nucleus and organelles. Some fungi are useful, such as those to produce beer and leavened bread; however, others cause disease, such as histoplasmosis and ringworm. Fungi can cause disease to the skin and nails, the circulatory system, and the lymphatic system.

4. Protozoans (parasites) are complex, singled-celled animals that can live independently. Parasites are eukaryotic but have no cell wall. Parasites are classified as motile (moving) or nonmotile, often called *sporozoans* (unable to move). Motile parasites, sometimes also called *amoeboid*, can be pseudopods (change shape), flagella (whip-like formations), or cilia (fine hair-like projections). Parasites can be transmitted by vehicles or vectors to humans.

Prions are believed to be infectious proteins that cause irreversible neurologic damage. Little is known about this pathogen, but it does not have DNA or RNA and is resistant to the human body's natural defense mechanisms.

Fomites, Vehicles, and Vectors[1,2,4,5]

The spreading of disease can occur through human contact such as sneezing, coughing, and sexual contact. In addition, pathogens can be spread by numerous others means such as water, equipment, and animals.

- Fomites are objects that are contaminated with pathogens. Fomites are inanimate objects such as imaging plates, stretchers, and examination tables.
- Vectors are animals and arthropods that host or develop pathogens. Examples of vectors include mosquitoes, fleas, and ticks.
- Vehicles transport pathogens and include such things as water, food, blood, and drugs.

Nosocomial Infections

Nosocomial infections are hospital-acquired infections, meaning the patient must contract the pathogen for the disease while being treated in a hospital. A similar type of infection is iatrogenic; however, this occurs as a result of treatment by a physician and does not have to occur in the hospital setting.[1,2] Nosocomial infections are opportunistic, meaning they cause disease in individuals who are susceptible. Examples of those who are susceptible include the immunosuppressed, such as those on chemotherapy, transplant patients on anti-rejection drugs, burn victims, and the elderly. Sources of nosocomial infections include the following[1,2,4]:

- Medical personnel through direct or indirect contact with patients, contact with food or items the patient ingests (e.g., medication), and inhalation (airborne or droplet transmission).
- Patient's normal flora, located on the skin, in the genitourinary tract, gastrointestinal tract, or respiratory tract can be infectious if transmitted to other parts of the body where they are not normally found.
- Hospital environment if surfaces or objects are not clean or through contamination of food, liquids, or medications.
- Blood-borne pathogens including, but not limited to, hepatitis B and HIV through exposure with infected blood or body fluids.
- Invasive procedures including, but not limited to, the placement of indwelling urinary catheters, surgical procedures, and use of invasive equipment and needles. Most common nosocomial infection is a urinary tract infection due to urinary catheters.

Cycle of Infection[1,2,4]

The cycle of infection outlines the process by which a microorganism infects an individual and causes disease. When discussing the cycle of infection, it is important to be familiar with specific terminology related to microorganisms:

- *Pathogenicity* is the ability of an organism to produce disease.
- *Virulence* is the degree of pathogenicity or likelihood the microorganism will cause disease.
- *Specific microorganisms* are those that are attracted only to a particular host.
- *Invasive microorganisms* have the ability to invade or enter a host.
- *Infection* is the invasion and multiplication of a microorganism that does result in cellular injury.
- *Colonization* is the multiplication of a microorganism that does not result in cellular injury.

The cycle of infection has six essential links that must be continuous for infection to occur. A break in the cycle at any point can hinder or prevent disease from occurring. The cycle of infection is as follows:

1. Pathogen or infectious agent is present and capable of causing disease
2. Reservoir or host is carrying the infectious pathogen
3. Portal of exit: The pathogen must exit the host through a mode of transmission
4. Mode of transmission is how the infectious microorganism travels from the reservoir to the susceptible host; modes of transmission are discussed below
5. Portal of entry is how the infectious microorganism gains access to the susceptible host; this can occur through the skin, mucous membranes, genitourinary tract, gastrointestinal tract, or respiratory tract
6. Susceptible host is a person who has a compromised immune system or lacks resistance to the disease and is vulnerable to the infection

It is important to understand the cycle of infection because it impacts how radiographers protect both themselves and their patients from disease-causing microorganisms. One specific point in the cycle of infection where the radiographer can hinder the spread of infection is the mode of transmission. Personal protective equipment (PPE) is used to inhibit the mode of transmission of infectious agents.

Modes of Transmission

In order for a microorganism to leave the reservoir and infect a susceptible host, there has to be a bridge between the two. This bridge is the mode of transmission of that microorganism. Transmission can occur through numerous methods including contact, droplet, airborne, vehicle, and vector methods. For the radiographer, is it important to have knowledge of how a microorganism is transmitted so the correct PPE can be worn to inhibit the transmission.[1,2,4]

- Contact transmission can be either direct or indirect. Direct contact is when the susceptible host comes in contact with the reservoir carrying the infectious microorganism. This occurs commonly through touching. Indirect contact is when the susceptible host comes in contact with a fomite that has the infectious microorganism present, for example, an unclean imaging plate or door handle. The best types of PPE to prevent contact transmission are gloves and gowns; in addition, hand-washing is a vital step to preventing infection.
- Airborne transmission occurs when the droplet nuclei of an infectious microorganism travel through the air. For a microorganism to be infectious by airborne transmission, it must be 5 micrometers (μm) or less in size and have the ability to be suspended in air for a long period of time. Diseases spread by airborne transmission enter through the respiratory tract. Examples include tuberculosis. The best method of PPE to prevent airborne transmission is a mask.
- Droplet transmission is similar to airborne except droplet nuclei are larger in size and cannot stay suspended in air for long distances. Infectious droplet nuclei are larger than 5 μm and can only travel approximately 3 ft. Examples include the common cold and influenza. The types of PPE that are used to prevent droplet transmission are masks and face shields.
- Vehicle transmissions are achieved through a medium for transport. Such mediums include food, water, and blood. Examples include cholera.
- Vector transmissions occur through contact with animals or arthropods such as ticks, mosquitoes, and fleas. Examples include Lyme disease and malaria.

Standard Precautions[1,2,4,5]

Standard precautions reduce the risk of transmission of infectious microorganisms, including blood-borne microorganisms. Standard precautions apply to blood, all body fluids, all secretions and excretions (excluding sweat) regardless if there is visible blood present, nonintact skin (open wounds), and mucous membranes. The type of standard precaution(s) employed is commonly related to the mode of disease transmission; however, standard precautions are to be used for all patients regardless of condition.

Hand-washing is the primary method of reducing the spread and risk of infection from a pathogen. Hand-washing should occur before and after contact with patients regardless of glove use, before and after using the restroom, after cleaning equipment, and after coming in contact with an item that may harbor infectious microorganisms. The best method to clean hands is to use soap, water, and friction. Alcohol-based hand rubs can be used but are not effective against all types of microorganisms. The proper procedure for washing hands is as follows[1]:

1. Turn on water with foot or knee lever. If no lever is available, use a paper towel to turn on water. Avoid touching the sink area.
2. Wet hands; apply soap and rub together vigorously to produce lather. Clean all hand surfaces, between fingers, and nails.
3. Rinse hands and repeat the process.

4. Turn off water with the lever or clean paper towel.
5. Dry hands beginning at elbows and working down toward fingers.

As stated previously, hand-washing should occur before and after each patient regardless of whether gloves are worn. However, gloves should be worn for all patients regardless of health condition.

Protective gowns are worn for patients who have stated disease precautions due to disease type or when there is a risk of splattering of fluids such as blood or feces. Gowns should be removed after each patient; radiographers should not keep a gown on and travel to different patient rooms.

Masks are worn when there is a risk of infection from airborne or droplet diseases. Masks should be discarded after each patient. Face shields are worn when there is a risk of being splattered by droplets from sneezing or coughing or from splattering of body fluids including blood. Face shields should be removed after each patient contact.

Additional or Transmission-Based Precautions

Patients with infections with known modes of transmission are identified with specific types of precautions. These precautions are posted on the patient chart and outside the patient room. This method of identification is meant to protect health-care workers and visitors from becoming infected or spreading the infectious disease. Although each facility may have specific protocols regarding how to address precautions, below is a general overview of each[1,2,4]:

- Airborne precautions are for those diseases that are spread by airborne transmission. Airborne transmission is by droplets that are 5 μm in size or less and have the ability to stay suspended in the air for long periods of time. Patients under these precautions are placed in private rooms with negative air ventilation systems. The rooms have a minimum of six air exchanges per hour, and the exchanged air is vented outside the building or through a filtration system. All health-care workers who enter must wear a particulate air filter mask that filters particles as small as 1 micron with 95% efficiency. In addition, if the patient is transported to another department, the patient must also wear a particulate air filter mask. The door to the room must remain closed at all times.
- Droplet precautions are for patients with diseases spread by droplet transmission. Droplet transmis-

sion is by microorganisms larger than 5 μm and that cannot travel farther than 3 ft in the air. Patients under these precautions can share a room with another person infected with the same disease or with a person who will not be closer than 3 ft. The room does not require special air handling or ventilation. Health-care workers should wear a mask when entering the room and a face shield if they will be in close proximity to the patient.
- Contact precautions are for patients with diseases spread by contact transmission (direct or indirect). Patients with these precautions should be placed with another patient with the same disease or in a private room. Health-care workers entering the room must wear, at a minimum, gloves and gown.

Disposal of Contaminated Materials[2]

Materials that are contaminated by blood or body fluids must be discarded in appropriate receptacles. It is important to know and follow the specific protocol of a facility regarding hazardous waste disposal.

- Linens should be folded with the edges toward the center. Linens should not be shaken because doing so can distribute certain infectious microorganisms in the air. Linens should be placed in the appropriate container. Some facilities separate linens soiled with blood or body fluids from those without; however, many hospitals do not segregate linens and all are placed in the same container.
- Needles are disposable and are for one-time use only. Needles should never be recapped by the radiographer once used. All needles and syringes should be discarded in labeled sharps containers provided by the facility. If a sharps container is filled to the maximum line, it is not appropriate to force the needle or syringe inside or attempt to push down the contents to make additional room; begin using a new container.
- Patient supplies such as emesis basins can be rinsed and reused for the same patient only. Once the patient no longer uses the supply, it can be discarded in the trash according to facility protocol.
- Bandages and dressings that are soiled with blood or fluids should be placed in a biohazard bag, sealed, and discarded in a biohazard container.

PHYSICAL ASSISTANCE AND TRANSFER

Patient Transfer and Movement

Part of the job responsibilities of a radiographer is to assist with patient transfers. Patient transfers can consist of helping a patient out of a wheelchair, lifting a nonambulatory patient from the stretcher to the x-ray table, or simply helping a patient ambulate to the restroom. The key to performing patient transfers safely is to remember the key components to good body mechanics. Body mechanics is the proper alignment, movement, and balance of a person to prevent injury when moving/lifting something.[1,2,4] The first part of proper body alignment is having a wide base of support in full contact with the floor. This broad base can be with the feet parallel to each other slightly apart or with one leg slightly in front of the other with feet apart. The separation of feet should be approximately shoulder width. Another important aspect of body mechanics to remember is the location of the center of gravity. The center of gravity is the center of a person's body weight and is commonly around the level of the second sacral segment (S2). When performing any type of patient transfer or movement of an object, there are five rules to remember[1,2,4]:

1. Have a broad base of support
2. Work at a comfortable height if possible
3. If lifting, bend knees and keep back straight at all times
4. Make sure the load is well balanced and kept close to the body during moving
5. Always roll or push an object if possible; avoid pulling or lifting

In addition, if a patient or load is too heavy for you to move, it is best to ask for assistance. This can prevent injury to yourself and possibly the patient.

Patient Transfer

The transferring of patients in the radiology department occurs when a patient is either transported by wheelchair or gurney (stretcher). Inpatients (those receiving care in the hospital) are always transported to the department by wheelchair or gurney. Outpatients (those not being treated in the hospital) may come to the department by wheelchair or gurney depending on health status. If a patient arrives in the department by wheelchair or gurney, it is better to assume the patient cannot ambulate independently and will require assistance when being transferred to the x-ray table.

The first step in a patient transfer is to properly identify the patient. For inpatients, this can be done by comparing the patient (medical record) number on the requisition to the number on the patient's wristband. Do not use the chart for verification of patient identification because charts can be misplaced. The second step is to assess the patient's ability to ambulate, for example: Is the patient conscious? Is there a visible injury? Did the

patient just have a procedure performed? Third, it is important to identify any equipment that the patient is connected to, such as an IV or oxygen. Also note if the patient has an indwelling urinary catheter. Finally, the key to a successful transfer is to make sure to have constant communication with the patient. Explain what is going to occur, how it is going to occur, and when. The process of being transferred is frightening for a patient and that fear can impede the process. Communication with the patient can result in the patient's assistance with the process and a successful transfer.

The list below provides examples of how to successfully transfer a patient to/from a wheelchair or gurney. Be sure to explain the transfer technique to the patient prior to beginning.

- Wheelchair: bed or table to chair[1]
  1. Lower the bed or table to level of chair
  2. Elevate the head of the bed slightly to assist the patient with sitting up
  3. Place the chair parallel to the bed or table and lock the brakes
  4. Put one arm under the shoulders of the patient, the other under the knees
  5. In one motion swing the patient to a sitting position with legs off bed/table
  6. Stand facing the patient and wrap arms around patient to the scapulae
  7. Have the patient grasp your shoulders with the hands
  8. Instruct the patient to assist as you lift the patient upward
  9. Instruct the patient to pivot so back of knees are against the wheelchair
  10. Assist the patient to sit in the wheelchair
- Wheelchair: x-ray table to chair[1]
  1. If possible, lower table to the height of the wheelchair
  2. Place chair parallel to the table and lock the brakes
  3. If table cannot be lowered, use a stool and place handle between chair and table
  4. Put one arm under the shoulders of the patient, the other under the knees
  5. In one motion swing the patient to a sitting position with legs off bed/table
  6. Stand facing the patient and wrap arms around patient to the scapulae
  7. Have the patient grasp your shoulders with the hands
  8. Instruct the patient to assist as you lift the patient upward

9. Instruct the patient to pivot so back of knees are against the wheelchair
10. Assist the patient to sit in the wheelchair
11. If using a stool, have patient place one hand on the stool while seated
12. Have patient stand on the stool when elevated to a standing position
13. Assist patient into chair

- Wheelchair: stroke patients or patients with fractures to chair[1]
  1. Place bed or table at same height as the chair
  2. Position chair parallel with bed or table on the strong or uninjured side of the patient
  3. Once patient is in a seated position (follow steps above), brace your knee against patient's weak or injured leg
  4. Stand facing the patient and wrap arms around patient to the scapulae
  5. Have the patient grasp your shoulders with the hands
  6. Instruct the patient to assist as you lift the patient upward
  7. Instruct the patient to pivot so back of knees are against the wheelchair
  8. Assist the patient to sit in the wheelchair

- Wheelchair: chair to table or bed[1]
  1. If possible, lower bed/table to the height of the wheelchair
  2. Place chair parallel to the bed/table and lock the brakes
  3. If table cannot be lowered, use a stool and place handle between chair and table
  4. Stand in front of patient with one leg in between patient's legs
  5. Instruct patient to put hands on your shoulders
  6. Wrap your arms around the patient under the patient's axilla
  7. Instruct the patient to stand and assist with standing
  8. Assist the patient onto the foot stool
  9. Instruct patient to pivot to put back against the table
  10. Assist the patient onto the table in a sitting position
  11. Support the patient's upper body and raise legs onto the table and place patient supine

- Wheelchair: two-person lift; the stronger person is considered the primary lifter[1]
  1. Lower table/bed to height of the chair if possible
  2. Place chair parallel to the table/bed
  3. Remove arm rest closest to table/bed if possible
  4. Instruct patient to cross both arms across chest
  5. Primary lifter stands behind the patient and reaches around patient, grasping around chest and holding onto patient's forearms
  6. Secondary person places hands under legs
  7. Primary and secondary people lift the patient in unison onto table/bed

- Wheelchair: three-person lift; the strongest person is the primary lifter[1]

Procedure is same as two-person lift except third person assists by placing hands under patient's waist and buttocks to assist with lift.

- Stretcher transfer: two-person lift to bed/table[1]
  1. Lower the head of the gurney flat
  2. Lower side rails
  3. Have patient place arms across chest
  4. One person lifts and supports the head, neck, and shoulders
  5. Second person lifts and supports the pelvis and knees
  6. Lift is done in unison in a lift-pull motion

- Draw-sheet transfer[1]
  1. Single sheet is under patient and over middle third of the bed
  2. Sheet is rolled up at edges against patient to provide "handles" for transfer
  3. Side rail closest to bed/table is down
  4. Instruct patient to put arms across chest
  5. Two people lift and pull patient across from stretcher to table/bed

- Slideboard transfer[1]
  1. Patient rolled onto side
  2. Slideboard is placed under draw-sheet and under half of the patient
  3. Slideboard closes gap between table/bed and stretcher
  4. Patient is slid onto Slideboard and across to the table/bed using the draw-sheet technique

Assisting Patients with Medical Equipment

When transferring a patient with medical equipment, it is important to make sure that during the transfer no tubes, wires, or lines are disrupted. For patients with infusion catheters or pumps, make sure the pump is placed in such a position that, when the patient is transferred, there is enough slack on the tubing to prevent pulling or dislodging. For patients on oxygen therapy, move the tank if needed to allow for sufficient slack of the tubing during transfer. When a patient has a urinary catheter, move the bag along with the patient and then place it on the floor next to the patient during the examination. Be sure to keep the bag below the level of the patient at all times. For all other types of equipment, make sure you do not pull, twist, or kink any tubes, lines, or wires. If you believe something was altered, notify a physician or nurse immediately. All assessments of patients need to be documented by the radiographer with time, date, and radiographer name. In addition, the name of the physician or nurse who responds should also be documented.

Routine Monitoring

As part of their scope of practice, radiographers must be able to obtain a patient's vital signs. Vital signs indicate how the body is functioning and provide a quick assessment of patient condition. The vital signs a radiographer is responsible for obtaining include temperature, pulse, respiratory rate, and blood pressure.

Vital Signs[1,2,4]

- Temperature is indicative of the body's heat loss and heat production in the tissues. Temperature is regulated by the hypothalamus and can fluctuate in response to numerous factors including metabolic rate, infection, or exertion. A normal oral temperature in an adult is between 96.8° and 99.8°F. A normal rectal temperature is approximately 0.5° to 1.0°F higher than the normal oral temperature, and a normal axillary temperature is 0.5° to 1.0°F below the normal oral temperature.
- The sites used to determine temperature include oral, rectal, axillary, tympanic, and temporal. Oral temperature should not be taken if the patient recently ate or drank, is unconscious, or is mouth breathing; it also should not be performed on patients with facial injuries or history of seizures or young children. Oral thermometers are digital with disposable covers. Glass is no longer used in the clinical setting. Rectal temperature is fast and accurate but is no longer the preferred method due to patient discomfort. Rectal temperature should not be performed on patients with rectal pathology; in addition, it should not be performed on cardiac patients as it can stimulate the vagus nerve and alter blood pressure and pulse. Axillary temperatures are slower and less accurate. The temperature is taken under the patient's axilla and is dependent on thermometer placement for accuracy. Tympanic is performed using a special thermometer inserted into the external ear canal. Temporal is performed using a special thermometer slid across the patient's forehead across the temporal artery.
- Patients whose temperature is above normal have a fever or pyrexia (100.4° to 104°F). Patients with pyrexia often have an increased pulse rate and respiratory rate, flushed skin, and chills. If a patient's temperature is between 105.8° and 111.2°F, the patient has hyperpyrexia; it is unlikely a person can survive with a temperature higher than 111.2°F. Temperature 95°F or lower is termed *hypothermia*; patients are unlikely to survive if the temperature is at or below 93.2°F.
- Other methods to take temperatures that are less accurate include disposable oral thermometers. These thermometers are plastic with heat-sensitive areas. Also, there are forehead patches that remain in place to evaluate temperature over a period of time.
- Pulse is the pressure wave in an artery when blood is expelled from the left ventricle. A normal pulse rate in an adult is 60 to 80 beats per minute (bpm). Pulse rates higher than 100 are termed *tachycardia*, and rates lower than 60 are termed *bradycardia*. Pulse rate can be monitored by assessing superficial arteries; these sites include the following: radial, apical, carotid, femoral, popliteal, temporal and dorsal pedis, posterior tibial, and brachial. The rate should be evaluated for 1 full minute regardless of location assessed. The most common sites for assessing the pulse include the radial, carotid, temporal, and femoral arteries and the apical pulse.
- The radial, temporal, femoral, and carotid pulses can be evaluated using your fingers and applying pressure against the artery. The thumb should not be used because it has a pulse. The apical pulse requires the use of a stethoscope. If the pulse using the fingers is irregular, the apical pulse should be evaluated. For pulses taken at the brachial, dorsal pedis, posterior tibial, and popliteal sites, the assessment should be bilateral. Pulse rate is recorded in bpm as well as assessed for strength and rhythm.
- Respiration is the exchange of oxygen and carbon dioxide (CO_2) between the external environment and the circulating blood. The average respiratory rate in an adult is 10 to 20 breaths per minute. Respiration rates below 10 for adults can lead to cyanosis, restlessness, apprehension, and loss of consciousness. Normal respirations are quiet, effortless, and uniform. Factors such as illness, medication, exercise, or age can alter a respiratory rate. If a patient is using more than a normal effort to breathe and is having difficulty breathing, it is termed *dyspnea*. The use of accessory muscles for breathing, including the use of

the abdominals, intercostals, or neck muscles, can indicate dyspnea.

- The evaluation of respiratory rate needs to occur with the patient either seated or supine. In addition, the patient should not be told breathing will be assessed as it will alter the pattern. Assessment should take place immediately before or after the pulse to prevent patient from realizing the breathing is being watched. Respiratory rate should be assessed for 1 full minute. In addition to counting respirations, the pattern, body position, and movement of the chest and abdomen need to be evaluated. Patients having difficulty breathing often lean forward and place hands on knees. Respiratory rate (breaths per minute) and characteristics of breathing should be documented with an R to distinguish from pulse rate.
- Blood pressure is the product of blood flow and resistance to that blood flow. When blood pressure is assessed, two different numbers are reported as a fraction: The top number is the systolic pressure and the bottom number is the diastolic pressure. Systolic pressure is the highest pressure point reached by the left ventricle during contraction. Diastolic pressure is the lowest pressure exerted against the arterial walls during ventricle relaxation. Normal blood pressure is less than 120 millimeters of mercury (mm Hg) for systolic and less than 80 mm Hg for diastolic. Patients with blood pressure readings in the range of 120 to 139 over 80 to 89 mm Hg are considered prehypertensive. Ranges of 140 to 159 over 90 to 99 mm Hg are considered stage I hypertensive; 160 to 169 over 100 to 109 are stage II hypertensive; and pressures greater than 180 mm Hg systolic or greater than 110 mm Hg diastolic mean the patient is in hypertensive crisis.
- Blood pressure is commonly assessed using a stethoscope and a sphygmomanometer. The values of the numbers are reported in mm Hg; however, mercury sphygmomanometers are no longer used. Currently, aneroid (air pressure) or digital blood pressure machines are used, but the values are still reported in mm Hg. The blood pressure is influenced by numerous factors including, but not limited to, age, gender, level of physical activity, last meal, and medications. A patient's blood pressure should be taken with the patient either seated or supine and using the left arm if available. When using a stethoscope, the systolic pressure is the first audible sound heard, and the diastolic pressure is the last audible sound heard. If the pressure needs to reassessed, the opposite arm should be used.

Physical Signs and Symptoms

During the course of performing a diagnostic examination, the radiographer should also be assessing a patient's physical condition. Radiographers should be aware of changes in skin color such as bluish lips, mouth, and nails, which are signs of cyanosis. Patients who appear pale and claim to be light-headed need to be seated because they could faint. Patients with hot, dry skin may have a fever; contrarily, patients who are diaphoretic or in a cold sweat may also have a fever. Radiographers need to also monitor levels of consciousness and changes to those levels. Note if the patient is alert, drowsy but responsive, unconscious but reactive to touch, or comatose. In addition, the radiographer needs to report any changes in the patient's pain level or discomfort.

MEDICAL EMERGENCIES

Medical emergencies can occur in the radiography department regardless of whether it is a hospital or outpatient setting. A radiographer must be aware of the signs and symptoms of a medical emergency and know how to respond accordingly. Quick, appropriate, and efficient responses to medical emergencies can be the difference between life and death. It is important for the radiographer to know the facility's procedures for calling for assistance (calling a code) and the location of the crash cart. Below is a list of common medical emergencies seen in the radiography department.

Allergic Reactions

Patients can have allergic reactions to medications, contrast agents, and even equipment (latex-based items) in the radiography department. Allergic reactions can vary from mild to severe; a person's first-time reaction can be either be mild or severe. If a person had a previous mild allergic reaction to something, it is anticipated the next reaction would be severe in nature. It is important to ask a patient if he or she has any allergic history to foods, animals, or common allergens (e.g., hay fever) as these may be precursors for reactions to other allergens.

In the radiology department, common allergens patients come in contact with are contrast agents. Allergic reactions to contrast agents can be mild and include mild urticaria (hives), itching, and a scratchy throat. These can also occur with reactions to other substances, including latex. Severe allergic reactions are called anaphylactic shock and can be life threatening. Anaphylactic shock can occur after a mild reaction or the first time a person has a reaction to an allergen. When a person goes into anaphylactic shock, the response is usually extremely quick and severe. The body releases histamine which results in a full systemic reaction to the allergen.

The full systemic reaction includes the following symptoms[1,2,3,4]:

- Hives
- Throat swelling and itching
- Swelling of the tongue and upper airway
- Wheezing
- Difficulty breathing
- Inspiratory stridor
- Low blood pressure
- Increased respiratory rate
- Pulmonary edema

Treatment of anaphylactic shock includes the use of epinephrine to open the airway and increase blood pressure and the use of antihistamines to reduce the body's allergic reaction. If the patient is not treated promptly, the prognosis is poor and may result in death; with prompt and appropriate treatment, the patient can recover fully.

Cardiac or Respiratory Arrest (Cardiopulmonary Resuscitation)

Cardiac arrest occurs when there is damage to the heart muscle. A patient who suffers from cardiac arrest suffers from a myocardial infarction (MI). An MI is a result of damage to the ventricle(s); the heart cannot adequately pump blood through the circulatory system. Patient suffering from MI may also go into cardiogenic shock. When this occurs, the blood backs up into the lungs causing pulmonary edema (fluid in the lungs). Signs and symptoms of both cardiogenic shock and cardiac arrest include[2]:

- Chest pain
- Left arm and/or jaw pain
- Shortness of breath
- Increased respiratory rate
- Irregular heartbeat
- High blood pressure
- Increased heart rate

Cardiac arrest can also occur because of other reasons including, but not limited to, myocardial contusion or severe valve prolapse.

For patients in cardiac arrest, it is necessary to begin CPR and call for help (code). The radiographer should continue CPR until the code team or other medical personnel arrive. The only time CPR should not begin is if a patient has a DNR order.

Respiratory arrest can occur as a result of cardiac arrest. Respiratory arrest occurs when the lungs do not receive adequate oxygen. In addition to an MI, respiratory arrest can occur as a result of restriction of the airway such as asthma, airway obstructions, trauma, congestive heart failure, pulmonary edema, and chronic obstructive pulmonary disease. Patients in respiratory arrest will appear cyanotic; have cool and clammy skin, wheezing, stridor on inspiration; and use accessory muscles to breathe. As with cardiac arrest, CPR should begin with those in respiratory arrest.

Physical Injury or Trauma[1,2,4]

Radiographers often must conduct examinations on patients suffering from severe traumatic injuries. It is important for the radiographer to understand the complexity of the injury and methods to properly perform the radiographic procedure. Modifications to routine projections are often necessary to maintain the safety of the patient and prevent further injury from occurring during the examination. When performing an exam on a patient with a traumatic injury, it is important to wear PPE (gloves, gown, face shield); if performing in the emergency department, it is important to also work quickly and efficiently. It is important to never remove any immobilization devices (e.g., collars, splints, dressings) without an order from a physician. The radiographer will need to modify how the exam is performed to compensate for the immobilization devices.

Patients suffering from head injuries can present with either open or closed injuries. Closed injuries do not show any visible signs of injury, such as bleeding or wound. Although a closed head injury is not visible, the effects of such an injury can be life threatening. Signs and symptoms of head injuries include:

- Varied levels of consciousness
- Loss of reflexes
- Changes in vital signs
- Headache
- Vision changes
- Dizziness
- Giddiness
- Gait disturbances
- Unequal pupil dilation
- Seizures
- Nausea and vomiting

Open head injuries present with a visible wound or abrasion. Although the visible injury site may be small in size, this does not correlate to the severity of the injury. Signs and symptoms of an open head injury include:

- Halo sign: visible cerebrospinal fluid due to injury to the base of the skull

- Varying levels of consciousness
- Subconjunctival hemorrhage
- Hearing loss
- Periorbital ecchymoses
- Facial nerve injury

The radiographer when performing diagnostic examinations on patients with open or closed head injuries must keep the patient immobilized at all times. The patient's head elevation should not be adjusted; if the patient arrives to the department or is in the emergency room (ER) with head elevated, keep patient in that position. This also holds true for patients in the fully supine position. Do not flex, twist, or move the patient. Also, be aware of patient's respirations and notify medical staff if any changes occur.

Spinal cord injuries require the radiographer to be extremely cautious during radiographic examinations. Injuries to the spinal cord can result in severe neurologic injury, paralysis, or death. Often, a spinal cord injury is not fully realized until imaging examinations are performed; however, patients with suspected injuries are immobilized for precautionary purposes. A patient's cervical collar should never be removed unless directed by a physician. A patient on a backboard should not be transferred to an x-ray table. For a patient with a spinal cord injury, some signs and symptoms include:

- Flaccid paralysis of the skeletal muscles
- Loss of sensation
- Respiratory distress
- Unstable blood pressure
- Bradycardia
- Incontinence (bowel or bladder)
- Priapism

A radiographer performing images on a suspected or diagnosed patient with a spinal cord injury must be aware of any changes in vital signs, especially respiratory changes. The radiographer should employ assistance when possible to aid in the examination.

Patients with fractures often require numerous radiographs to aid in diagnosis and treatment. Fractures of the extremities require special handling during imaging. When moving a fractured part, it is necessary to hold the injured part above and below the fracture site. This will allow the part to be moved safely and prevent any dislocation of the fracture. Patients with a fracture may demonstrate the following:

- Pain and swelling of the affected part
- Loss of function
- Deformity
- Grating sound with movement

- Discoloration of the skin (ecchymosis)
- Bleeding
- Open wound

Abdominal injuries can present themselves with open, visible wounds or with closed injuries. Patients with severe abdominal injuries may have internal bleeding that can be life threatening. Patients with abdominal injuries may present with the following:

- Lacerations or open wounds to the abdomen
- Bleeding
- Rigid abdomen
- Pain, sometimes severe
- Nausea and vomiting
- Extreme thirst

It is important for the radiographer during imaging of an abdominal injury patient to monitor the patient's vitals and report any changes. It is also important to assist the patient if vomiting occurs, to keep the patient as immobile as possible, and to not provide the patient any fluids, including water or ice.

Other Medical Disorders

Other medical problems that radiographers may encounter include pulmonary embolism (PE), seizures, strokes, and diabetic emergencies. PEs occur when one or more of the pulmonary arteries are occluded by a thrombus. Patients with PE may present with the following:

- Chest pain
- Rapid/weak pulse
- Dyspnea
- Tachycardia
- Hyperventilation
- Apprehension
- Cough
- Hemoptysis
- Diaphoresis
- Syncope
- Cyanosis

Some patients with a PE may have very nonspecific signs and symptoms. Causes of a PE include surgery, pelvic trauma, extremity trauma, pregnancy, and long periods of immobilization. Patients with a PE require immediate medical attention.

Patients who present with sudden weakness, numbness to a part of the body, loss of or difficulty with vision, difficulty speaking, a severe headache, or changes in their gait may be suffering from a stroke. The radiographer needs to get immediate medical attention for the patient.

Patients who suffer from epilepsy may suffer a seizure while in the radiography department. There are numerous different types of seizures; however, they all present with similar signs and symptoms. Patients often present with early warning signs of a seizure, but it is important to note that some seizures occur with no warning signs. The signs and symptoms of a seizure can be broken into three categories: sensory/thought, emotional, and physical.

1. Sensory/thought
   - Blackout
   - Confusion
   - Deafness or intense sounds
   - Feeling of an electric shock
   - Loss of consciousness
   - Strong sense of smell; often odors no one else smells
   - Visual loss or blurring
   - Out-of-body experience
   - Spacing out
2. Emotional response is usually fear or panic
3. Physical
   - Chewing movements
   - Convulsions
   - Difficulty talking
   - Drooling
   - Eyelid fluttering
   - Eyes rolling upward
   - Falling down; loss of balance
   - Foot stomping
   - Hand waving
   - Inability to move
   - Incontinence
   - Lip smacking
   - Shaking
   - Staring
   - Stiffening of the body
   - Excessive swallowing
   - Profuse sweating
   - Teeth clenching or grinding
   - Tongue biting
   - Tremors
   - Twitching
   - Difficulty breathing
   - Racing heart

If a patient is suffering from a seizure, it is important that the radiographer not touch the patient unless the patient is in danger of falling. Any items near the patient that could harm him or her should be moved away. The radiographer should call for medical assistance.

Diabetes is another type of medical condition that can result in a medical emergency in the radiology department. It is important for the radiographer to be aware of the types of diabetic conditions, signs and symptoms of different diabetic emergencies, and the appropriate response for those emergencies. Patients with diabetes can either have Type 1 or Type 2. Type 2 diabetes, previously termed *adult-onset* or *non–insulin-dependent*, is the most common type. Patients with Type 2 diabetes either do not produce enough insulin or the cells do not use the insulin produced. The cause of Type 2 diabetes is not known, but obesity, heart disease, and other conditions are thought to be contributory factors. If Type 2 diabetes is not properly treated, the condition can be life threatening. It is important to note that Type 2 diabetes can occur in children as well as adults.

Type 1 diabetes, previously referred to as *juvenile-onset* or *insulin-dependent*, is a chronic condition. Patients with this form do not produce enough or produce no insulin in the pancreas, prohibiting cells from using glucose. Although Type 1 diabetes often occurs in children, it can be diagnosed at any age. The causative factors may include genetics or viral infections; however, the primary causes are unknown.

Patients with either type of diabetes can suffer from dangerous medical emergencies as a result of their insulin and glucose levels.

- Diabetic hypoglycemia[6]: This condition occurs when there is an excess amount of insulin and blood glucose levels are low. The causes include taking excess insulin or dose of diabetes medications and skipping meals. If diabetic hypoglycemia is not treated promptly, it can result in seizures, loss of consciousness, and coma. The signs and symptoms include: tremors, dizziness, sweating, hunger, irritability, nervousness, headache, and rapid heartbeat. Other signs and symptoms include blurred vision, confusion, drowsiness, muscle weakness, and slurred speech. The initial treatment for this condition is the administration of food or, preferably, glucose tablets. If the condition does not improve, emergency treatment is required. The radiographer should call for medical assistance immediately if diabetic hypoglycemia is suspected. This condition can occur especially for diabetics who are having gastrointestinal or genitourinary studies which require fasting and preprocedure bowel preparations.
- Diabetic ketoacidosis[7]: Diabetic ketoacidosis occurs when the body produces high levels of ketones, which are blood acids. The production of ketones

occurs when there is an insufficient amount of insulin in the body; consequently, cells cannot use glucose for energy. As an alternative, cells begin breaking down fats, which produces a toxic byproduct: ketones. The signs and symptoms of diabetic ketoacidosis occur quickly and, if left untreated, can be life threatening. These include: excessive thirst, frequent urination, nausea, vomiting, abdominal pain, loss of appetite, weakness, shortness of breath, fruity-smelling breath, and confusion. Patients will also have high blood sugar levels and ketone levels in their urine. The causes of diabetic ketoacidosis may include illness, infections, surgery, or problems with insulin administrations. Treatment for the condition includes administration of insulin, potassium, sodium, and chloride. A radiographer should call for medical assistance immediately if this condition is suspected.

- Diabetic hyperosmolar syndrome[8]: Diabetic hyperosmolar syndrome occurs when a patient's blood sugar is in excess of 600 milligrams per deciliter. When blood sugar reaches this point, the blood becomes viscous and results in excess fluid being drawn from the body. This condition is more common in those with Type 2 diabetes but can also occur with Type 1. If left untreated or not treated properly, this condition can result in death. Signs and symptoms of this condition usually do not develop quickly but occur over an extended period of time (days to weeks). However, a radiographer should be aware of the signs and symptoms especially in older patients, those who fasted for an examination, and those with chronic illness. The signs and symptoms may include: excessive thirst, dry mouth, increased urination, warm skin with no sweating, fever, vision loss, and one-sided body weakness. A radiographer should call for immediate medical assistance.

PHARMACOLOGY[3]

Radiographers often are required to administer pharmaceutical agents during the course of a diagnostic procedure. In addition, radiographers need to be knowledgeable of patient's medication history, current medications, contraindications to the administration of radiopaque contrast media, and complications during administration of contrast media. First, it is important for a radiographer to understand basic information regarding pharmacology.

- *Pharmacokinetics* refers to the study of how drugs are absorbed, metabolized, and excreted by the body.
- *Absorption* refers to how the drug enters the circulatory system. Some drugs are absorbed through the mucosal lining (oral medications), others are absorbed through blood vessels, muscle tissue, subcutaneously, or through the dermis. If medication is directly injected into a vein or artery, there is no method of absorption required.
- *Metabolism* refers to how the body changes the drug from the form in which it was introduced into a form that can be used by the body. The metabolism of drugs commonly occurs in the liver.
- *Excretion* refers to how the drug, once it has been metabolized, exits the body. Methods by which a drug can be excreted include through urine, feces, breathing, breast milk, and exocrine glands.

Drugs can be administered in various forms, referred to as *dosage forms*; drugs can be solid, liquid, gas, and any combination of these forms. Solid dosages of drugs include tablets, capsules, suppositories, and troches. Troches are drugs in solid form in a hard sugar or glycerinated gelatin base. Troches are designed to dissolve in the mouth like a lozenge.

Patient History

Prior to performing any radiologic procedure that will require the administration of a radiopaque contrast material, it is important to gather a comprehensive medical history. This medical history is vital when deciding contrast type to administer, identifying possible drug interactions and complications, and determining the appropriate treatment if an adverse complication occurs.

Medication Reconciliation (Current Medications)

A comprehensive list of all medications being taken by the patient must be recorded. This medication list must include all prescription drugs, over-the-counter drugs, and any herbal supplements the patient is taking. For all medications, the correct name of the medication, the dose, the number of times per day taken, and the duration of the therapy must be recorded. In addition, the radiographer should record any over the counter medications that the patient takes on an as-needed basis even if they were not taken immediately prior to the procedure.

Premedications[1]

One medication that is given prior to a diagnostic procedure is glucagon. Glucagon is used to slow peristaltic activity in the gastrointestinal tract and also helps prevent cramping. Another medication that may be given prior to a radiographic examination includes an antianxiety medication such as diazepam (Valium). Patients who are required to do a preparation prior to the procedure may use a cathartic (strong laxative), suppository to initiate bowel movements, and/or cleansing enemas.[1,2,4]

Patients who might be sensitive to the administration of radiopaque contrast material may also be given antihistamine medications such as diphenhydramine (Benadryl), H_2 blockers (Tagamet), or corticosteroids (cortisone) prior to IV injection.

Contraindications

For patients who are to receive radiopaque contrast media, it is important to note any current medications that may be contraindications. Patients who are taking metformin (Glucophage) should stop the medication at least 1 day before any contrast procedure and not resume until at least 2 days postprocedure. This will reduce the risk of kidney damage due to lactic acidosis.

Scheduling and Sequencing of Examinations

The following should be the schedule of diagnostic examinations for patients undergoing multiple examinations[1,4]:

1. Any radiographic examination that DOES NOT require the use of contrast media or use of radioactive iodine
2. Radiographic examinations of the genitourinary tract
3. Radiographic examinations of the biliary system
4. Barium enema
5. Examinations of the upper gastrointestinal system including small bowel series and upper gastrointestinal tract

It is important to remember that all computed tomography (CT) examinations requiring IV contrast should be performed after any radioactive iodine studies. In addition, CT examinations of the abdomen or pelvis should be performed prior to barium procedures.

Complications/Reactions

Patients who receive radiopaque contrast media may have complications as a result of the administration of the drug or the drug itself. A radiographer needs to be able to identify administration complications as well as drug complications, specifically, allergic reactions.

Local Effects

A common method of administering drugs in the radiographic department is through IV route. Complications from this method of contrast administration include[1]:

- Infiltration—leakage/diffusion of contrast media into the surrounding tissues
- Extravasation—contrast media outside the vessel; condition is painful and dangerous
- Phlebitis—inflammation of a vein

Infiltration and *extravasation* are sometimes used interchangeably. Regardless of the terminology, the condition, when it occurs, can be dangerous. It is important to stop the injection immediately if the patient complains of discomfort or you notice swelling at the site. The radiographer should apply pressure to the area, then apply a cold pack to the area for 20 to 60 minutes. An incident report should be completed by the radiographer documenting where the infiltration occurred, the medication that was given, the dosage, and the treatment provided.

Other complications that can occur with the administration of radiopaque contrast media include aspiration during upper gastrointestinal procedures and perforation of the bowel during barium enemas. The radiographer should seek medical assistance if either of these complications occurs.

Systemic Effects

Reactions to radiopaque contrast media that do not involve the administration usually are systemic in nature. Systemic reactions to radiopaque contrast media usually occur with iodinated contrast. Rarely do patients have systemic reactions to the use of barium sulfate. Systemic reactions to iodinated contrast media can range from mild to severe; it is important for the radiographer to recognize the symptoms and respond quickly and appropriately. A systemic reaction to contrast media, if not treated properly, can result in serious medical problems or death. Reactions to contrast material generally occur within the first few seconds of administration, but some may take up to 30 minutes after injection to appear. A radiographer must continually monitor the patient throughout the procedure for signs of a reaction.

Mild[1,2]

Many patients may experience a mild reaction to contrast administration. Symptoms of mild reaction may include warmth at the site of injection, flushing, coughing, nausea, vomiting, or a metallic taste in the mouth. If a patient experiences a mild reaction, the radiographer needs to document the occurrence and monitor the patient. The symptoms usually resolve quickly and do not require any medical attention.

Moderate[1,2]

A moderate reaction to contrast media is a concern for the radiographer and requires medical attention. Signs of a moderate reaction include erythema, urticaria, and bronchospasm. Treatments for a moderate contrast reaction include antihistamines and, if needed, a bronchodilating medication. In a situation when a patient is suffering from a moderate contrast reaction, the appropriate response for the radiographer is to seek medical assistance.

Severe

If a patient suffers from the following symptoms, it is indicative of a severe reaction to contrast media: warmth, tingling, itching, dysphasia, and throat constriction. The patient will completely progress to bronchial edema, respiratory arrest, cardiac arrest, and possible seizures. This reaction, termed *anaphylactic shock*, can be fatal if the patient does not receive prompt and appropriate treatment. The radiographer needs to call for medical assistance immediately. In addition, the radiographer needs to maintain the patient's airway until medical assistance arrives. The primary medication that is administered is epinephrine.

Emergency Medications[1,2]

In all radiography departments, a crash cart is available. The content of crash carts vary, but all contain common items such as emergency medications and artificial ventilation equipment. Some common drugs found in crash carts include:

- Adrenaline (epinephrine)
- Atropine
- Glucagon
- Sodium bicarbonate
- Valium
- Sterile water

When accessing medications in a crash cart, it is vital to first verify the medication is not expired and then identify the medication with the physician prior to using. Once a crash cart is used, it must be restocked immediately.

Documentation

For all emergencies, a radiographer needs to document all aspects of the event. The information that should be documented includes: patient information, procedure name, contrast media used and amount, time reaction occurred postinjection, reaction symptoms, and treatment given.

CONTRAST MEDIA

Contrast media are used to allow visualization of structures not normally visible on radiographic images. Types of contrast media that are used in imaging include barium sulfate, air, gas, and iodinated/noniodinated contrast agents. It is important for radiographers to know the different types of contrast media used in imaging, the properties of each, the exams they are used for, and complications that can result from their use.

Types and Properties

Air and Gas[1]

Air and gas are used in imaging as a negative contrast agent. Air and gas appear black on images and allow structures to be outlined for better visualization. Air and gas are often used in conjunction with other positive contrast agents such as barium to assist in the visualization of structures. When air or gas is used with a positive contrast agent for an imaging study, the examination is termed *double contrast*. An example of a procedure that uses air for negative contrast visualization is an arthrogram. The gas that is commonly used for imaging studies is CO_2, as in myelography.

Barium Sulfate[1]

Barium sulfate is used for examinations of the gastrointestinal tract. Barium sulfate is made from a compound of inorganic salt and barium; it can be supplied in various forms: powdered, premixed solutions, concentrated solutions, and paste. Manufacturer directions regarding administration must be followed for each type of barium sulfate product. Barium sulfate may be mixed with a flavor to make it palatable to patients. For barium enema procedures, the barium sulfate is administered rectally. A primary concern for the administration of barium sulfate is the thickness or viscosity of the barium. Barium sulfate is a positive contrast agent, meaning it appears light on a radiograph. Different procedures require different viscosities; for studies of the esophagus, thicker barium, and for the colon, thinner barium. Barium sulfate does not commonly cause allergic reactions; however, once administered, it can cause problems in the bowel. Barium sulfate is *hygroscopic* (absorbs liquid) and slowly solidifies. Patients can develop impactions in the colon due to solidified barium sulfate. Prevention of impaction can be achieved with increased fluid intake after the procedure as well as administration of a laxative.

Iodinated Contrast[1]

To assist in the visualization of internal structures, iodinated contrast media can be used. Iodinated contrast media absorb more radiation than tissue or blood, thus demonstrating the structure. An iodinated contrast medium appears light on a radiograph and is termed a positive contrast agent. Iodine-based contrast media are water soluble or aqueous, meaning they can mix easily with blood or other liquids in the body. Water-soluble iodine-based contrast media are administered by injection into a blood vessel, duct, or joint.

A water-soluble iodine-based contrast medium is formed by a combination of iodine and other chemicals. The concentration of the iodine directly influences the absorption property of the material. The higher the concentration, the higher or greater amount of radiation the material can absorb. Different iodine-based contrast media with different concentrations are used for various imaging procedures.

Iodine-based contrast media is divided into two primary types, *ionic* and *nonionic*. The determination of type is based on the dissociative properties of the material. If the material dissociates into two charge particles, called *ionization*, it is termed *ionic*. Materials that do not dissociate are termed *nonionic*. The importance of this dissociation is directly related to the risk of adverse reactions in patients. Ionic water-soluble contrast media that dissociate will have a higher osmolality versus nonionic contrast media. *Osmolality* is defined as the number of particles dissolved in a solution per kilogram of water. If the osmolality of a solution is higher than blood, it changes the body's osmotic pressure and can be dangerous. An ionic contrast medium is also termed *hyperosmolar*; when it dissociates, it increases the number of particles in the blood. The lower the osmolality of a contrast medium, the less risk associated.

Another characteristic of a water-soluble iodine-based contrast medium is its viscosity. *Viscosity* is not related to whether the material is ionic or nonionic; it is primarily related to the concentration of iodine. The viscosity of the material needs to be considered when selecting needle size, rate of flow, and injection method.

Appropriateness of Contrast Media to Exam

The selection of contrast media to be used in an examination is determined by various factors including the type of examination, patient's medical condition, and laboratory values. It is important for the radiographer to recognize when alternate or modified contrast media should be used for imaging exams. The radiographer should confirm with the radiologist the type, dose, and preparation of the contrast medium being used for each individual examination prior to preparation and administration.

Patient Condition

It is important for the radiographer to review the patient's medical chart for conditions that may warrant a modification of the requested procedure. This review should occur for all contrast media examinations including barium studies. Patient conditions can alter the type, dose, or preparation of the contrast medium or may result in cancellation of the examination. If a medical condition is identified by the radiographer, it should be brought to the radiologist's attention prior to examination preparation. The following are examples of common patient conditions that affect the preparation and procedure of contrast media examinations.

Barium Studies[1]

Barium sulfate is safe to administer; however, it can cause major problems due to impaction or if it escapes beyond the confines of the gastrointestinal tract. For patients undergoing a barium enema with a diagnosis of an enlarged colon, congenital megacolon, or Hirschsprung disease, the increased surface area of the colon results in more rapid water absorption. This can lead to severe impaction. An alternative to barium sulfate for such patients is a water-based iodinated contrast medium. In addition, patients with congestive heart failure who also have megacolon are at risk for excessive fluid in the blood (*hypervolemia*). Adding normal saline instead of water to the barium when mixing can reduce the risk.

Another patient condition that can influence the choice of contrast media in gastrointestinal studies is *ostomies*. An ostomy is when a portion of the intestine is removed and the patient has an artificial opening in the abdomen called a *stoma*. The administration of the contrast is performed through the stoma, commonly using a Foley catheter instead of a rectal catheter. The amount of barium used for the procedure is commonly less than a normal barium enema examination.

Patients at risk for bowel perforation, such as the elderly or patients with ulcerative colitis, are at increased risk for perforation during barium enema examinations. For the colon, a perforation can cause barium to enter the peritoneal cavity, resulting in barium peritonitis. To reduce the risk, the enema bag can be lowered to decrease the pressure or a water-soluble contrast medium can be used instead of barium.

Laboratory Values[1]

Prior to the injection of IV contrast media, patients must have completed a series of laboratory tests. These tests are primarily done to evaluate kidney function to determine type of contrast to be administered. The common laboratory values that are evaluated are blood urea nitrogen (BUN) or serum urea nitrogen, creatine, and glomerular filtration rate (GFR). Each of these tests evaluates the function of the kidneys. If a patient is suffering from compromised kidney function, the laboratory values will be higher than normal. When evaluating laboratory values, it is important to reference the normal range as provided by the laboratory conducting the test; normal ranges can vary by laboratory.

Patient Education

It is the responsibility of the radiographer to provide patient education before, during, and after contrast media procedures. The radiographer should maintain constant communication with the patient throughout the procedure, assessing the patient's condition and relating any concerns to the radiologist. Prior to the procedure, it is important for the radiographer to explain what will occur throughout the examination. It is also important for the radiographer to verify the patient understands the procedure and respond to any questions or concerns. The radiographer should answers questions related to the procedure; however, if a question is beyond the radiographer's scope of practice or the radiographer is not sure of the answer, the radiologist should be consulted before continuing with the examination. Prior to discharging the patient, the radiographer should educate the patient on postprocedural care and what to do in case any problems arise postprocedure. Examples of postprocedural instructions may include increasing fluid intake after a barium enema procedure, monitoring the injection site for signs of infection post-IV contrast administration, and being aware of signs of impaction after administration of barium sulfate. The radiographer should provide the patient with appropriate contact information in case a problem arises.

Verify Informed Consent

Prior to the administration of contrast media, it is required for the patient to be thoroughly informed of the procedure, including the risks, benefits, and alternatives of having the procedure performed. Each facility varies regarding who is responsible for providing this information to the patient; however, it is the responsibility of the radiographer to ensure the patient fully understands the procedure prior to beginning the examination. It is also the radiographer's responsibility to verify that a properly completed and signed consent form is in the patient's chart prior to beginning the procedure. If a consent form is not in the chart or the patient is still unsure about any aspect of the procedure, the examination should be stopped and the radiologist consulted.

Instructions Regarding Preparation, Diet, and Medications

Patients who will be undergoing diagnostic examinations that require contrast media administration have to be properly prepped prior to the examination. Instructions for patient preparation are commonly provided at the time the appointment is scheduled; however, the radiographer needs to be aware of appropriate preparation for each examination.

For examinations that involved imaging of the abdomen, a patient must follow a low-residue diet prior to the examination. In addition, patients should be encouraged to increase fluid intake several days before the examination. The day prior to the examination, the patient should follow a clear liquid diet, and 8 to 12 hours prior to the examination, patients are asked to fast. For patients undergoing barium enema examinations, a cathartic is commonly administered to cleanse the bowel. A complement to a cathartic, and sometimes used as an alternative, is a cleansing enema. Administration of a cleansing enema may be performed at home by the patient or in the department by the radiographer prior to the examination.

It is common for facilities to provide patients written instructions that include appropriate preparation for the examination. In addition, facilities commonly provide instructions regarding medication prior to the procedure. Most often, patients are instructed to not take any medications the morning of the procedure.

Venipuncture

IV administration of contrast media requires access to a vein. State laws and individual facilities vary regarding who is permitted to inject IV contrast media during diagnostic examinations. All radiographers should be aware of venous anatomy, the supplies required for IV injection, and how to perform venipuncture.

Venous Anatomy[1,3]

Veins are used for the injection of contrast media because their superficiality makes them easier to access. The veins that are commonly used are located in the arm or hand. Common veins used include:

- Cephalic vein
- Basilic vein
- Brachial vein
- Accessory cephalic vein
- Median cubital vein
- Median antebrachial vein

The selection of a vein should be based on viability and size. The antecubital veins located in the arm are commonly used for contrast administration; however, overuse of these veins can cause them to be scarred and difficult to use. A thorough assessment of available veins should be performed prior to choosing a site; this should include visual inspection, palpation, and questioning of the patient to determine which veins are commonly used for blood draw or other procedures.

Supplies

The equipment used for IV contrast administration may vary by facility, examination type, or patient condition. Common supplies needed for contrast administration include the following:

- Gloves
- Alcohol wipes
- Disinfectant for the skin (per facility protocol)
- Syringe
- Needle for drawing contrast media
- Needle for venipuncture (commonly a butterfly set)
- Tubing if not included with butterfly needle
- Tape

It is important for radiographers to verify at each facility what supplies are used for IV contrast injection. Variations may also be required for different types of contrast media used, patient size, age, or radiologist preference.

Procedural Technique

When a patient is to undergo IV contrast injection, a strict technique should be followed to prevent infection. The following is an example of how to access for IV contrast administration[1]:

Drawing of contrast agent:

1. Check the label on the contrast agent to verify name, dose, and expiration date
2. Record lot number in chart for contrast agent
3. Attach the needle to the syringe if required
4. Pull back on the syringe to the desired dose
5. Insert needle into vial and inject air
6. Tip vial and draw out appropriate dose of contrast into the syringe
7. Remove needle from vial
8. Place syringe on sterile surface

Accessing vein for contrast administration:

1. Gather all required materials for IV access
2. Locate vein to be accessed
3. Apply tourniquet
4. Put on gloves
5. Disinfect area
6. Insert needle at an angle, bevel up, into vein
7. Verify blood return
8. Secure needle to arm with tape

Administration

Contrast media can be administered numerous ways including oral, IV, and instilled. The method of contrast media administration is determined by examination type and, sometimes, also patient condition. Radiographers must be familiar with all forms of contrast administration.

Routes

Contrast for IV studies is administered through injection into a vein. Injection of contrast can also be done for other examinations, including intrathecal, as is done in myelography. Oral contrast administration is achieved by mouth; instilled contrast can be done through the rectum, stoma, or nasogastric/nasoenteric tubes.

Supplies

For contrast administration for barium enemas, the following supplies are required:

- Barium sulfate (usually premeasured in a bag)
- Water for mixing barium sulfate
- Tubing
- Enema catheter with a retention balloon
- Gloves
- Lubricant to aid in catheter insertion
- IV pole
- Sheet to cover the patient
- Bedpan if needed

REVIEW QUESTIONS

1. A patient presents to the emergency department after a motor vehicle accident (MVA) by ambulance; she is conscious but has multiple injuries. The patient seems disoriented and confused regarding her whereabouts. She cannot tell the ER staff her name or date of birth (DOB). The patient requires medical treatment to stabilize her injuries. What type of consent would this situation result in?

   a. Informed
   b. Oral
   c. Implied
   d. None, she cannot be treated

2. What legal doctrine requires the burden of proof to be on the defendant?

   a. Malpractice
   b. Res ipsa loquitur
   c. Respondeat superior
   d. Civil tort

3. Which of the following would be considered a block to good communication?

   a. Standing 3 ft from the patient
   b. Using gentle touch when speaking with a patient
   c. Using nonmedical terminology to explain a procedure
   d. Providing advice regarding medical care

4. Which of the following is an example of positive nonverbal communication?

   a. Looking puzzled in response to a patient's answer to a question
   b. Standing with arms tightly crossed across the chest
   c. Not providing direct eye contact
   d. Standing very close to the person

5. The virulence of a microorganism to a person is defined as:

   a. How likely pathogen will infect the patient
   b. Severity of the infection
   c. Multiplication of the infection
   d. Immune response required to fight the microorganism

6. The most common nosocomial infection occurs in the _____.

   a. Gastrointestinal tract
   b. Respiratory tract
   c. Urinary tract
   d. Lymphatic system

7. To aid in the transfer of a nonambulatory patient, which of the following devices can be used to move the patient from the gurney to the radiography table when a gap is present between them?

   a. Pigg-O-Stat
   b. Hoyer lift
   c. Log roller
   d. Slideboard

8. When performing a patient transfer, there are five rules to follow. Which one of the following is not one of these rules?

   a. Use a broad base of support
   b. Lift with the knees
   c. Keep heavy loads close to the body
   d. Pull an object if possible

9. Confusion, blacking out, and sensing strong smells can all be signs of which of the following medical emergencies?

   a. Seizure
   b. Stroke
   c. MI
   d. Cyanosis

10. After a contrast emergency in the radiography department, the radiographer must do which of the following?

    a. Document the type of contrast given
    b. Document the reaction
    c. Document the response to the emergency
    d. All listed should be done

11. This refers to how a drug is removed from the body.

    a. Pharmacokinetics
    b. Metabolism
    c. Excretion
    d. Pharmaceuticals

12. Prior to a radiographic contrast procedure, patients are commonly asked to refrain from taking metformin _____ prior to the procedure.

    a. 8 to 12 hours
    b. 1 day
    c. 3 days
    d. 2 hours

13. A severe reaction to contrast media may be indicated by which of the following:

    a. Cirrhosis
    b. Atelectasis
    c. Giardiasis
    d. Bronchial edema

14. Patients with a suspected perforated bowel should have which of the following modifications to the procedure?

    a. Raising the enema bag to increase flow
    b. Use of oil-based contrast
    c. Use of water-soluble contrast
    d. Use of standard barium sulfate but without air contrast

15. Ionic contrast material increases the number of particles dissolved in the blood and is termed:

    a. Hyperosmolar
    b. Hypo-osmolar
    c. Water soluble
    d. Hypervolemic

REFERENCES

1. Ehrlich RA, Daly JA. *Patient Care in Radiography with an Interlocution to Medical Imaging.* 7th ed. St. Louis, MO: Mosby; 2009.

2. Torres LS, Linn-Watson Norcutt T, Dutton AG. *Basic Medical Techniques and Patient Care in Imaging Technology.* 7th ed. Baltimore, MD: Lippincott Williams & Wilkins; 2003.

3. Jensen SC, Peppers MP. *Pharmacology and Drug Administration for Imaging Technologists.* 2nd ed. St. Louis, MO: Mosby; 2006.

4. Adler AM, Carlton RR. *Introduction to Radiologic Sciences and Patient Care.* 4th ed. St. Louis, MO: Saunders; 2007.

5. Trolley Gurley L, Callaway WJ. *Introduction to Radiologic Technology.* 6th ed. St. Louis, MO: Mosby; 2006.

6. Living with diabetes: hypoglycemia (low blood glucose). American Diabetes Association Web site. http://www.diabetes.org/living-with-diabetes/ treatment-and-care/blood-glucose-control/ hypoglycemia-low-blood.html. Accessed February 5, 2011.

7. Living with diabetes: ketoacidosis (DKA). American Diabetes Association Web site. http://www.diabetes .org/living-with-diabetes/complications/ketoacidosis- dka.html. Accessed February 5, 2011.

8. Living with diabetes: hyperosmolar hyperglycemic nonketotic syndrome (HHNS). American Diabetes Association Web site. http://www.diabetes.org/living- with-diabetes/complications/hyperosmolar- hyperglycemic.html. Accessed February 5, 2011.

APPENDIX A

Answers to Review Questions

Note: There are no questions in Chapter 1.

CHAPTER 2

1. **B**

   When irradiation occurs in the human body, the resulting effect will either be a direct or indirect action. The human body is composed of approximately 80% water and therefore is more prone to damaging effects caused by radiation. Indirect action indicates that the x-ray photon interacts with a water molecule, which results in the creation of ions and reactive free radicals. These resulting ions and free radicals have the ability to produce toxic substances to cause biologic damage.

2. **D**

   Photoelectric absorption produces ionizing radiation through the interaction of the incoming x-ray photon and an inner-shell electron and energy transfer. Movement of electrons through this interaction results in ionization and therefore useful radiation to produce x-ray images. Compton scattering results in scatter of radiation in all directions, which becomes a consideration for the protection of patients and medical personnel during radiologic procedures.

3. **C**

   Through ionization of water molecules, x-ray photons in the human body may cause separation of these molecules into other components. With a positive water molecule (HOH+), the resulting smaller molecules will produce H+ (hydrogen ion) and OH*. With a negative water molecule (HOH−), the smaller molecules will produce an OH− and an H*. The free radicals OH* and H* are volatile for the short time that they are present and have the ability to break chemical bonds, resulting in further biologic damage.

4. **B**

   The phase of cell division in which damage to chromosomes can be evaluated is metaphase. At no other phase can this damage be seen to chromosomes.

5. **A**

   In vivo refers to changes occurring in the living human body.

6. **C**

   Through observations of populations who have experienced an acute exposure to radiation, studies have shown that survivors and descendents of survivors demonstrate genetic mutations, develop cancer, and may not be able to reproduce.

7. **B**

   Immature cells and tissues with a high metabolic rate are at a higher risk for genetic mutation because of their increased ability to enter into the cell division cycle.

8. **A**

   LET is the amount of energy that is transferred from ionizing radiation to soft tissue and is another method for expressing the quality of the radiation as it relates to radiation protection. As LET increases, so does the ability of the radiation used to cause a damaging biologic response.

9. **A**

   When radiation is administered over a long period of time, the effect of a large dose is lessened. The continual dosing of radiation through protraction allows for less effect because the body is allowed time for repair of cellular organisms as well as recovery of tissues affected.

10. **A**

    Bone marrow contains stem cells which are more immature than epithelial cells of the skin. Immature cells are more available to enter into the cell cycle through rapid cell division.

11. C

Generally speaking, tissue that is irradiated in a fully oxygenated environment is more radiosensitive than tissue in an anoxic environment.

12. A

The response that is seen is directly related to the dose that is administered. In a nonthreshold dose-response relationship, any dose that is given is expected to produce a response. A radiation dose that is doubled will result in a response to that dose doubling as well.

13. D

Lethal dose administered to a population resulting in 50% of population dying within 60 days is referred to as $LD_{50/60}$. It is expected that if death is to occur postirradiation, it will happen within 60 days of exposure. Acute radiation lethality in humans is approximately 350 rad (3.5 Gy).

14. B

In terms of administering compounds that would protect human beings from acute radiation exposure, the amount that would have to be administered to a human in an acute event would be considered toxic to humans and would be worse than the radiation exposure itself.

15. D

Leakage radiation must be minimized within the protective tube housing. Federal regulation mandates that leakage radiation must not exceed 100 mR/h at a distance of 1 m from the protective tube housing.

CHAPTER 3

1. B

mA controls the quantity of radiation produced.

2. B

The charge of the anode is positive.

3. A

The filament produces electrons.

4. C

The outer edge of the anode is constructed of tungsten.

5. D

AEC measures the amount of radiation reaching the image detector.

6. A

Proper patient positioning is specifically important when using AEC because the part being imaged must be over the selected detector for the AEC to work properly and to not underexpose or overexpose the anatomy.

7. A

The collimator is the most common device used by the RT.

8. D

When x-radiation is produced, there are critical elements that must occur in order for radiation to be emitted from the x-ray tube. These three elements include:

1. The source of the free electrons, which are released from the focusing cup of the tube as a result of thermionic emission
2. The focusing of these electrons to be accelerated from the cathode to the anode through use of kV
3. The target of the anode, which acts as the site of the interaction of projectile electrons, which results in deceleration and causes them to either slow down as they come close to the nuclear field or to interact with the orbital electrons located in the target atom

9. C

At the target, the projectile electrons do not have enough energy to knock the outer-shell electrons out of orbit or to ionize them; rather, the interaction is enough to cause excitation of these outer-shell electrons and raise their energy levels. With this excitation and need to level off their raised energy level, outer-shell electrons emit a large amount of infrared heat or radiation, which is equal to approximately 99% of the kinetic energy of the initial projectile electrons. The remaining less than 1% of kinetic energy is available for the production of x-radiation.

10. B

The remaining less than 1% of kinetic energy is available for the production of x-radiation. Bremsstrahlung radiation refers to the interaction of the projectile electron that is influenced by the nuclear field of the target atom. Characteristic radiation refers to the interaction of the projectile electron with a k-orbit electron in the target that results in ionization.

11. **A**

Characteristic radiation refers to the interaction of the projectile electron with an inner-shell electron and results in ionization and production of x-radiation.

12. **D**

Bremsstrahlung radiation refers to the interaction of the projectile electron that is influenced by the nuclear field of the target atom.

13. **A**

The amount of energy that comes from Bremsstrahlung radiation is dependent on what kV is used for the exposure; brems can be produced at any projectile electron energy. Therefore, the range of energies is wide when associated with these types of interactions and depends on electron speed and proximity to nucleus.

14. **B**

The greater the brems, the closer the projectile electron is to the nuclear field of the target atom.

15. **B**

The majority of radiation that is produced at the target atom is classified as Bremsstrahlung because of its wide range of energies at various kV values.

CHAPTER 4

1. **D**

Spatial resolution can be defined as the amount of detail in a digital image which is measured in pixels.

2. **B**

Sampling rate describes how many times along a scan line the information is sampled in pixels per millimeter.

3. **A**

DEL is a term used in DR to determine the size of the electronic charge detector.

4. **C**

Each pixel has a numerical value and is represented as a brightness level on a digital image.

5. **D**

Quantum mottle is displayed as image noise or grainy appearance and is caused by lack of photons reaching the image receptor.

6. **A**

Signal-to-noise is expressed as a ratio comparing two components of an image (image and noise). The higher the signal-to-noise ratio, the better the image.

7. **D**

Contrast-to-noise ratio refers to the overall grayscale quality of an image and how an image is perceived by the viewer.

8. **D**

Film sensitivity is a result of grain size; finer-grained films are less sensitive than larger-grained films.

9. **A**

The process for capturing a digital radiographic image is similar to the digital photographic process where an image is exposed to radiation on a flat plate called a detector. In CR, the image is then extracted by a system with a photomultiplier tube; in DR, the image is directly connected electronically and converted to a digital image.

10. **B**

Patient information is available and is entrusted to the radiographer and should be kept confidential.

11. **D**

Radiographs should be able to be stored indefinitely if processed in the correct temperature and dilution of film-processing solutions. Also, films should be stored in low humidity, free of warm and cold temperatures.

12. **C**

During film processing, developer reacts with emulsion, turning halide crystals of a latent image to black metallic silver.

13. **B**

Water is used to wash the film after it comes out of the fixer and also is used to help maintain the proper development temperature by heat exchangers.

14. **A**

Grayscale rendition records all intensity values in a radiographic image; these values form an LUT.

15. **C**

Histogram equalization is where the digital system attempts to normalize the image to help increase the contrast.

16. **B**

Edge enhancement increases the brightness along edges of the pixels, which increases the spatial resolution.

17. **A**

It takes nearby pixel values and averages them, which also can lower the image contrast and reduce noise.

18. **B**

The process of changing contrast will reflect on the number of shades of gray that is displayed. The number of shades of gray is reduced when the displayed contrast of the image is increased.

19. **D**

Ghosting occurs when the IP is exposed and is processed; a faint image of a previous exam is shown along with a normally exposed image.

20. **D**

DICOM GSDF is a standard within DICOM to derive a common (consistent) grayscale standard that can be used between different manufacturers when viewing images.

21. **A**

PACS in radiography is an abbreviation for picture archiving and communication system. It is a system where digital images, patient data, and other information can be stored and delivered to various sites through a digital network.

22. **B**

HL7 is a standard (universal language) that is networked for the exchanging, sharing, and retrieval of electronic health information such as clinical, administrative, and financial information in a medical center.

23. **D**

In CR, the imaging plate is subject to problems on rollers, which can contain dirt and dust that can accumulate on the IP, imaging optics, and guide plates. Film artifacts are also caused by physical handling.

24. **C**

Once a film is exposed and processed, there can be no further changes to the film, whereas a digital image can be manipulated and therefore has a larger acceptable range of exposure.

CHAPTER 5

1. **D**

The heart is closer to the IR in the PA projection, which reduces OID, therefore reducing magnification of the cardiac shadow and enabling a truer representation of heart size versus the AP position.

2. **A**

Patient is already in upright position, so begin with the upright projections followed by the supine projections.

3. **C**

The medial oblique would best demonstrate the trochlea located medially in the elbow.

4. **C**

A 15-degree to 20-degree internal rotation of the ankle brings the intermalleolar line parallel to the IR and opens the mortise.

5. **A**

A shorter person would have a wider pelvis.

6. **B**

The head and neck are rotated anteriorly 15 degrees to 20 degrees. Internally rotating the entire leg will place the neck parallel for a true AP hip.

7. **D**

The 45-degree oblique allows the intervertebral foramina to open because the foramina are situated 45 degrees to the MSP.

8. **A**

Unlike the cervical obliques, the T-spine obliques demonstrate the superior/inferior articulating joint.

9. **C**

Flexion/extension laterals will demonstrate the mobility of the spine status post (s/p) fusion.

10. **D**

A 25-degree caudal angle exiting the nasion will demonstrate the petrous ridges below the orbital floor.

11. **B**

The LPO position allows the stomach to move away from the spine, barium to settle in the fundus, but air in the body and pylorus.

12. **B**

The RPO position would open the left splenic flexure, and the LPO position would open the right hepatic flexure.

13. **A**

Obliques demonstrate the up side kidney and the down side ureter.

14. **C**

When barium fills the ileocecal valve, barium has traveled through the entire small bowel.

15. **D**

The RAO would best demonstrate the esophagus between the heart and spine because rotating the patient moves the esophagus away from the spine and placing the patient PA rather than AP brings the esophagus closer to the IR.

CHAPTER 6

1. **C**

   The patient cannot provide written, informed consent because of her injuries but is present in the hospital and needs to have immediate care to treat her injuries.

2. **B**

   Res ipsa loquitur requires the defendant to prove he or she was not negligent.

3. **D**

   Providing advice regarding medical care can disrupt proper communication with a patient.

4. **A**

   A puzzled look can be helpful when a patient responds to a question.

5. **A**

   Virulence is the degree of pathogenicity of a microorganism or how likely it is that it will cause disease.

6. **C**

   The most common nosocomial infection occurs in the urinary tract due to urinary catheters.

7. **D**

   Slideboard is used to close the gap between the patient and the x-ray table.

8. **D**

   It is best not to pull an object but to push an object.

9. **A**

   Confusion, blacking out, and sensing strong smells are all indicative of a seizure.

10. **D**

    After a contrast reaction the radiographer should document the type of contrast given, the reaction that occurred, and what response (treatment) was done.

11. **C**

    Excretion is how a drug is removed from the body.

12. **B**

    Metformin (Glucophage) should be stopped 1 day prior to the procedure.

13. **D**

    Bronchial edema occurs with a severe reaction to contrast media.

14. **C**

    Water-soluble contrast should be used for patients with a suspected perforated bowel.

15. **A**

    Hyperosmolar means that, when it dissociates, it increases the number of particles in the blood.

APPENDIX B
Comprehensive Exam 1

1. Renal calculi will be better demonstrated when the patient is _____?

   a. Supine
   b. Prone
   c. Lateral
   d. Erect

2. For radiographic procedures, radiographers should don proper protective shielding, including:

   a. Lead apron of minimum 0.25 millimeter (mm) lead equivalent
   b. Lead gloves of minimum 0.5 centimeter (cm) lead equivalent
   c. Thyroid shields of minimum 0.5 mm lead equivalent
   d. Lead glasses of minimum 0.25 cm lead equivalent

3. A consent form must contain which of the following?

   a. Name of the facility
   b. Name of the physician
   c. Name of the procedure
   d. All of the choices must be present on a consent form

4. When performing an image of an axial sacroiliac (SI) joint, what degree of angulation is appropriate for women?

   a. No angle is necessary
   b. 35-degree angle
   c. 30-degree angle
   d. 25-degree angle

5. The component that controls the amount of penetrating energy in an x-ray is:

   a. Kilovoltage (kV) controller
   b. Milliampere (mA) controller
   c. Timer
   d. kV and timer controller

6. Which of the following is described as the degree of blackening on a radiograph?

   a. Density
   b. Contrast
   c. Recorded detail
   d. Distortion

7. The National Council on Radiation Protection and Measurements (NCRP) mandates which of the following?

   a. Source-to-image distance (SID) should be no less than 15″ (inches) for stationary fluoroscopes
   b. SID should be no less than 12″ for mobile fluoroscopes
   c. Source-skin distance (SSD) should be no less than 12″ for mobile fluoroscopes
   d. SSD should be no less than 10″ for stationary fluoroscopes

8. Why should a patient remain erect for a minimum of 5 minutes when having imaging of an erect abdomen performed?

   a. Demonstrate calculi
   b. Demonstrate air-fluid levels
   c. Demonstrate the diaphragm
   d. Demonstrate the psoas muscles

9. The type of radiation that is responsible for the formation of an image is:

   a. Leakage
   b. Primary
   c. Scatter
   d. Remnant

10. What angle direction is appropriate for the axial SI joint view when the patient is supine?

    a. Cephalic
    b. Caudal
    c. Tangential
    d. Transverse

11. The anode in an x-ray tube:

    a. Is a rotating disk and is charged negatively
    b. Is a rotating disk and is charged positively
    c. Is a rotating disk and contains a filament
    d. Is a rotating disk and has no charge

12. Assault is defined as:

    a. Threatening to restrain a patient if he or she does not cooperate
    b. Applying a tourniquet to a patient without obtaining consent for an intravenous injection
    c. Using positioning aides during the exam
    d. Physically harming a patient

13. What angle direction is appropriate for the axial SI joint view when the patient is prone?

    a. Tangential
    b. Transverse
    c. Caudal
    d. Cephalic

14. The action from irradiation of water molecules in the human body that results in the creation of ions and reactive free radicals is known as:

    a. *Direct effect*
    b. *Indirect effect*
    c. *Target theory*
    d. None of these

15. Most x-ray tubes contain two different-sized wires that emit electrons, called _____.

    a. A *focusing cup*
    b. *Filaments*
    c. The *target*
    d. A *cathode*

16. A three-way abdomen consists of:

    a. Erect abdomen, decubitus, and supine abdomen
    b. Lateral abdomen, decubitus, and erect abdomen
    c. Posteroanterior (PA) chest, lateral abdomen, and left lateral decubitus abdomen
    d. PA chest, erect abdomen, and supine abdomen

17. The outer edge of an anode contains the target, which is made of _____.

    a. Tungsten
    b. Copper
    c. Steel
    d. Nickel

18. Useful ionizing radiation that is produced through the energy transfer between the incoming x-ray photon and inner-shell electron is known as:

    a. Characteristic
    b. Coherent
    c. Compton
    d. Photoelectric effect

19. Which of the following does not affect radiographic density?

    a. Milliamperes per second (mA/s)
    b. Kilovoltage peak (kVp)
    c. Object-to-image distance (OID)
    d. None listed

20. Which of the following would not be demonstrated on a soft tissue analog neck radiograph?

    a. Adenitis
    b. Epiglottitis
    c. Vertebral fracture
    d. Foreign body

21. When a patient has a DNR, which of the following is true?

    a. No efforts can be made to assist the patient once the patient has gone into cardiac or respiratory arrest
    b. All lifesaving methods can be done until the patient dies
    c. Patient can be given oxygen via a respirator only
    d. If the patient's heart stops, he or she cannot receive CPR but can be given defibrillator paddles

22. A rotating anode is an:

    a. Induction motor made of low-heat-resistance material
    b. Induction motor containing a stator and rotor
    c. Induction motor containing aluminum bars
    d. Induction motor containing the filament

23. A major consideration during radiologic procedures associated with protection of patients and medical personnel is:

    a. Characteristic
    b. Compton
    c. Coherent
    d. Photoelectric

24. At what level will you center for an antero-posterior (AP) axial SI joint?

    a. At the level of the anterior superior iliac spine (ASIS)
    b. At the level of the crest
    c. Directed to the apex of the sacrum
    d. 2″ below the ASIS

25. A pathogen that is contracted and starts to multiply is termed a(n):

    a. *Normal flora*
    b. *Colonized pathogen*
    c. *Infectious pathogen*
    d. *Transient pathogen*

26. A _____ angle is required to open the metatarsophalangeal (MTP) joints.

    a. 10-degree posterior
    b. 10-degree caudal
    c. 15-degree caudal
    d. 20-degree posterior

27. With a positive water molecule (HOH+) from radiolysis, the smaller molecules will produce the following:

    a. Hydrogen radical (H*) and hydroxyl radical (OH*)
    b. Hydroxyl ion (OH−) and H*
    c. Hydrogen ion (H+) and OH*
    d. OH* and H*

28. *Pes cavus* refers to _____.

    a. Pes planus
    b. Flat feet
    c. Pigeon chest
    d. A high arch

29. Which of the following is true of automatic exposure control (AEC)?

    a. Measures the correct amount of radiation reaching an image detector
    b. Doesn't use a backup timer
    c. Cannot be adjusted in small increments
    d. Usually has one sensor

30. The virulence of a microorganism to a person is defined as:

    a. Severity of the infection
    b. How likely it is that the pathogen will infect the patient
    c. Immune response required to fight the microorganism
    d. Multiplication of the infection

31. Proper positioning is an important factor when using AEC.

    a. True
    b. False

32. Patients with pes cavus require _____ when having a dorsoplantar foot radiograph performed.

    a. No angle
    b. 5-degree angle
    c. 10-degree angle
    d. 15-degree angle

33. As mA/s increases, what happens to density?

    a. Density does not change
    b. Density decreases
    c. Density increases

34. With a negative water molecule (HOH−) from radiolysis, the smaller molecules will produce the following:

    a. H* and OH*
    b. H+ and H*
    c. OH* and H*
    d. OH− and H*

35. What positioning error has been made if the occipital bone is superimposed over the odontoid, for the open mouth view?

    a. The head was flexed too much
    b. The head was extended too much
    c. The tube wasn't angled
    d. The patient was prone

36. False imprisonment is:

    a. Using a Pigg-O-Stat to restrain a child
    b. Unlawful touching of a patient
    c. Failing to assist a patient during an exam
    d. Applying a vest restraint without written medical order

37. The control that allows an imaging specialist the ability to determine and adjust exposure values is:

    a. AEC
    b. Manual exposure control
    c. Backup timer
    d. Automatic collimation

38. The PA method for imaging the dens is the _____.

    a. AP axial
    b. AP oblique
    c. Judd
    d. Wagging jaw

39. The resulting free radicals that have the ability to break chemical bonds and result in biologic damage are:

    a. H* and OH*
    b. OH− and H*
    c. H+ and OH*
    d. H− and OH*

40. Which of the following is a beam restriction device?

    a. Aperture diaphragm
    b. Collimator
    c. Cone
    d. All of these

41. Patients with pes planus require _____ when having a dorsoplantar foot radiograph performed.

    a. No angle
    b. 5-degree angle
    c. 10-degree angle
    d. 15-degree angle

42. This type of interview is based on simple, one-answer questions.

    a. Open
    b. Closed
    c. Structured
    d. Unstructured

43. The main controlling factors of density are:

    a. mA and mA/s
    b. kVp and mA/s
    c. mA and time
    d. kVp and SID

44. Tissues that are _____ with a _____ metabolic rate are more radioresistant.

    a. Mature, low
    b. Mature, high
    c. Immature, low
    d. Immature, high

45. On a dorsoplantar radiograph, what anatomy should appear free of superimposition?

    a. 1st metatarsal only
    b. 1st and 2nd metatarsals
    c. 3rd through 5th metatarsals
    d. 5th metatarsal only

46. Health Insurance Portability and Accountability Act (HIPAA) consent can be used to cover all medical procedures.

    a. True
    b. False

47. A beam restriction device _____.

    a. Reduces patient exposure and improves image quality
    b. Reduces patient exposure and can be a manual or automatic collimator
    c. Improves image quality and can be a manual or automatic collimator
    d. Reduces patient exposure, improves image quality, and can be a manual or automatic collimator

48. Why would PA cervical obliques be preferred over AP?

    a. Decreases the thyroid dose
    b. Better demonstrates the odontoid
    c. Better demonstrates fractures
    d. Opens the joint space

49. Tissues that are _____ with a _____ metabolic rate are less radiosensitive.

    a. Immature, low
    b. Immature, high
    c. Mature, low
    d. Mature, high

50. The basis for res ipsa loquitur states:

    a. Facility is responsible for the employee
    b. Negligence caused the resulting injury
    c. Employee is protected against malpractice when working at a facility
    d. All patients must be treated equally

51. What should be done to place the femoral neck parallel for a true AP hip/femur?

    a. The neck is naturally parallel
    b. Externally rotate the leg
    c. Internally rotate the entire leg
    d. Rotate the leg and angle to tube

52. What allows the selection of voltages to produce an x-ray?

    a. Step-up transformer
    b. Step-down transformer
    c. Direct current (DC) transformer
    d. Autotransformer

53. "Different combinations of mA and time that produce the same mA/s will produce the same density" describes which law?

    a. The law of linearity
    b. The law of reciprocity
    c. The law of reproducibility
    d. None of these

54. What view would best demonstrate the cuboid?

    a. Medial oblique foot
    b. Lateral oblique
    c. Axial view
    d. It is difficult to demonstrate the cuboid

55. Tissues that are _____ with a _____metabolic rate are less radioresistant.

    a. Immature, high
    b. Immature, low
    c. Mature, high
    d. Mature, low

56. The time when symptoms of the illness begin to disappear and the patient returns to a normal state of health is termed:

    a. *Incubation*
    b. *Prodromal*
    c. *Convalescence*
    d. *Transient*

57. What is the angle of the neck to shaft on a femur in the average adult?

    a. 10 degrees
    b. 15 degrees to 20 degrees
    c. 90 degrees
    d. 125 degrees

58. For an x-ray tube to generate an x-ray, the incoming power needs to be converted from _____ to _____.

    a. DC to alternating current (AC)
    b. AC to DC
    c. AEC to _____ meson exchange current (MEC)
    d. Single phase to three phase

59. As linear energy transfer (LET) increases, _____ increases.

    a. Megaelectron voltage (MeV)
    b. Relative biologic effectiveness (RBE)
    c. K-edge
    d. Oxygen enhancement ratio (OER)

60. What radiograph would best demonstrate anterior/posterior displacement?

    a. Lateral obliques
    b. Medial obliques
    c. Lateral radiographs
    d. Tangentials

61. Acquired infections in a health-care setting are termed:

    a. *Iatrogenic*
    b. *Transmitted*
    c. *Nosocomial*
    d. *Pathogenic*

62. "Doubling the mA/s doubles the amount of density on the resulting image" describes which law?

    a. The law of linearity
    b. The law of reciprocity
    c. The law of reproducibility
    d. None of the above

63. What view is appropriate to visualize the common sesamoid bones of the foot?

    a. 30-degree axial
    b. 45-degree axial
    c. Tangential
    d. Craniocaudal oblique

64. The power source in the United States uses _____.

    a. 50-hertz (Hz) DC
    b. 50-Hz AC
    c. 60-Hz DC
    d. 60-Hz AC

65. Gas plasma sterilization uses which of the following?

    a. Low-moisture hydrogen peroxide
    b. Toxic gases
    c. Vaporized hydrogen peroxide
    d. High temperature and dry air

66. What is the correct radiographic positioning obliquity for the thoracic spine?

    a. 70 degrees
    b. 45 degrees
    c. 30 degrees
    d. 15 degrees

67. Three-phase x-ray systems generally are used in the main radiology department for _____.

    a. Portable units only
    b. General x-ray, fluoroscopy, and angiography
    c. Fluoroscopy and angiography only
    d. General x-ray only

68. As LET decreases, _____ decreases.

    a. MeV
    b. K-edge
    c. OER
    d. RBE

69. A fracture of the vertebral body and spinous process that results from a hyperflexion force is known as _____.

    a. *Spina bifida*
    b. *Chance fracture*
    c. *Spondylolysis*
    d. *Herniated nucleus pulposus* (HNP)

70. A digital fluoroscopic unit uses flat-panel detectors that replace _____.

    a. Grids
    b. Automatic brightness control
    c. An image intensifier
    d. Three-phase power

71. The common cold is classified as what type of disease transmission?

    a. Droplet
    b. Airborne
    c. Contact
    d. Vector

72. How would a patient be positioned for the Holly method?

    a. Axial
    b. Sagittal
    c. Supine
    d. Prone

73. When continual dosing of radiation is provided at a lower rate over a long period of time, the body is allowed time for cellular repair and tissue recovery. This type of dosing is referred to as:

    a. Protraction
    b. Refraction
    c. Retraction
    d. Fractionation

74. How would a patient be positioned for the Lewis method?

    a. Supine
    b. Prone
    c. Sagittal
    d. Axial

75. When an action can have two effects, it is termed *fidelity*.

    a. True
    b. False

76. A digital imaging system that uses reusable imaging plates instead of image detectors is called _____.

    a. *Image detector array*
    b. *Indirect panel radiography*
    c. *Direct radiography*
    d. *Computed radiography* (CR)

77. Weight-bearing feet require a _____ angle.

    a. 10-degree posterior
    b. 15-degree posterior
    c. 20-degree posterior
    d. 15-degree anterior

78. What pathology involves forward slipping of one vertebra onto another?

    a. Compression fracture
    b. Chance fracture
    c. Spondylolisthesis
    d. Spondylolysis

79. Which of the following affects the quality of radiation?

    a. Time
    b. kVp
    c. mA/s
    d. mA

80. When dosing of radiation is administered in equal portions separated by 24-hour time frames, the body is allowed time for cellular repair and tissue recovery. This type of dosing is used frequently in radiation oncology and is referred to as:

    a. *Fractionation*
    b. *Protraction*
    c. *Retraction*
    d. *Refraction*

81. Pes planus and cavus are best demonstrated on _____ radiographs.

    a. Medial oblique
    b. Lateral oblique
    c. Lateral weight-bearing
    d. Tangential

82. A patient has a blood pressure (BP) of 145 over 95 millimeters of mercury (mm Hg). How would this be classified?

    a. Stage I hypertensive
    b. Stage II hypertensive
    c. Normal hypertensive
    d. Normal

83. A dedicated chest unit can be a _____.

    a. Computed, digital, and conventional film system
    b. Computed and digital radiography system
    c. Computed and conventional film system
    d. Digital and conventional film system

84. Why must the base of the 5th metatarsal be included on an ankle radiograph?

    a. The 5th metatarsal isn't required for an ankle radiograph
    b. The entire foot is required
    c. Only the mortise is required
    d. It is a common fracture site

85. Tissue that is in an environment rich in oxygen will be _____ to the effects of radiation.

    a. Unaffected
    b. Less sensitive
    c. Radioresistant
    d. Radiosensitive

86. A right posterior oblique (RPO) lumbar image will demonstrate _____.

    a. The intervertebral foramina
    b. The left zygapophyseal joints
    c. The right zygapophyseal joints
    d. The spinous processes

87. One of the differences between young and elderly patients is:

    a. Young patients have decreased cognitive impairment
    b. Young patients have increased resilience
    c. Elderly patients have a greater support system
    d. There is no difference between young and elderly patients as it pertains to health-care needs

88. The tissue in the _____ is more radioresistant than _____ tissue.

    a. Brain, bone marrow
    b. Brain, muscle
    c. Bone marrow, skin
    d. Muscle, gonadal

89. Which oblique is appropriate to demonstrate the entire mortise joint open?

    a. 45-degree internal oblique
    b. 30-degree internal oblique
    c. 15-degree to 20-degree internal rotation
    d. 5-degree internal oblique

90. A tomography unit is a system where the x-ray tube and image receptor (IR) _____.

    a. Create a pivot point or fulcrum
    b. Are stationary
    c. Move side to side
    d. Work only with film

91. Which of the following are inversely proportional?

    a. mA/s and density
    b. kVp and density
    c. Relative speed index (RSI) and density
    d. SID and density

92. Which oblique opens the distal tibiofibular joint?

    a. 15-degree to 20-degree internal rotation
    b. 30-degree internal oblique
    c. 45-degree internal oblique

93. For the cycle of infection, once a pathogen is present in an infected person, what are next steps required for the pathogen to infect a new person?

    a. Susceptible host, mode of transmission, portal of entry
    b. Portal of exit, mode of transmission, portal of entry
    c. Mode of transmission, portal of exit, susceptible host
    d. Mode of transmission, portal of entry, susceptible host

94. Which of the following accurately defines grids?

    a. They are devices that filter scatter radiation
    b. They reduce image quality
    c. They reduce image detail
    d. They are made up of aluminum strips

95. What images would assess the mobility of the lumbar spine?

    a. Axial
    b. AP
    c. Flexion/extension laterals
    d. Obliques

96. Tissue is _____ radiosensitive under low oxygen conditions and _____ radiosensitive under aerobic conditions.

    a. Less, more
    b. Less, equally
    c. More, less
    d. More, equally

97. Which of the following statements is true regarding quality assurance testing for light field and radiation field testing?

    a. Quality assurance testing is not required with digital systems
    b. Testing would include radiopaque markers on the edges of the light field, a fluorescent plate, and a plastic or aluminum tube for beam alignment
    c. Testing would include radiopaque markers on the edges of the light field and a fluorescent plate
    d. Testing would include a fluorescent plate and a plastic or aluminum tube for beam alignment.

98. A correctly positioned lateral ankle is demonstrated radiographically by:

    a. The distal fibula being free of superimposition from the tibia
    b. The proximal fibula being free of superimposition
    c. Superimposing the distal fibula over the posterior three-quarters of the tibia
    d. Superimposing the distal fibula over the posterior one-third of the tibia

99. Human responses to radiation that are considered to be a result of early or acute exposure are referred to as:

    a. *Stochastic*
    b. *Deterministic*
    c. *Hormesis*
    d. *Recovery*

100. Cultural competency requires _____ elements.

    a. Three
    b. Five
    c. Six
    d. Ten

101. When imaging a knee, what is the correct degree of angulation for a patient who measures 17 cm from ASIS to tabletop?

    a. 5 degrees caudal
    b. 5 degrees cephalic
    c. 10 degrees cephalic
    d. No angle is required

102. When x-ray equipment malfunctions:

    a. It can endanger both the patient and the operator
    b. It can endanger the operator; the error should be reported to maintenance
    c. The procedure should be stopped immediately and the error should be reported to maintenance
    d. It can endanger the patient and the operator; the procedure should be stopped immediately, and the error should be reported to maintenance

103. Human responses to radiation that are considered to be a result of late or chronic exposure are referred to as:

    a. *Stochastic*
    b. *Deterministic*
    c. *Hormesis*
    d. *Recovery*

104. What specialized view of the ankle demonstrates ligament rupture?

    a. Mortise view
    b. Lateral view
    c. Stress view
    d. Tangential

105. "The intensity of radiation is inversely proportional to the square of the distance from the x-ray source" describes which principle?

    a. Direct square law
    b. Inverse square law
    c. Radiation intensity law
    d. Density maintenance formula

106. The dose-response relationship that produces a response in a radiated population regardless of size or dose is known as:

    a. Linear, nonthreshold
    b. Linear, threshold
    c. Nonlinear, threshold
    d. Nonlinear, nonthreshold

107. What is demonstrated on an internal oblique knee?

    a. Medial tibial plateau
    b. Distal tibiofibular joint
    c. Medial condyle
    d. Head of the fibula free of superimposition

108. Aerobes require _____ to survive.

    a. Carbon dioxide
    b. Oxygen
    c. Host cell
    d. Capsule

109. Stress views performed while the patient is placed in inversion demonstrate _____.

    a. Medial ligament tear or rupture
    b. Anterior ligament tear or rupture
    c. Posterior ligament tear or rupture
    d. Lateral ligament tear or rupture

110. Digital IRs are subject to artifacts as in conventional radiography.

    a. True
    b. False

111. In high-dose fluoroscopy, skin effects are assessed using this dose-response relationship:

    a. Linear, threshold
    b. Linear, nonthreshold
    c. Nonlinear, threshold
    d. Nonlinear, nonthreshold

112. What is demonstrated on the external oblique knee?

    a. Superimposed fibula over tibia
    b. Femoral lateral condyle
    c. Tibial lateral condyle
    d. Proximal tibiofibular joint space is open

113. _____ is the normal respiratory rate for adults.

    a. 5 to 10 breaths per minute
    b. 10 to 20 breaths per minute
    c. 25 to 35 breaths per minute
    d. 60 to 80 breaths per minute

114. The dose of radiation that causes 50% of irradiated subjects to die within 30 days is referred to as:

    a. $LD_{30/50}$
    b. $LD_{50/30}$
    c. $LD_{50/50}$
    d. $LD_{30/30}$

115. A large outpouching of the esophagus would refer to:

    a. Polyp
    b. Barrett
    c. Zenker diverticulum
    d. Gastroesophageal reflux disease (GERD)

116. What is the minimum amount of air gap required to result in a visible change in density?

    a. 6″
    b. 10″
    c. 12″
    d. 14″

117. Digital imaging artifacts such as debris on IRs are usually _____.

    a. Not visible
    b. Seen as fingerprint marks
    c. Seen as dark densities
    d. Seen as light densities

118. The human application of radiosensitizing agents would _____.

    a. Be fatally toxic
    b. Double the radiation damage
    c. Decrease the effect of radiation by a ratio of 2
    d. Increase the effect of radiation by a ratio of 2

119. What are the two esophageal indentations caused by?

    a. Aorta and left primary bronchus
    b. Superior vena cava and heart
    c. Descending aorta and inferior vena cava
    d. Articulation with the stomach

120. To aid in the transfer of a nonambulatory patient, which of the following devices can be used to move the patient from the gurney to the radiography table when a gap is present between them?

    a. Pigg-O-Stat
    b. Hoyer lift
    c. Log roller
    d. Slideboard

121. Which of the following is not a location to properly take a pulse with the hands?

    a. Femoral
    b. Apical
    c. Tympanic
    d. Radial

122. What is the proper knee flexion when performing a lateral knee image?

    a. 5 degrees to 10 degrees of flexion
    b. 20 degrees to 30 degrees of flexion
    c. 45 degrees of flexion
    d. Full extension

123. Incomplete system erasures on CR and direct radiography systems can contribute to an imaging artifact.

    a. True
    b. False

124. Federal regulation mandates that _____ radiation must not exceed 100 milliroentgens per hour (mR/hr) at a distance of 1 meter from the tube housing.

    a. Primary
    b. Scatter
    c. Leakage
    d. Remnant

125. During a barium enema exam, the enema bag should be hung _____ above the table.

    a. 15"
    b. 18" to 24"
    c. 30"
    d. 40"

126. If possible, the knee should be flexed _____ degrees for a lateral trauma knee.

    a. 5 degrees to 10
    b. 10 degrees to 15
    c. 20 degrees to 25
    d. 45

127. What two aspects of the knee should be seen in profile?

    a. Intercondylar eminence
    b. Femur
    c. Patella and tibial tubercle
    d. Fibular head

128. Digital imaging monitors are subject to artifacts and display issues. A _____ can be used to check sharpness, distortion, and luminescence.

    a. Line pair gauge
    b. Fluorescent plate
    c. Focused grid
    d. Society of Motion Picture and Television Engineers (SMPTE) pattern

129. The stage of mitosis in which resulting chromatids are separate, complete, and distinct sets of chromosomes is referred to as:

    a. *Anaphase*
    b. *Prophase*
    c. *Metaphase*
    d. *Telophase*

130. Fluoroscopy is the most commonly used method to check for holes and cracks in lead shielding and aprons.

    a. True
    b. False

131. Proper preparation for a barium enema exam is important. Patients are asked to adhere to a clear liquid diet for _____ hours before the exam.

    a. 2 to 4
    b. 4 to 6
    c. 8 to 12
    d. 24

132. What space should open on a properly positioned lateral knee?

    a. Intercondylar eminence
    b. Femoropatellar joint space
    c. Proximal tibia/fibula space
    d. There is no open joint space

133. The stage of mitosis in which the nuclear membrane disappears and visibility of the nucleolus is absent is referred to as:

    a. *Prophase*
    b. *Metaphase*
    c. *Anaphase*
    d. *Telophase*

134. When the adductor tubercle is visualized on a lateral knee, the knee is _____.

    a. Positioned correctly
    b. Overrotated
    c. Underrotated
    d. Positioned with too much flexion

135. A patient with a disease spread by droplet transmission should be placed _____.

    a. In a private room with negative air pressure
    b. 3 feet away from another patient
    c. In complete isolation
    d. With no specific precautions

136. A common pathology found on a lateral knee radiograph is:

    a. Torn anterior cruciate ligament (ACL)
    b. Sinding-Larsen-Johansson
    c. Tripod fracture
    d. Unhappy triad

137. Rapidly moving electrons originate from the _____ end of the x-ray tube.

    a. Target
    b. Rotor
    c. Anode
    d. Cathode

138. The stage of mitosis in which there is complete disappearance of the nuclear membrane and division of the centromeres occurs is referred to as:

    a. *Anaphase*
    b. *Telophase*
    c. *Metaphase*
    d. *Prophase*

139. A common pathology found on a lateral knee radiograph is:

    a. Torn ACL
    b. Osgood-Schlatter
    c. Tripod fracture
    d. Unhappy triad

140. The stage of mitosis in which two daughter cells are formed is referred to as:

    a. *Prophase*
    b. *Metaphase*
    c. *Anaphase*
    d. *Telophase*

141. When administering contrast media intravenously, it is important to position the needle:

    a. Bevel down
    b. Bevel up
    c. At a 90-degree angle to the vein
    d. At a 45-degree angle to the vein

142. The purpose of intercondylar fossa views is to:

    a. Possibly demonstrate degenerative joint disease
    b. Create a more costly charge for patients
    c. Better demonstrate a fracture of the patella
    d. Demonstrate a stellate fracture

143. In a lateral knee image, the femoral epicondyles are _____.

    a. Not visualized
    b. 45 degrees to IR
    c. Perpendicular to the IR
    d. Parallel to the IR

144. For the focused electrons to be accelerated within the tube for x-radiation, a force must be applied. This force is referred to as:

    a. *mA*
    b. *mA/s*
    c. *kVp*
    d. *Kiloelectron volt* (keV)

145. Cells that are considered to be highly radiosensitive include:

    a. Endothelial cells
    b. Muscle cells
    c. Chondrocytes
    d. Lymphocytes

146. Having a patient roll the shoulders forward during chest radiography:

    a. Moves the diaphragm inferiorly
    b. Moves the scapula laterally
    c. Allows deeper inhalation
    d. Is unnecessary

147. The _____, located in the arm, is commonly used for contrast injection.

    a. Median cubital vein
    b. Jugular vein
    c. Renal vein
    d. Popliteal vein

148. The majority of interactions that occur in the x-ray tube result in:

    a. Kinetic energy available for x-ray production
    b. Kinesthetic energy available for infrared radiation production
    c. Kinesthetic energy available for x-ray production
    d. Kinetic energy available for infrared radiation production

149. Double inhalation during a chest x-ray:

    a. Moves the diaphragm superiorly
    b. Demonstrates inferior rib fractures
    c. Obscures vascular markings
    d. Allows for greater lung expansion

150. Which of the following may be used when a grid is not available?

    a. Decreased kVp
    b. Decreased mA/s
    c. Air-gap technique
    d. Compression bands

151. The correct IR orientation for a PA projection on a hypersthenic patient would be:

    a. $14'' \times 17''$ crosswise
    b. $14'' \times 17''$ lengthwise
    c. $10'' \times 12''$ crosswise
    d. $10'' \times 12''$ lengthwise

152. The phase of the cell cycle that is considered to be the most radioresistant is:

    a. Early G_1
    b. Late G_1
    c. Late S
    d. Interphase

153. Patients are commonly asked to refrain from taking metformin _____ before a radiographic contrast procedure.

    a. 3 days
    b. 1 day
    c. 8 to 12 hours
    d. 2 hours

154. The central ray is directed to the level of _____ for a PA chest.

    a. C6–C7
    b. T6–T7
    c. T1–T2
    d. Sternal angle

155. The interaction of the projectile electron and the nuclear field of the target atom is referred to as:

    a. *Characteristic*
    b. *Coherent*
    c. *Compton*
    d. *Bremsstrahlung*

156. The phase of the cell cycle that is considered to be the most radiosensitive is:

    a. Interphase
    b. Early G_1
    c. Late G_1
    d. Late S

157. For an AP image of the chest, the central ray is placed:

    a. At the xiphoid tip
    b. At the acromioclavicular joint
    c. $2''$ below the jugular notch
    d. $4''$ below the jugular notch

158. Patients who have abnormal glomerular filtration rate (GFR) cannot undergo which of the following procedures?

    a. Small bowel series
    b. Myelogram
    c. Intravenous urography
    d. Barium enema

159. The irradiation of the human body may result in lesions at the molecular level. When there is a break in the backbone of the long-chain macromolecule and a reduction in viscosity, the injury is known as:

    a. *Cross-linking*
    b. *Point lesions*
    c. *Main-chain scission*
    d. *Translocation*

160. What is the purpose of using a $72''$ SID?

    a. To decrease the mA/s
    b. To reduce heart magnification
    c. To increase magnification of the thoracic structures
    d. To demonstrate the ribs

161. The majority of radiation that is produced at the target atom is classified as:

    a. Bremsstrahlung
    b. Characteristic
    c. Compton
    d. Coherent

162. What is the appropriate contrast scale for chest radiography?

    a. Short-scale contrast
    b. Medium-scale contrast
    c. Long-scale contrast
    d. Contrast isn't important

163. Patients with a suspected perforated bowel should have which of the following modifications to the procedure?

    a. Raising the enema bag to increase flow
    b. Use of oil-based contrast
    c. Use of standard barium sulfate but without air contrast
    d. Use of water-soluble contrast

164. A projectile electron interacts with an inner-shell electron and is successful in totally removing it from its orbital shell. This process is often referred to as:

    a. *Transformation*
    b. *Transition*
    c. *Ionization*
    d. *Iodination*

165. What kVp range would demonstrate long-scale contrast?

    a. Long-scale contrast is demonstrated by higher mA/s
    b. ≥100 kVp
    c. 50 to 65 kVp
    d. 70 to 80 kVp

166. The irradiation of the human body may result in lesions at the molecular level. When there are small, spurlike structures that develop as a result of this irradiation, the main chain becomes sticky, thereby increasing viscosity. The injury that is described here is known as:

    a. *Cross-linking*
    b. *Main-chain scission*
    c. *Point lesions*
    d. *Translocations*

167. What alternate chest view would demonstrate the apices free of superimposition?

    a. AP lordotic
    b. Left anterior oblique (LAO)
    c. Right anterior oblique (RAO)
    d. Decubitus

168. A surgically created external opening in the bowel is termed:

    a. *Enteroclysis*
    b. *Diverticula*
    c. *Perforation*
    d. *Stoma*

169. The irradiation of the human body may result in lesions at the molecular level that are not detectable but will result in disruptions in single chemical bonds that may cause cell malfunction. The injury that is described here is known as:

    a. *Main-chain scission*
    b. *Point lesions*
    c. *Cross-linking*
    d. *Translocations*

170. The products of ionization within the orbital shells are:

    a. Characteristic and transition
    b. Characteristic and translation
    c. Coherent and translation
    d. Coherent and transition

171. What is the correct degree of obliquity necessary when a chest oblique is ordered, in terms of tissue superimposition?

    a. Obliquity isn't necessary for superimposition
    b. 10 degrees to 15 degrees
    c. 45 degrees oblique
    d. 60 degrees oblique

172. The thickness of a contrast agent is known as:

    a. *Durability*
    b. *Osmolarity*
    c. *Osmolality*
    d. *Viscosity*

173. The following statements are true as it relates to radiation damage to DNA EXCEPT:

    a. May not be visibly detected
    b. May be transferred through high LET radiations to daughter cells
    c. May result in rapid and uncontrolled cell proliferation
    d. May produce nondetectable responses at the cellular or whole-body level

174. As the atomic number (Z) of the target element decreases, the effective energy of the characteristic x-rays:

    a. Decreases
    b. Increases
    c. Stays the same

175. A 60-degree oblique is appropriate for:

    a. Apical superimposition
    b. View of the costophrenic angles
    c. A heart study
    d. None of the choices is correct

176. A patient presents with right anterior rib pain. Which oblique would be appropriate to best demonstrate potential pathology?

    a. Left posterior oblique (LPO)
    b. LAO
    c. RAO
    d. RPO

177. Body temperature is regulated by which of the following?

    a. Thyroid
    b. Hypothalamus
    c. Skin
    d. Heart

178. Which of the following is not a principal observable effect resulting from irradiation of cells?

    a. Apoptosis
    b. Neoplastic disease
    c. Radiolysis
    d. Transition

179. A patient presents with left posterior rib pain. Which oblique position would best demonstrate potential pathology?

    a. LPO
    b. LAO
    c. RPO
    d. RAO

180. Characteristic x-rays that occur in orbital shells are vital to the production of radiation that is useful in general diagnostic imaging. These rays must be produced from which element and which orbital shell?

    a. Molybdenum, k-shell
    b. Molybdenum, l-shell
    c. Tungsten, k-shell
    d. Tungsten, l-shell

181. The insulating oil surrounding the x-ray tube is a form of _____ filtration.

    a. Total
    b. External
    c. Added
    d. Inherent

182. What is the correct breathing technique when imaging lower ribs?

    a. Autotomography
    b. Inhalation
    c. Exhalation
    d. It doesn't matter

183. A complication of barium sulfate after a barium enema procedure is:

    a. Diarrhea
    b. Impaction
    c. Ecchymosis
    d. Erythema

184. What is the correct SID for rib radiography?

    a. 72″ SID
    b. 56″ SID
    c. 40″ SID
    d. 30″ SID

185. Aluminum sheets that may be placed outside of the tube housing to aid in absorption of lower-energy x-rays are a form of _____ filtration.

    a. Added
    b. Total
    c. Inherent
    d. External

186. As frequency decreases, wavelength _____ as a result of a(n) _____ type of relationship.

    a. Decreases, inverse
    b. Decreases, direct
    c. Increases, inverse
    d. Increases, direct

187. Which of the following is a common drug found in a crash cart?

    a. Lipitor
    b. Lidocaine
    c. Tylenol
    d. Epinephrine

188. What is the correct breathing technique when imaging the upper ribs?

    a. Exhalation
    b. Inhalation
    c. Autotomography
    d. It doesn't matter

189. As the distance from the source of radiation is decreased by one-half, the intensity of the radiation is increased by _____ based on the _____.

    a. 25%; inverse square law
    b. 25%; direct square law
    c. 50%; inverse square law
    d. 50%; direct square law

190. A severe reaction to contrast media may be indicated by which of the following?

    a. Cirrhosis
    b. Atelectasis
    c. Bronchial edema
    d. Giardiasis

191. When imaging the lateral sternum, what breathing technique is appropriate?

    a. Inhalation
    b. Exhalation
    c. Autotomography
    d. Stop breathing

192. Mobile and fluoroscopic radiographic units require total permanent filtration of:

    a. 1.5 cm aluminum equivalent
    b. 1.5 mm aluminum equivalent
    c. 2.5 cm aluminum equivalent
    d. 2.5 mm aluminum equivalent

193. The proper medical term for hives is:

    a. *Ecchymosis*
    b. *Erythema*
    c. *Urticaria*
    d. *Tinnitus*

194. Which oblique is preferred for imaging the sternum?

    a. 15-degree to 20-degree RAO
    b. 15-degree to 20-degree LAO
    c. 45-degree RAO
    d. 45-degree LAO

195. What medical term describes a funnel (sunken) chest?

    a. *Pectus carinatum*
    b. *Pectus excavatum*
    c. *Convex*
    d. *Pigeon chest*

196. An increase in kVp will result in all of the following EXCEPT:

    a. Increase in amplitude
    b. Change in discrete spectrum
    c. Increase in energy
    d. Increase in quantity

197. The metal that is most frequently used in filters because of its ability to effectively remove low-energy x-rays without decreasing beam intensity is:

    a. Aluminum
    b. Zinc
    c. Copper
    d. Molybdenum

198. A patient's reaction to contrast material can occur up to _____ after injection.

    a. 5 minutes
    b. 10 minutes
    c. 15 minutes
    d. 30 minutes

199. In mobile C-arm fluoroscopy, the minimal source-to-end of collimator assembly distance is:

    a. 15 cm
    b. 30 cm
    c. 6″
    d. 10″

200. The medical term describing a protruding chest is _____.

    a. *Pectus carinatum*
    b. *Pectus excavatum*
    c. *Funnel chest*
    d. *Concave*

201. An increase in mA/s will result in which of the following?

    a. Decrease in energy
    b. Decrease in amplitude and energy
    c. Increase in amplitude
    d. Change in discrete spectrum

202. Which of the following statements is not true of the control-booth barrier?

    a. Intercepts only remnant and scatter radiation
    b. Diagnostic x-rays must scatter at least two times before reaching any area behind the barrier
    c. Exposure cord must be short enough that it can only be operated from behind the control-booth barrier
    d. Must extend 7 feet upward from the floor and be secured to it

203. Do hypersthenic patients require more or less obliquity when oblique imaging of the sternum is being performed?

    a. More
    b. Less
    c. No modification is needed

204. The medical term for fever is:

    a. *Hypervolemia*
    b. *Hypoglycemic*
    c. *Isotonic*
    d. *Pyrexia*

205. Do asthenic patients require more or less obliquity when oblique imaging of the sternum is being performed?

    a. More
    b. Less
    c. No modification is needed

206. The attenuation properties of the protective devices used in control-booth construction should include the following EXCEPT:

    a. Secondary barriers should overlap the primary barrier by ½″
    b. Secondary barriers consist of ¹⁄₃₂″ lead or lead equivalent
    c. Primary barriers consist of ¹⁄₁₆″ lead or lead equivalent
    d. Primary barriers should be 5 to 7 feet from the secondary wall

207. Added filtration is most effective at low energies and will result in:

    a. An increase in energy and change in discrete spectrum
    b. An increase in amplitude and decrease in energy
    c. A decrease in amplitude and increase in energy
    d. A decrease in energy and change in discrete spectrum

208. What is the recommended breathing technique for imaging of the oblique sternum?

    a. Exhalation
    b. Autotomography
    c. Slight inhalation
    d. Stop breathing

209. Moving a partially ambulatory patient from a gurney to a wheelchair involves:

    a. Using two people to lift the patient into the chair
    b. Allowing the patient to sit up without assistance and get into the chair
    c. Helping the patient turn onto his or her side, then assisting the patient to sit upright
    d. Assisting the patient into an upright position from a fully supine position

210. A change in the Z of the target material will be represented by the following:

    a. Change in discrete spectrum and filtration
    b. Change in discrete spectrum and amplitude
    c. Change in discrete spectrum and waveform
    d. Change in discrete spectrum and energy

211. Diaphoretic patients may be experiencing which of the following?

    a. Cold sweats
    b. Bleeding
    c. Dehydration
    d. Vomiting

212. Which sternoclavicular (S-C) joint will be demonstrated when the patient is placed in an RAO position?

    a. Right S-C joint
    b. Left S-C joint
    c. Both the left and right S-C joints are well demonstrated
    d. An oblique position isn't necessary

213. Why is an anterior oblique position, rather than a posterior oblique position, recommended for S-C views?

    a. It increases thyroid dose
    b. The joint appears open
    c. The anterior oblique position is not recommended
    d. Magnification, and therefore distortion, is decreased

214. Hospice provides which of the following types of care?

    a. Curative
    b. Cancer treatment
    c. Palliative
    d. Preventive

215. Voltage waveform and generator type has an effect on quantity and quality of the resulting beam. Of the following, identify the TRUE statement.

    a. The more efficient the generator, the greater the voltage ripple
    b. The greater the efficiency of the generator, the less voltage ripple will occur
    c. The greater the voltage ripple, the greater the intensity and energy of the x-ray beam produced
    d. The lesser the voltage ripple, the lesser the intensity and energy of the x-ray beam produced

216. What should be demonstrated on a _____ Kidneys Ureter Bladder (KUB) to monitor accurate technical factors?

    a. Xiphoid process
    b. The psoas muscles
    c. Stones
    d. Air-fluid level

217. The metabolism of drugs occurs in which of the following organs?

    a. Stomach
    b. Pancreas
    c. Small intestine
    d. Liver

218. The type of radiation that is produced when the target is bombarded with projectile electrons is referred to as:

    a. *Primary*
    b. *Leakage*
    c. *Remnant*
    d. *Scatter*

219. What is the correct breathing technique for abdominal imaging?

    a. Exhalation
    b. Inhalation
    c. Cease breathing
    d. It doesn't matter

220. A misrepresentation of either the size or shape of an object is known as _____?

    a. *Recorded detail*
    b. *Unsharpness*
    c. *Distortion*
    d. All of the answers are correct

Comprehensive Exam 2

1. _____ results from the irradiation of water molecules in the human body that results in the creation of ions and reactive free radicals.

   a. Indirect effect
   b. Direct effect
   c. Target theory
   d. None of the above

2. This type of useful ionizing radiation is produced through the energy transfer between the incoming x-ray photon and inner-shell electron.

   a. Characteristic
   b. Coherent
   c. Compton
   d. Photoelectric effect

3. This type of radiation is a major consideration during radiologic procedures associated with protection of patients and medical personnel.

   a. Characteristic
   b. Coherent
   c. Compton
   d. Photoelectric effect

4. What is produced by radiolysis of positive water molecule (HOH+)?

   a. Hydrogen radical (H*) and hydroxyl radical (OH*)
   b. Hydroxyl ion (OH−) and H*
   c. Hydrogen ion (H+) and OH*
   d. OH* and H*

5. What is produced by radiolysis of negative water molecule (HOH−)?

   a. H* and OH*
   b. OH− and H*
   c. H+ and H*
   d. OH* and H*

6. _____ and _____ are the resulting free radicals that have the ability to break chemical bonds and result in biologic damage.

   a. H* and OH*
   b. H+ and OH*
   c. OH− and H*
   d. H− and OH

7. Tissues that are mature with a _____ metabolic rate are more radioresistant.

   a. High
   b. Low
   c. Static
   d. Varied

8. Tissues that are _____ with a low metabolic rate are less radiosensitive.

   a. Thin
   b. Thick
   c. Mature
   d. Immature

9. Tissues that are immature with a _____ metabolic rate are less radioresistant.

   a. Weak
   b. Strong
   c. Low
   d. High

10. As linear energy transfer (LET) _____, relative biologic effectiveness (RBE) increases.

    a. Increases
    b. Decreases
    c. Strengthens
    d. Stays the same

11. As _____ transfer decreases, RBE decreases.

    a. K-edge
    b. Linear energy
    c. Megaelectron volt (MeV)
    d. Oxygen enhancement ratio (OER)

12. _____ is continual dosing of radiation at a lower rate provided over a long period of time; the body is allowed time for cellular repair and tissue recovery.

    a. Fractionation
    b. Refraction
    c. Retraction
    d. Protraction

13. _____ is dosing of radiation administered in equal portions separated by 24-hour time frames, during which the body is allowed time for cellular repair and tissue recovery.

    a. Fractionation
    b. Refraction
    c. Retraction
    d. Protraction

14. Radiosensitive tissue that is in an environment rich in _____ will be radiosensitive to the effects of radiation.

    a. Carbon dioxide
    b. Iron
    c. Magnesium
    d. Oxygen

15. Brain tissue is _____ when compared to bone marrow.

    a. Equally radiosensitive
    b. More radiosensitive
    c. More radioresistant

16. Tissue is _____ radiosensitive under low oxygen conditions and _____ radiosensitive under aerobic conditions.

    a. Less, equally
    b. More, equally
    c. Less, more
    d. More, less

17. _____ radiation responses refer to human responses to radiation that are considered to be a result of early or acute exposure.

    a. Deterministic
    b. Stochastic
    c. Hormesis
    d. Recovery

18. _____ radiation responses refer to human responses to radiation that are considered to be a result of late or chronic exposure.

    a. Deterministic
    b. Stochastic
    c. Hormesis
    d. Recovery

19. The _____ dose-response relationship produces a response in a radiated population regardless of size or dose.

    a. Linear, nonthreshold
    b. Linear, threshold
    c. Nonlinear, threshold
    d. Nonlinear, nonthreshold

20. A _____ relationship is used to assess skin effects in high-dose fluoroscopy.

    a. Linear, nonthreshold
    b. Linear, threshold
    c. Nonlinear, threshold
    d. Nonlinear, nonthreshold

21. The dose of radiation that causes _____% of irradiated subjects to die within _____ days is referred to as:

    a. 20; 50; $LD_{20/50}$
    b. 30; 50; $LD_{30/50}$
    c. 50; 50; $LD_{50/50}$
    d. 50; 30; $LD_{50/30}$

22. The human application of radiosensitizing agents _____.

    a. Increases the enhancement of radiation by 2
    b. Decreases the radiation by 2
    c. Is fatally toxic
    d. Doubles the radiation damage

23. Federal regulation mandates that _____ radiation must not exceed 100 milliroentgens per hour (mR/hr) at a distance of 1 meter from the tube housing.

   a. Primary
   b. Leakage
   c. Scatter
   d. Remnant

24. _____ is the third stage of mitosis where centromeres divide.

   a. Prophase
   b. Anaphase
   c. Metaphase
   d. Telophase

25. The stage of mitosis in which the nuclear membrane disappears and visibility of the nucleolus is absent is referred to as:

   a. *Prophase*
   b. *Anaphase*
   c. *Metaphase*
   d. *Telophase*

26. _____ is the _____ stage of mitosis.

   a. Anaphase; first
   b. Metaphase; second
   c. Prophase; third
   d. Telophase; fourth

27. The _____ of mitosis results in the formation of two daughter cells.

   a. Prophase
   b. Anaphase
   c. Metaphase
   d. Telophase

28. Which of the following cells are greatly affected by radiation exposure?

   a. Chondrocytes
   b. Endothelial cells
   c. Lymphocytes
   d. Muscle cells

29. Which of the following is the most radioresistant phase of the cell cycle?

   a. Early G_1
   b. Late G_1
   c. Interphase
   d. Late S

30. The most sensitive phase of the cell cycle is _____.

   a. Early G_1
   b. Late G_1
   c. Interphase
   d. Late S

31. When there is a break in the backbone of the long-chain macromolecule and a reduction in viscosity, the injury that is determined is known as _____.

   a. Cross-linking
   b. Main-chain scission
   c. Point lesions
   d. Translocation

32. Cross-linking results in _____ structures.

   a. Main-chain scission
   b. Spur-like
   c. Crescent-shaped
   d. Round

33. The irradiation of the human body may result in lesions at the molecular level that are not detectable but will result in disruptions in single chemical bonds that may cause cell malfunction. This injury is known as _____.

   a. Cross-linking
   b. Main-chain scission
   c. Point lesions
   d. Translocations

34. The following statement is true as it relates to radiation damage to DNA EXCEPT:

   a. May be transferred through high LET radiations to daughter cells
   b. May result in rapid and uncontrolled cell proliferation
   c. May produce nondetectable responses at the cellular or whole-body level
   d. May not be visibly detected

35. Which of the following is not a principal observable effect resulting from irradiation of cells?

   a. Apoptosis
   b. Neoplastic disease
   c. Radiolysis
   d. Transition

36. The _____ surrounding the x-ray tube is/are a form of inherent filtration.

    a. Insulation oil
    b. Aluminum sheets
    c. Copper panels
    d. Water

37. _____, which may be placed outside of the tube housing to aid in the absorption of lower-energy x-rays, is/are a form of added filtration.

    a. Tungsten
    b. Aluminum sheets
    c. Iron
    d. Copper

38. The permanent filtration required for mobile and fluoroscopic radiographic units is _____.

    a. 1.5 millimeter (mm) aluminum equivalent
    b. 1.5 centimeter (cm) aluminum equivalent
    c. 2.5 mm aluminum equivalent
    d. 2.5 cm aluminum equivalent

39. Aluminum is most frequently used in filtration because of its ability to _____.

    a. Remove low-energy x-rays
    b. Absorb all radiation
    c. Be molded

40. In mobile C-arm fluoroscopy, the minimal source-to-end of collimator assembly distance is _____.

    a. 15 cm
    b. 6″ (inches)
    c. 10″
    d. 12″

41. Which of the following statements is not true of the control-booth barrier?

    a. Diagnostic x-rays must scatter at least two times before reaching any area behind the barrier
    b. Exposure cord must be short enough so that it may only be operated from behind the control-booth barrier
    c. Intercepts only remnant and scatter radiation
    d. The barrier must extend 7 feet up from the floor and be secured to it

42. The attenuation properties of the protective devices used in control-booth construction should include all of the following EXCEPT:

    a. Primary barriers consist of ¹⁄₁₆″ lead or lead equivalent
    b. Secondary barriers consist of ¹⁄₃₂″ lead or lead equivalent
    c. Secondary barriers should overlap the primary barrier by ½″
    d. Primary barriers should be 5 to 7 feet from the secondary wall

43. For radiographic procedures, radiographers should don proper protective shielding, including:

    a. Thyroid shields of minimum 0.5 mm lead equivalent
    b. Lead apron of minimum 0.25 mm lead equivalent
    c. Lead gloves of minimum 0.5 cm lead equivalent
    d. Lead glasses of minimum 0.25 cm lead equivalent

44. Which of the following is required for fluoroscopes per the National Council on Radiation Protection and Measurements (NCRP)?

    a. Source-to-skin distance (SSD) should be no less than 10″ for stationary fluoroscopes
    b. SSD should be no less than 12″ for mobile fluoroscopes
    c. Source-to-image distance (SID) should be no less than 12″ for mobile fluoroscopes
    d. SID should be no less than 15″ for stationary fluoroscopes

45. Why is the angle of female sacroiliac (SI) joints 35 degrees?

    a. Because of the narrow shape of the pelvis
    b. Because the pelvis is deep compared with that of men
    c. Because of the thoracic curve
    d. Because of the lumbosacral curve

46. What angle is used for imaging the SI joints of a male?

    a. 20 degrees
    b. 30 degrees
    c. 35 degrees
    d. 40 degrees

47. What angle direction is appropriate for the axial view of the SI joint when the patient is supine?

    a. Cephalic
    b. Caudal
    c. Tangential
    d. Transverse

48. At what level will you center for an antero-posterior (AP) axial SI joint?

    a. 2″ below the anterior superior iliac spine (ASIS)
    b. At the level of the ASIS
    c. At the level of the crest
    d. Directed at the apex of the sacrum

49. What positioning error has been made in the open mouth view if the lower margin of the front teeth is superimposed over the odontoid?

    a. The head was extended too much
    b. The head was flexed too much
    c. The tube was not angled
    d. The patient was prone

50. The posteroanterior (PA) method for imaging the dens is the _____?

    a. AP axial
    b. AP oblique
    c. Judd
    d. Wagging jaw

51. To decrease dose to a patient, how should cervical obliques be performed?

    a. At a 72″ SID
    b. At a 40″ SID
    c. PA
    d. AP

52. When performing AP imaging of the pelvis, how should the patient's legs be positioned to best demonstrate the femoral necks in a nontrauma situation?

    a. Naturally (the neck is always demonstrated on AP images of the pelvis)
    b. Rotate the leg and angle to the tube
    c. Externally rotated
    d. Internally rotated

53. What is the angle of the neck to the shaft of a femur in the average adult?

    a. 10 degrees
    b. 15 degrees to 20 degrees
    c. 90 degrees
    d. 125 degrees

54. To demonstrate the zygapophyseal joints of the thoracic spine, _____ degrees of obliquity should be performed.

    a. 70
    b. 45
    c. 30
    d. 15

55. When the nucleus pulposus extrudes from the annulus fibrosis, the condition is termed _____.

    a. *Herniated nucleus pulposus (HNP)*
    b. *Chance fracture*
    c. *Spina bifida*
    d. *Spondylolysis*

56. A lateral radiography of the lumbar spine would best demonstrate which of the following pathologies?

    a. Spondylolysis
    b. Spondylolisthesis
    c. Burst fracture
    d. Jefferson fracture

57. To demonstrate the right zygapophyseal joints of the lumbar spine, which of the following should be performed?

    a. Left posterior oblique (LPO)
    b. Right posterior oblique (RPO)
    c. Right anterior oblique (RAO)
    d. AP

58. Flexion/extension laterals of the spine are performed to evaluate _____.

    a. Mobility
    b. Disk space height
    c. Spinal cord integrity
    d. Fractures

59. What is the correct degree of angulation for a patient whose ASIS to tabletop (TT) measures 28 cm when imaging a knee?

    a. No angle is required
    b. 5-degree cephalic angle
    c. 5-degree caudal angle
    d. 10-degree cephalic angle

60. To demonstrate the head of the fibula, which of the following should be performed?

    a. Lateral knee
    b. Mortise projection
    c. 45-degree medial oblique of the knee
    d. 45-degree medial oblique of the ankle

61. What is demonstrated on the medial oblique knee?

    a. Superimposed tibia fibula
    b. Femoral lateral condyle
    c. Tibial lateral condyle
    d. Proximal tibiofibular joint space open

62. Which of the following is not the proper flexion for a lateral of the knee?

    a. 5-degree to 10-degree flexion
    b. 20-degree to 30-degree flexion
    c. 45-degree flexion
    d. 90-degree flexion

63. A patient had a traumatic injury to the knee. To demonstrate if there is an effusion, which of the following areas should be imaged?

    a. Cross-table lateral knee
    b. Medial oblique
    c. Weight-bearing knee
    d. Intercondylar fossa view

64. On an image of the lateral knee, what two structures are seen in profile?

    a. Patella and tibial tubercle
    b. Intercondylar eminence
    c. Femur
    d. Fibular head

65. Which of the following indicate properly positioned lateral knee radiography?

    a. Intercondylar eminence visible without superimposition
    b. Proximal tibia/fibula space
    c. Open femoropatellar joint space
    d. There is no open joint space

66. Which of the following is indicative of an underrotated lateral knee?

    a. Visualization of the abductor tubercle
    b. Visualization of the adductor tubercle
    c. Visualization of the base of the patella
    d. Superimposition of the condyles

67. Which of the following is a disorder of the apex of the patella?

    a. Unhappy triad
    b. Torn anterior cruciate ligament (ACL)
    c. Tripod fracture
    d. Sinding-Larsen-Johansson

68. Which of the following projections will best demonstrate Osgood-Schlatter disease?

    a. AP oblique of the shoulder
    b. Lateral knee
    c. Mortise
    d. Medial oblique of the foot

69. To demonstrate degenerative joint disease of the knee, especially the area around the tibial eminences, which of the following should be performed?

    a. Settegast
    b. Intercondylar fossa view
    c. Lateral knee
    d. AP knee

70. To properly position for a lateral knee, how should the femoral condyles be positioned in relation to the image receptor (IR)?

    a. Not visualized
    b. In profile
    c. Perpendicular
    d. Parallel

71. What is the purpose of instructing a patient to drop the shoulders during chest radiography?

    a. Moves the clavicles inferiorly from the apices
    b. Moves the diaphragm inferiorly
    c. Moves the scapula out of the lung field
    d. Allows deeper inhalation

72. To have greater lung expansion, which of the following techniques should be used by the radiographer when instructing the patient?

    a. Double inhalation
    b. Single inhalation
    c. Full exhalation
    d. Breathe normally

73. The correct IR orientation for a PA projection on a hyposthenic patient is _____.

    a. 10″ × 12″ crosswise
    b. 10″ × 12″ lengthwise
    c. 14″ × 17″ crosswise
    d. 14″ × 17″ lengthwise

74. The central ray is directed to the level of _____ for a PA image of the chest.

    a. T1–T2
    b. T6–T7
    c. C6–C7
    d. Sternal angle

75. The central ray placement for an AP image of the chest should be directed at _____?

    a. T6–T7
    b. T10–T12
    c. C7–T2
    d. At the sternoclavicular (S-C) joints

76. To reduce the magnification of the heart, which of the following techniques is used by the radiographer?

    a. Automatic exposure control (AEC)
    b. 40″ SID
    c. 72″ SID
    d. High kilovoltage peak (kVp)

77. Why is long-scale contrast important when performing chest radiography?

    a. Demonstrates thoracic structures in black and white
    b. Best demonstrates the ribs
    c. Allows for visualization of the thoracic structures in shades of white, gray, and black
    d. Allows for a short exposure time

78. What kVp would be necessary when performing radiography of the lungs?

    a. 50–65 kVp
    b. 70–80 kVp
    c. ≥100 kVp
    d. Long-scale contrast is demonstrated by higher milliamperes per second (mA/s)

79. A patient is suspected of having a tumor in the right apical region of the lungs. Which of the following positions could be performed to better visualize this area?

    a. AP lordotic
    b. Decubitus
    c. Left anterior oblique (LAO)
    d. RAO

80. A 10-degree to 15-degree oblique image of the chest may be performed for which of the following reasons?

    a. Study the heart
    b. Visualize the hilum
    c. Demonstrate the mediastinum
    d. Remove superimposed tissue

81. When performing oblique imaging for a study of the heart, the degree of obliquity should be which of the following?

    a. 30 degrees
    b. 40 degrees
    c. 45 degrees
    d. 60 degrees

82. A patient presents with right posterior rib pain. Which oblique position would best demonstrate potential pathology?

    a. RAO
    b. RPO
    c. LAO
    d. LPO

83. A patient presenting with left posterior rib pain at the level of the 10th rib would require _____ breathing instructions.

    a. Inhalation
    b. Exhalation
    c. Autotomography
    d. Breathe normally

84. A patient complains of left posterior rib pain at the level of the body of the sternum. What is the best projection to demonstrate a possible injury?

    a. RPO
    b. RAO
    c. LPO
    d. LAO

85. A patient complains of right anterior rib pain at the level of the sternum. What is the best projection to demonstrate a possible injury?

    a. RPO
    b. RAO
    c. LPO
    d. LAO

86. What is the correct breathing technique when imaging the lower ribs?

    a. Exhalation
    b. Inhalation
    c. Autotomography
    d. Cease breathing

87. Why is inhalation used when imaging the lateral sternum?

    a. Halts peristalsis
    b. Temporarily stops the heartbeat to reduce motion
    c. Pushes the sternum away from the thoracic cavity
    d. Pushes the diaphragm up

88. A 15-degree to 20-degree RAO position of the sternum is performed for which of the following reasons?

    a. It pulls the sternum away from the spine and into the heart shadow
    b. It pulls the sternum away from the spine and away from the heart
    c. It places the sternum over the right lung field
    d. It is easiest for the patient to perform

89. The medical term describing a funnel (sunken) chest is best demonstrated on which of the following radiographs?

    a. Oblique sternum
    b. Lateral sternum
    c. PA chest
    d. RAO of the S-C joints

90. The medical term describing a sunken positioned chest is _____?

    a. *Funnel chest*
    b. *Concave*
    c. *Pectus carinatum*
    d. *Pectus excavatum*

91. Do hypersthenic patients require more or less obliquity when oblique imaging of the sternum is being performed?

    a. Less
    b. More
    c. No modification is needed

92. Do asthenic patients require more or less obliquity when oblique imaging of the sternum is being performed?

    a. Less
    b. More
    c. No modification is needed

93. An oblique of the sternum is best demonstrated when which of the following techniques are employed?

    a. Slight inhalation
    b. Stop breathing
    c. Autotomography
    d. Exhalation

94. Which S-C joint will be demonstrated when the patient is placed in a LAO position?

    a. Both joints are best demonstrated
    b. An oblique is not necessary
    c. Left S-C joint
    d. Right S-C joint

95. When performing S-C joint projections, which of the following is the primary reason for positioning the patient in a RAO or LAO?

    a. The joint appears magnified
    b. It increases thyroid dose
    c. The joint appears closed
    d. There is no recommendation

96. When imaging of a kidney, ureter, and bladder (KUB) is being performed, what anatomical landmark can be used to ensure that the bladder will be visualized on the radiograph?

    a. ASIS
    b. Iliac crests
    c. Xiphoid process
    d. Symphysis pubis

97. When performing erect abdominal radiographs, which of the following anatomical structures must be present?

    a. Diaphragm
    b. Bladder
    c. Rectum
    d. Sigmoid

98. Pathology in the small intestines will be better demonstrated when the patient is _____?

    a. Lateral
    b. Supine
    c. Prone
    d. Erect

99. An ambulatory patient arrives for two-way abdominal imaging. In what order should the projections be taken to best demonstrate whether there is free air?

    a. Left lateral decubitus, then erect abdomen
    b. Erect abdomen, then AP supine abdomen
    c. AP supine abdomen, then erect abdomen
    d. AP abdomen, then left lateral decubitus

100. To best demonstrate free air in the abdomen in a nonambulatory patient, which of the following projections should be performed?

    a. Erect abdomen
    b. Decubitus
    c. AP abdomen
    d. PA abdomen

101. Which of the following would not be demonstrated on a soft tissue analog neck radiograph?

    a. Vertebral fracture
    b. Epiglottitis
    c. Foreign body
    d. Adenitis

102. To *best* demonstrate a posteriorly displaced fracture of the ankle, which of the following projections should be performed?

    a. AP
    b. Mortise
    c. Mediolateral lateral
    d. Lateromedial lateral

103. A common fracture of the foot occurs at which anatomical site?

    a. Second cuneiform
    b. Lateral cuneiform
    c. 5th metatarsal
    d. Navicular

104. Patients with pes cavus require a _____ when performing a dorsoplantar foot radiograph.

    a. 5-degree angle
    b. 10-degree angle
    c. 15-degree angle
    d. No angle is required

105. Patients with pes planus require a _____ when performing a dorsoplantar foot radiograph.

    a. 5-degree angle
    b. 10-degree angle
    c. 15-degree angle
    d. No angle is required

106. On a medial oblique radiograph of the foot, what anatomy should appear free of superimposition?

    a. 1st and 2nd metatarsals
    b. 3rd through 5th metatarsals
    c. 5th metatarsal only
    d. Navicular

107. What view would best demonstrate the lateral cuneiform?

    a. Lateral oblique
    b. Medial oblique foot
    c. Axial view
    d. It is difficult to demonstrate the cuboid

108. What radiograph would best demonstrate medial/lateral displacement of a calcaneus fracture?

    a. Tangential
    b. Medial oblique
    c. Lateral oblique
    d. Dorsoplantar axial

109. When positioning a patient for a weight-bearing projection of the foot, it is necessary to instruct the patient to do which of the following?

    a. Put full weight onto the affected foot
    b. Put equal weight on both feet
    c. Distribute weight onto the toes of both feet
    d. Lean backward to place weight on the calcaneus

110. When a patient is positioned prone to demonstrate the sesamoids, how is the central ray directed?

    a. Perpendicular
    b. Tangential
    c. Caudal
    d. Cephalic

111. How would a patient be positioned in the Holly method to demonstrate the sesamoids?

    a. Axial
    b. Prone
    c. Supine
    d. Sagittal

112. A dorsoplantar foot projection requires what angle?

    a. 7-degree to 10-degree anterior angle
    b. 7-degree to 10-degree posterior angle
    c. 15-degree to 20-degree posterior angle
    d. 25-degree to 30-degree posterior angle

113. Lateral weight-bearing projections of the feet best demonstrate which of the following pathologies?

    a. Tendonitis
    b. Hallux valgus
    c. Pes planus
    d. Osgood-Schlatter disease

114. When performing ankle radiography, which anatomic structure of the foot should be demonstrated?

    a. Base of the 5th metatarsal
    b. Lateral cuneiform
    c. Cuboid
    d. Navicular

115. A 15-degree to 20-degree internal rotation of the ankle will demonstrate which of the following structures?

    a. Posterior malleolus
    b. Lateral malleolus
    c. Medial malleolus
    d. Mortise

116. The correct degree of rotation for an internal oblique of the ankle to demonstrate the distal tibiofibular joint space is?

    a. 15 degrees to 20 degrees
    b. 30 degrees
    c. 45 degrees
    d. 90 degrees

117. To demonstrate the posterior malleolus of the ankle, which of the following projections should be performed?

    a. Lateral (external) oblique
    b. Medial oblique
    c. Lateral
    d. Mortise

118. What view of the ankle most accurately demonstrates the ankle joint?

    a. AP ankle
    b. 15-degree mortise
    c. Stress
    d. Lateral

119. To demonstrate a medial ligament tear of the ankle, which of the following views can be performed?

    a. Eversion stress
    b. Posterior obliques
    c. Inversion
    d. Broden

120. Zenker diverticulum is an outpouching of what anatomical structure?

    a. Anus
    b. Ascending colon
    c. Duodenum
    d. Esophagus

121. The aorta and left primary bronchus result in indentations in what anatomical structure?

    a. Heart
    b. Stomach
    c. Esophagus
    d. Superior vena cava

122. The component that controls the duration of the x-ray exposure is the _____.

    a. Milliampere (mA) controller
    b. Kilovoltage (kV) controller
    c. kV controller and timer
    d. Timer

123. Which of the following correctly defines the anode in an x-ray tube?

    a. Is a rotating disk and is positively charged
    b. Is a rotating disk and is negatively charged
    c. Is a rotating disk and contains a filament
    d. Is a rotating disk and has no charge

124. Most x-ray tubes contain two different-sized wires that emit electrons during which process?

    a. Primary radiation production
    b. Luminescence
    c. Thermionic emission
    d. Ionization

125. Tungsten makes up which of the following parts of the x-ray unit?

    a. Cathode
    b. Anode
    c. Bucky tray
    d. Oscillating grid

126. A rotating anode includes which two mechanical parts?

    a. Aluminum bars and a rotor
    b. Stator and rotor
    c. Filament and target
    d. Hard iron and copper bars

127. Which of the following is true of AEC?

    a. Does not use a backup timer
    b. Measures the correct amount of radiation reaching an flat panel detector
    c. Usually has one sensor
    d. Can be adjusted in small increments

128. An automatic exposure system has _____ different ionization chambers the radiographer can select prior to patient exposure.

    a. Two
    b. Three
    c. Four
    d. Five

129. This system uses detectors to determine the appropriate amount of radiation to produce during an imaging study.

    a. Automatic collimation
    b. Backup timer
    c. Manual exposure control
    d. AEC

130. Which of the following is NOT considered a beam restriction device?

    a. Filter
    b. Rectifier
    c. Aperture diaphragm
    d. Image intensifier

131. Which of the following can describe a beam restriction device?

    1. Reduces patient exposure
    2. Improves image quality
    3. Can be a manual or automatic collimator

    a. 1 and 3
    b. 1 and 2
    c. 2 and 3
    d. All of these

132. What allows the current to be changed from alternating current (AC) to direct current (DC)?

    a. Rectifier
    b. Autotransformer
    c. Step down transformer
    d. Multiplier

133. For an x-ray tube to generate an x-ray, the incoming power needs to be converted from AC to _____.

    a. DC
    b. Indirect current
    c. Automatic current
    d. Simple current

134. _____ is the power source in the United States.

    a. 60 hertz (Hz) DC
    b. 60 Hz AC
    c. 50 Hz DC
    d. 50 Hz AC

135. General x-ray, _____, and _____ are commonly three-phase x-ray systems.

    a. Portable units; digital radiography (DR)
    b. Fluoroscopy; portable units
    c. Fluoroscopy; angiography
    d. General x-ray is the only three-phase system

136. In digital fluoroscopy, the _____ is/are replaced with a flat panel detector.

    a. Grids
    b. Image intensifier
    c. Automatic brightness control
    d. Three-phase power

137. _____ is an imaging system that uses flat panel detectors.

    a. Image detector array
    b. Indirect panel radiography
    c. Computed radiography (CR)
    d. DR

138. A dedicated chest unit can be which of the following types of units?

    a. CR system
    b. Conventional film-type system
    c. DR system
    d. All of these

139. A pivot point and fulcrum is produced between the x-ray tube and IR with which imaging procedure?

    a. Tomography
    b. Fluoroscopy
    c. Image intensification
    d. DR

140. Which of the following accurately defines grids?

    a. Grids are devices that filter primary radiation
    b. Grids reduce image detail
    c. Grids increase image quality
    d. Grids are made up of aluminum strips

141. Which of the following statements are true regarding quality assurance testing for light field and radiation field testing?

    1. Radiopaque markers on the edges of the light field
    2. A fluorescent plate
    3. A plastic or aluminum tube for beam alignment
    4. Not required with digital systems

    a. 1, 2, and 3
    b. 2 and 4
    c. 3 and 4
    d. 4 only

142. What occurs when x-ray equipment malfunctions?

    1. It can endanger the patient.
    2. It can endanger the operator.
    3. The procedure does not need to be stopped.
    4. The error should be reported to maintenance only if the patient is harmed.

    a. 1 and 2
    b. 2 and 4
    c. 3 and 4
    d. All of these occur

143. True or False? Unlike conventional radiography, digital imaging receptors are not subject to artifacts.

    a. True
    b. False

144. A digital imaging artifact called a _____ can occur if a previous exposure is trapped.

    a. Fingerprint mark
    b. Ghost image
    c. Dark density
    d. Light density

145. Incomplete system erasures on CR and DR systems can contribute to _____.

    a. An increase in mA
    b. A decrease in exposure time
    c. An imaging artifact
    d. No effect on the image

146. Digital imaging monitors are subject to artifacts and display issues. A Society of Motion Picture and Television Engineers (SMPTE) pattern can be used to check for which of the following?

    a. Alignment
    b. Efficiency
    c. Exposure settings
    d. Luminescence

147. _____ exposure setting(s) should be used to check for holes or cracks in lead aprons.

    a. Manual
    b. Automatic
    c. Short time
    d. High kVp

148. The _____ is made of soft iron and copper bars.

    a. Anode
    b. Cathode
    c. Rotor
    d. Target

149. For the focused electrons to be accelerated within the tube for x-radiation, a force must be applied. This force is referred to as:

    a. *mA*
    b. *mA/s*
    c. *kVp*
    d. *Kiloelectron volt (keV)*

150. _____ makes up 99% of the kinetic energy of projectile electrons.

    a. Characteristic radiation
    b. Infrared radiation
    c. Primary radiation
    d. Bremsstrahlung radiation

151. The interaction of the projectile electron and the nuclear field of the target atom is referred to as:

    a. *Coherent*
    b. *Compton*
    c. *Characteristic*
    d. *Bremsstrahlung*

152. The majority of radiation that is produced at the target atom is classified as _____.

    a. Coherent
    b. Compton
    c. Characteristic
    d. Bremsstrahlung

153. Ionization occurs when a(n) _____ interacts with a(n) _____ and is successful in totally removing it from its orbital shell.

    a. K-orbit electron; neutron
    b. Proton; inner-shell electron
    c. Projective electron; inner-shell electron
    d. Inner-shell proton; projectile electron

154. Characteristic radiation can occur in any orbital shell. However, which of the following is true regarding the radiation produced?

    a. It is not useful for imaging
    b. It can be used for imaging patients
    c. It has high energy
    d. The energy is higher when orbital shells other than k-shell electrons are used

155. The effective energy of the characteristic energy decreases when the atomic number (Z) _____.

    a. Increases
    b. Decreases
    c. Stays the same

156. Bremsstrahlung radiation is dependent on which of the following factors?

    a. The target material and the L-shell electron
    b. Electron speed and proximity to the nucleus
    c. Electron speed and the target material
    d. Proximity to the nucleus and the K-shell electron

157. As frequency decreases, wavelength _____ as a result of a(n) _____ relationship.

    a. Decreases; inverse
    b. Increases; inverse
    c. Increases; direct
    d. Stays the same; direct

158. As the distance from the source of radiation be doubled by 50%, the intensity of the radiation is reduced by _____ based on the _____.

    a. 25%; inverse square law
    b. 25%; direct square law
    c. 50%; inverse square law
    d. 50%; direct square law

159. An increase in kVp will result in all of the following EXCEPT:

    a. An increase in amplitude
    b. An increase in energy
    c. An increase in quantity
    d. A decrease in filtration of the x-ray beam

160. A decrease in mA/s will result which of the following?

    a. A decrease in amplitude
    b. A decrease in energy
    c. A change in discrete spectrum
    d. A decrease in electron speed

161. Added filtration results in which of the following?

    a. Increase in intensity of the x-ray produced
    b. Decrease in intensity of the x-ray produced
    c. Increase in energy and change in discrete spectrum
    d. No change in the intensity of the x-ray produced

162. A higher Z of the target material will result in which of the following effects on the brems radiation produced?

    a. The brems radiation will be less efficient
    b. The brems radiation produced will have greater efficiency
    c. There will be no effect on the brems radiation produced
    d. There will be a larger increase in low-energy radiation

163. Voltage waveform and generator type has an effect on quantity and quality of the resulting beam. Of the following, identify the FALSE statement:

    a. The lesser the voltage ripple, the greater the intensity and energy of the x-ray beam produced
    b. The lesser the voltage ripple, the lesser the intensity and energy of the x-ray beam produced
    c. The more efficient the generator, the less the voltage ripple
    d. The greater the efficiency of the generator, the more voltage ripple will occur

164. This type of radiation is defined by any radiation that is not considered a primary radiation:

    a. Primary
    b. Remnant
    c. Leakage
    d. Scatter

165. This type of radiation is produced when the target is bombarded by electrons:

    a. Primary
    b. Remnant
    c. Leakage
    d. Scatter

166. Which of the following statements are false regarding medical consent forms?

    a. Consent forms are transferrable to another date if the same procedure is rescheduled
    b. The name of the physician must appear on the consent form
    c. The correct name of the procedure must be written
    d. A witness must sign the consent form along with the patient and physician performing the procedure

167. Battery is defined as:

    a. Applying a tourniquet to a patient without obtaining consent for an intravenous injection
    b. Threatening to restrain a patient if he or she does not cooperate
    c. Physically touching a person without his or her consent
    d. Using positioning aides during an exam

168. The term *do not resuscitate* means which of the following?

    a. All life-saving methods can be continued until the patient dies
    b. No efforts can be made to assist the patient once he or she has gone into cardiac or respiratory arrest
    c. Patient can be given oxygen via a respirator only
    d. If the patient's heart stops, he or she cannot receive CPR, but defibrillator paddles can be applied

169. A pathogen that is present on a patient's skin and does not cause infection for the person is termed _____.

    a. *Infectious pathogen*
    b. *Colonized pathogen*
    c. *Transient pathogen*
    d. *Normal flora*

170. Which of the following defines the pathogenicity of a microorganism?

    a. Severity of the infection the pathogen will cause
    b. The ability of an organism to produce disease
    c. How quickly the pathogen will multiply
    d. The likelihood an organism will result in disease

171. Applying leg and arm restraints without a medical order may result in which of the following criminal charges?

    a. Libel
    b. Slander
    c. Malpractice
    d. False imprisonment

172. When interviewing a patient to gather specific information easily and quickly, which of the following interview types can be used?

    a. Open
    b. Closed
    c. Structured
    d. Unstructured

173. Which of the following legal documents is signed by the patient with regard to the physician's policies concerning personal health information?

    a. Health Insurance Portability and Accountability Act (HIPAA) privacy practices
    b. Consent form
    c. Insurance waiver
    d. Medicare release form

174. Which of the following legal doctrines states that the employer is responsible for the actions of the employee?

    a. Malpractice
    b. Negligence
    c. Respondeat superior
    d. Res ipsa loquitur

175. The likelihood a pathogen will result in active disease is termed _____.

    a. *Incubation*
    b. *Virulence*
    c. *Infection*
    d. *Transient*

176. _____ illness is acquired through the treatment prescribed by the physician.

    a. Iatrogenic
    b. Nosocomial
    c. Pathogenic
    d. Transmitted

177. Autoclave sterilization uses which of the following?

    a. Toxic gases
    b. Vaporized hydrogen peroxide
    c. High temperature and dry air
    d. High, moist heat (steam)

178. Influenza is classified as what type of disease transmission?

    a. Airborne
    b. Contact
    c. Vector
    d. Droplet

179. Which of the following defines the term *tort*?

    a. Restraining a person against his or her will
    b. An action not punishable by imprisonment
    c. An action punishable by imprisonment
    d. Violation of a federal law

180. A patient has a blood pressure (BP) of 110/70 mm Hg. How would this be classified?

    a. Normal
    b. Stage I hypertensive
    c. Stage II hypertensive
    d. Normal hypertensive

181. Which of the following does not describe the difference between a young patient and an elderly patient?

    a. There is no difference between young and elderly patients as it pertains to health-care needs
    b. Elderly patients have a greater support system
    c. Young patients have decreased resilience
    d. Young patients have increased cognitive impairment

182. When a person is infected with a contagious pathogen, which of the following in the cycle of infection is required before the pathogen can be transmitted to another person?

    a. Susceptible host
    b. Portal of entry
    c. Portal of exit
    d. Mode of transmission

183. Which of the following is one of the five cultural competencies?

    a. Valuing diversity
    b. Using language interpreters
    c. Fluency in a second language
    d. Understanding the basics of a second language as it pertains to the delivery of health care

184. _____ do not require oxygen to survive.

    a. Protozoans
    b. Capsules
    c. Anaerobes
    d. Aerobes

185. Ten to 20 breaths per minute is the normal respiratory rate for _____.

    a. Children
    b. Adults
    c. Those in a trauma situation
    d. Patients with COPD receiving oxygen therapy

186. To aid in the imaging of infants for chest radiographs, which of the following devices can be used?

    a. Slideboard
    b. Hoyer lift
    c. Log roller
    d. Pigg-O-Stat

187. Which of the following is the most common place to take a pulse with the hands?

    a. Femoral
    b. Radial
    c. Apical
    d. Tympanic

188. During the application of a barium enema, the enema bag should be hung 18″ to 24″ above the _____.

    a. Table
    b. Floor
    c. Patient
    d. X-ray tube

189. Preparation for a barium enema may include a(n) _____ administered to cleanse the bowel of any remaining fecal material.

    a. Antispasmodic
    b. Diuretic
    c. Cathartic
    d. Steroid

190. Patients with this type of precautions should be placed 3 feet away from another patient.

    a. Contact
    b. Airborne
    c. Vector
    d. Droplet

191. When injecting a patient with contrast media, it is important to insert the needle bevel up and _____.

    a. At a 90-degree angle to the arm
    b. At an angle of 45 degree
    c. Perfectly parallel to the arm
    d. None of these are appropriate

192. The median cubital vein is located in the _____ and is commonly used for contrast injection.

    a. Leg
    b. Wrist
    c. Arm
    d. Hand

193. Patients are commonly asked to refrain from taking this common diabetic drug 1 day before a radiographic contrast procedure.

    a. Lasix
    b. Metformin
    c. Paxil
    d. Diuretics

194. Patients who have abnormal blood urea nitrogen (BUN) levels may not undergo which of the following procedures?

    a. Intravenous urography
    b. Small bowel series
    c. Myelogram
    d. Barium enema

195. Patients with a suspected perforated bowel should have which of the following modifications to the procedure?

    a. Use an oil-based contrast
    b. Use standard barium sulfate without air contrast
    c. Decrease the height of the enema bag to reduce flow
    d. Increase the height of the enema bag to increase flow

196. A patient who is diagnosed with megacolon is at risk for what additional complication?

    a. Diverticula
    b. Enteroclysis
    c. Hypothermia
    d. Hypovolemia

197. Hygroscopic as it relates to barium sulfate is defined as a substance that _____.

    a. Dissociates into two charged particles
    b. Increases fluid in the blood stream
    c. Is viscous
    d. Absorbs liquid

198. The hypothalamus regulates which of the following vital signs?

    a. Blood pressure
    b. Temperature
    c. Respiratory rate
    d. Pulse rate

199. Which of the following is NOT a complication of instillation of barium sulfate after a barium enema procedure?

    a. Diarrhea
    b. Constipation
    c. Impaction
    d. Perforation of the bowel

200. Which of the following is a common drug found in a crash cart?

    a. Lipitor
    b. Lidocaine
    c. Glucagon
    d. Tylenol

201. A mild reaction to contrast media may be indicated by which of the following?

    a. Atelectasis
    b. Itchy throat
    c. Giardiasis
    d. Bronchial edema

202. Which of the following is the proper medical term for "black and blue"?

    a. *Urticaria*
    b. *Tinnitus*
    c. *Erythema*
    d. *Ecchymosis*

203. Besides iodinated contrast media, another severe allergic reaction in the radiography department can occur because patients are allergic to what commonly used material?

    a. Sodium chloride
    b. Gauze
    c. Nitrile
    d. Latex

204. The medical term for a patient with a body temperature below 95°F is _____.

    a. Hypervolemia
    b. Hypoglycemic
    c. Hypothermia
    d. Pyrexia

205. A patient with flaccid paralysis may have suffered which of the following traumatic injuries?

    a. Spinal cord trauma
    b. Myocardial infarction
    c. Asthmatic emergency
    d. Ecchymosis

206. Patients with pyrexia may be experiencing which of the following?

    a. Pale skin
    b. Decreased respiratory rate
    c. Decreased pulse rate
    d. Increased pulse rate

207. Palliative care commonly occurs in which of the following medical settings?

    a. Cancer center
    b. Hospice
    c. Primary care physician's office
    d. Radiology office

208. The secretion of drugs can occur through which of the following mechanisms?

    a. Urine
    b. Sweat
    c. Feces
    d. All of these

209. Which of the following is described as the visible difference between two densities on an image?

    a. Density
    b. Distortion
    c. Contrast
    d. Recorded detail

210. Which of the following affects radiographic density?

    a. mA/s
    b. kVp
    c. Object-to-image distance (OID)
    d. None of these

211. As mA/s decreases, what happens to density?

    a. Density decreases
    b. Density increases
    c. Density does not change

212. The main controlling factor(s) of contrast is/are _____.

    a. Time and SID
    b. kVp
    c. mA and time
    d. SID and mA/s

213. Which of the following describes the law of reciprocity?

    a. Every time the same combination of mA and time is set on the same x-ray unit, the resulting image will demonstrate the same density
    b. Doubling the mA will double the density on an image
    c. Different combinations of mA and time that produce the same mA/s will produce the same density
    d. The intensity of radiation is inversely proportional to the distance to the x-ray source

214. "Every time the same combination of mA and time is set on the same x-ray unit, the resulting image will demonstrate the same density" describes which of the following law?

    a. The law of linearity
    b. The law of reproducibility
    c. The law of reciprocity
    d. None of the above

215. Which of the following affects the quantity of radiation?

    a. SID
    b. OID
    c. mA
    d. kVp

216. Which of the following are directly proportional?

    a. Intensity of radiation and the square of the distance
    b. SID and density
    c. kVp and density
    d. Film-screen speed and density

217. The inverse square law is defined by which of the following statements?

    a. The intensity of radiation is inversely proportional to the square of the distance from the x-ray source
    b. The intensity of the radiation is directly proportional to the square of the distance from the x-ray source
    c. The magnification of an object is inversely proportional to the OID
    d. The grid frequency is inversely proportional to the distance from the x-ray source

218. A 6″ air gap will result in a change of which of the following factors?

    a. Motion
    b. Magnification
    c. Density
    d. Unsharpness

219. Which of the following techniques can be used as a replacement for a grid?

    a. Compression bands
    b. Air-gap technique
    c. Decreased mA
    d. Decreased kVp

APPENDIX C

Answers to Comprehensive Exam 1

1. **A**

   When the patient is placed supine, the kidneys are closest to the IR because the kidneys are located in the retroperitoneal region.

2. **C**

   While the radiographer should maintain appropriate distance and remain available for assistance during radiographic procedures, he or she should be dressed adequately. Protective aprons of 0.5 mm lead equivalent must be worn with protective lead gloves of 0.25 mm lead equivalent. In addition, thyroid shields of 0.5 mm lead equivalent should also be worn.

3. **D**

   A consent form must include the name of the facility, the name of the physician performing the procedure, and type of procedure being performed to be considered legal consent.

4. **B**

   A 35-degree angle is appropriate for women because of the lumbosacral curve.

5. **A**

   kV controls the amount of penetrating energy of an x-ray.

6. **A**

   Density is the degree of blackening on a radiograph.

7. **C**

   The NCRP mandates that the SSD should be no less than 15″ for stationary fluoroscopes and no less than 12″ for mobile fluoroscopes.

8. **B**

   The minimum time required to demonstrate air-fluid level is 5 minutes; however, 10 to 20 minutes is recommended.

9. **D**

   Remnant radiation is also known as *exit radiation* and refers to the primary beam that exits the patient onto the imaging receptor/plate. This type of radiation is responsible for the latent image that is formed on the imaging plate.

10. **A**

    A cephalic angle is appropriate when the patient is supine on the imaging table to open the SI joints.

11. **B**

    The anode rotates inside the x-ray tube and is positively charged.

12. **A**

    Assault is the threat of bodily harm to another person.

13. **C**

    A caudal angle is appropriate when the patient is prone on the imaging table in order to open the SI joints and L5–S1 junction.

14. **B**

    When irradiation occurs in the human body, the resulting effect will either be a direct or indirect action. The human body is composed of approximately 80% water and therefore is prone to damaging effects caused by radiation. *Indirect action* indicates that the x-ray photon interacts with a water molecule, which results in the creation of ions and reactive free radicals. These resulting ions and free radicals have the ability to produce toxic substances and cause biologic damage.

15. **B**

    The filaments are two different-sized wires that emit electrons.

16. **D**

    A three-way abdomen requires a PA chest to demonstrate anatomy superior to the diaphragm, the erect abdomen to include the diaphragm, and the supine abdomen to demonstrate down to the bladder.

17. **A**

The outer edge of the anode is made of tungsten.

18. **D**

Photoelectric absorption produces ionizing radiation through the interaction of the incoming x-ray photon and an inner-shell electron and energy transfer. Movement of electrons through this interaction results in ionization and therefore useful radiation to produce x-ray images.

19. **D**

All affect radiographic density.

20. **C**

The mA/s would be halved for a soft tissue neck radiograph, which would better demonstrate soft tissue rather than bone.

21. **A**

DNR stands for *do not resuscitate* and no efforts to restart the heart or respiratory function can be done on the patient.

22. **B**

The rotating anode is an induction motor that contains a stator and a rotor.

23. **B**

Compton scattering results in scatter of radiation in all directions, which becomes a consideration for the protection of patients and medical personnel during radiologic procedures.

24. **D**

Centering 2″ below the iliac crest will place the central ray at the midpoint of the SI joints.

25. **C**

An infectious pathogen is present in the body and is multiplying but is not causing disease processes.

26. **A**

A 10-degree posterior angle opens the MTP joints.

27. **C**

Through ionization of water molecules, x-ray photons in the human body may cause separation of these molecules into other components. With an HOH+, the resulting smaller molecules will produce H+ and OH*.

28. **D**

Pes cavus refers to high arches.

29. **A**

AEC measures the amount of radiation that reaches the detector.

30. **B**

Virulence is the degree of pathogenicity of a microorganism, or the likelihood it will cause disease.

31. **A**

Proper positioning is important when using AEC.

32. **D**

More angulation is required for a patient with high arches.

33. **C**

As mA/s increases, density increases as a result of increased thermionic emission.

34. **D**

Through ionization of water molecules, x-ray photons in the human body may cause separation of these molecules into other components. With an HOH−, the smaller molecules will produce an OH− and an H*.

35. **B**

When the head is extended too much, the occipital bone superimposes the odontoid.

36. **D**

Restraints cannot be applied without a medical order and are considered false imprisonment since patients cannot free themselves from the restraints.

37. **B**

Manual exposure control allows the technologist to select and adjust exposure values, including time, mA, and kVp.

38. **C**

The Judd view is performed PA and decreases thyroid dose when the dens is of interest.

39. **A**

The free radicals OH* and H* are volatile for the short time that they are present and have the ability to break chemical bonds, resulting in further biologic damage.

40. **D**

A collimator, aperture diaphragm, and cone are all types of beam restriction devices.

41. **B**

Less angulation is required for a patient with flat feet.

42. **C**

Structured interviews use simple, one-response questions to gather information.

43. **C**

mA and time are the main controlling factors of density.

44. **A**

Mature cells and tissues with a low metabolic rate are at a lower risk for genetic mutation because of their limited, if not nonexistent, ability to enter into the cell division cycle.

45. **B**

The 1st and 2nd metatarsals are free of superimposition, whereas the 3rd through 5th metatarsals are superimposed.

46. **B**

HIPAA consent only covers the dissemination of information and does not give permission to perform any medical procedure.

47. **D**

A beam restriction device reduces patient exposure, improves image quality, and can be a manual or automatic collimator.

48. **A**

Positioning the patient PA reduces thyroid dose to the patient.

49. **C**

Mature cells and tissues with a low metabolic rate are at a lower risk for genetic mutation because of their limited, if not nonexistent, ability to enter into the cell division cycle.

50. **B**

Injury was caused by a negligent act because the accident would not have occurred unless the person was negligent.

51. **C**

The head and neck are rotated anteriorly 15 degrees to 20 degrees. Internally rotating the entire leg will place the neck parallel for a true AP hip/femur.

52. **D**

The autotransformer selects the voltages to produce an x-ray.

53. **B**

The law of reciprocity states that different combinations of mA and time that produce the same mA/s will produce the same density.

54. **A**

A medial oblique will superimpose medial anatomy, whereas a lateral oblique will demonstrate lateral anatomy.

55. **A**

Immature cells and tissues with a high metabolic rate are at a higher risk for genetic mutation because of their increased ability to enter into the cell division cycle.

56. **C**

Convalescence is when the patient is no longer demonstrating symptoms of the illness and is returning to normal health.

57. **D**

The average angle of the neck to shaft is 125 degrees, with a possible 15-degree variance based on the width of the patient's pelvis.

58. **B**

Incoming power needs to be converted from AC to DC.

59. **B**

LET is the amount of energy that is transferred from ionizing radiation to soft tissue and is another method for expressing the quality of radiation as it relates to radiation protection. As LET increases, so does the ability of the radiation used to cause a damaging biologic response.

60. **C**

Lateral radiographs superimpose anatomy, demonstrating displacement more obviously.

61. **C**

Nosocomial infections are infections acquired by the patient in a health-care setting.

62. **A**

The law of linearity states that doubling the mA/s doubles the density on the resulting image, while halving the mA/s halves the density.

63. **C**

A tangential skims the anatomy of interest, allowing separation from other anatomy.

64. **D**

The power in the United States is 60-Hz AC.

65. **A**

Gas plasma sterilization uses low-moisture hydrogen peroxide plasma for sterilization.

66. **A**

70-degree oblique or 20 degrees off lateral would best demonstrate the zygapophyseal joints of the thoracic spine.

67. **B**

Three-phase x-ray systems are generally used in general radiography, fluoroscopy, and angiography units.

68. **D**

LET is the amount of energy that is transferred from ionizing radiation to soft tissue and is another method for expressing the quality of radiation as it relates to radiation protection. As LET decreases, ability of the radiation used to cause a damaging biologic response decreases as well.

69. **B**

A Chance fracture results from a hyperflexion force, resulting in a fracture of the vertebral body, spinous process, pedicles, and transverse processes.

70. **C**

In a digital fluoroscopic unit, the flat-panel detectors replace the image intensifier.

71. **A**

The common cold is transmitted in the air with large droplets that cannot travel farther than 3 feet.

72. **C**

A patient would be supine and would be instructed to dorsiflex the foot.

73. **A**

When radiation is administered over a long period of time but at a lower rate, the effect of a large dose is lessened. The continual dosing of radiation through protraction allows for less effect because the body is allowed time for repair of cellular organisms as well as recovery of tissues affected.

74. **B**

A patient would be prone and would be instructed to dorsiflex the foot, placing the 1st digit in contact with the IR.

75. **B**

An action that has two effects is termed *double effect*.

76. **D**

CR uses reusable imaging plates instead of image detectors.

77. **D**

A 15-degree posterior angle is required to open tarsal interspaces.

78. **C**

Spondylolisthesis involves forward slipping of one vertebra onto another, commonly due to a defect in the pars interarticularis.

79. **B**

kVp affects radiation quality.

80. **A**

When radiation is administered in equal fractions separated by 24 hours, the dose given is said to be *fractionated* and reduces effect because cells undergo repair and recovery between doses. This type of radiation dosing is most frequently used in radiation oncology.

81. **C**

Lateral weight-bearing radiographs demonstrate the true integrity of a patient's arch.

82. **A**

Stage I hypertension ranges from 140 to 159 over 90 to 99 mm Hg.

83. **A**

A dedicated chest unit can be a CR system, a digital radiography system, or a conventional film system.

84. **D**

The base of the 5th metatarsal is a common site of fracture.

85. **D**

Tissue is more radiosensitive when placed in an oxygen-rich environment. This response of tissue is a result of a characteristic referred to as the *oxygen effect*.

86. **C**

Posterior oblique positions demonstrate the down side zygapophyseal joints.

87. **B**

Young patients have increased resilience compared to elderly patients.

88. **A**

Bone marrow contains stem cells, which are more immature than the cells within the nervous system. Immature cells are more available to enter into the cell cycle through rapid cell division.

89. **C**

A 15-degree to 20-degree internal rotation of the ankle brings the intermalleolar line parallel to the IR and opens the mortise.

90. **A**

A tomography unit creates a pivot point or fulcrum between the x-ray tube and IR.

91. **D**

SID and density are inversely proportional. As SID increases, density decreases.

92. **C**

A 45-degree internal oblique allows the distal tibiofibular joint space to open.

93. **B**

The pathogen must have a means to exit the infected person, travel to a new host, and enter the new host in order to cause new infection.

94. **A**

Grids are devices that filter scatter radiation.

95. **C**

Flexion/extension laterals will demonstrate the mobility of the spine _____ status post (s/p) fusion.

96. **A**

Generally speaking, tissue that is irradiated in a fully oxygenated environment is more radiosensitive than tissues in an anoxic environment.

97. **B**

Quality assurance testing for light field and radiation field testing would include radiopaque markers on the edges of the light field, a fluorescent plate, and a plastic or aluminum tube for beam alignment.

98. **D**

Superimposition of the distal fibula over the posterior one-third of the tibia is an indicator of a correctly positioned lateral ankle.

99. **B**

Deterministic radiation responses result from a high-dose exposure that occurs in an acute exposure and presents as an early response. An example of this would be a radiation-induced skin burn.

100. **B**

The five elements of cultural competency include value diversity, capacity for self-assessment, understand cross-cultural interactions, applying cultural knowledge to medical care, and adapting patient services that reflect cultural understanding.

101. **A.**

The measurement of tabletop to ASIS allows the radiographer to angle the tube correctly and bring the tube parallel with the joint space.

102. **D**

When x-ray equipment malfunctions, it can endanger the patient and the operator; the procedure should be stopped immediately, and the issue should be reported to maintenance.

103. **A**

Stochastic radiation responses result from a low-dose exposure that occurs in chronic exposure and presents as a late response. Examples of this include cancer, leukemia, or genetic effects.

104. **C**

Stress views of the ankle demonstrate the integrity of lateral and medial ligaments.

105. **B**

The inverse square law states that the intensity of radiation is inversely proportional to the square of the distance from the x-ray source.

106. **A**

In a linear, nonthreshold dose-response relationship, a response will be exhibited regardless of size or dose.

107. **D**

A 45-degree medial oblique will move the fibula away from the tibia.

108. **B**

Aerobes require oxygen to survive.

109. **D**

Inversion places stress on the lateral compartment of the ankle, demonstrating possible lateral ligament tears.

110. **A**

Digital IRs are subject to artifacts.

111. **C**

The inflection point in a nonlinear, threshold relationship indicates that incremental doses, such as those used in fluoroscopy, become less effective at the uppermost level of the dose curve. Effects to the skin that result from high-dose fluoroscopy follow this sigmoid-type (or *S-type*) dose-response relationship, which may also be described as *nonlinear* and *threshold*.

112. **A**

The external oblique superimposes the fibula over the tibia.

113. **B**

A normal adult respiratory rate is 10 to 20 breaths per min.

114. **B**

A lethal dose administered to a population resulting in 50% of that population dying within 30 days is referred to as $LD_{50/30}$. It is expected that if death is to occur postradiation, it will happen within 30 days of exposure. Acute radiation lethal to humans is approximately 350 rad (3.5 gray [Gy]).

115. **C**

Zenker diverticulum is a large outpouching at the proximal esophagus.

116. **A**

A minimum air gap of 6″ is required to affect density.

117. **D**

Artifacts on digital IRs usually appear as light densities.

118. **D**

Radiosensitizing agents increase the effect of radiation by a ratio of 2.

119. **A**

The aorta and left primary bronchus cause two indentations in the esophagus.

120. **D**

A Slideboard is used to close the gap between the patient and the x-ray table.

121. **B**

The apical pulse requires the use of a stethoscope.

122. **B**

Flexing the knee 20 degrees to 30 degrees opens the femoropatellar joint space.

123. **A**

Incomplete system erasures on CR and direct radiography systems can contribute to imaging artifacts.

124. **C**

Leakage radiation must be minimized within the protective tube housing. Federal regulation mandates that leakage radiation must not exceed 100 mR/hr at a distance of 1 meter from the protective tube housing.

125. **B**

The enema bag should be hung 18″ to 24″ above the table during a barium enema.

126. **A**

Flexing the knee 5 degrees to 10 degrees opens the joint space.

127. **C**

The patella and tibial tubercle are seen in profile in a properly positioned lateral knee.

128. **D**

An SMPTE pattern can be used to check for sharpness, distortion, and luminescence.

129. **A**

Anaphase is the third stage of mitosis, in which centromeres divide and sister chromatids detach and are pulled to opposite poles. Resulting chromatids are now separate chromosomes and are two complete and distinct sets.

130. **A**

Fluoroscopy is commonly used to check for holes and cracks in lead aprons.

131. **D**

The day before the examination, the patient should follow a clear liquid diet.

132. **B**

The femoropatellar joint space should be open on a lateral knee.

133. **A**

Prophase is the first stage of mitosis, in which the chromosomes condense and spindle fibers that are formed between centrioles move toward opposite poles of the cell. In addition, the nuclear membrane disappears and there is no visible nucleolus.

134. **C**

The adductor tubercle will be demonstrated if the knee is underrotated.

135. **B**

Droplets are spread 3 feet or less, so the patient can be placed with another patient who is more than 3 feet away.

136. **B**

Sinding-Larsen-Johansson is a ligament disorder that pulls the apex of the patella.

137. **D**

The source of the free electrons is located in the focusing cup of the tube, which is at the cathode end of the x-ray tube.

138. **C**

Metaphase is the second stage of mitosis, in which spindle fibers from each centriole attach to the centromeres of the chromosomes and paired chromosomes line up at the cell's equator. In addition, there is complete disappearance of the nuclear membrane and centromeres divide.

139. **B**

Osgood-Schlatter is a patellar ligament disorder that attaches to the tibial tuberosity.

140. **D**

Telophase is the final stage of mitosis, in which the chromosome sets elongate and become thinner and indistinct as they reach the cell poles. DNA unravels to form chromatin and formation of new nuclear membranes occurs along with the reappearance of the nucleolus. Cell division is almost complete. The final steps include division of the cytoplasm with a new cell membrane and formation of two daughter cells.

141. **B**

The needle should always be positioned with the bevel up.

142. **A**

Intercondylar fossa views will better demonstrate pathology, such as osteochondritis dissecans in the knee joint space.

143. **C**

The femoral epicondyles are perpendicular to the IR in a lateral knee image.

144. **C**

There are three critical elements that must occur in order for radiation to be emitted from the x-ray tube. These elements include (1) the source of the free electrons, which are released from the focusing cup of the tube as a result of thermionic emissions; (2) the focusing of these electrons to be accelerated from the cathode to the anode through the use of kV; and (3) the target of the anode, which acts as the site of interaction of the projectile electrons, resulting in the projectile electrons either slowing down as they come close to the nuclear field or interacting with the orbital electrons located in the target atom.

145. **D**

Lymphocytes, spermatogonia, erythroblasts, and intestinal crypt cells are considered to be greatly affected by radiation exposure; endothelial cells, osteoblasts, spermatids, and fibroblasts are affected by radiation, but on a lesser scale. Finally, muscle cells, nerve cells, and chondrocytes have a low radiosensitivity; however, this sensitivity depends on where the cell is located within the cell cycle.

146. **B**

Rolling the shoulders forward moves the scapula laterally and out of the lung field.

147. **A**

The median cubital vein is located in the arm.

148. **B**

At the target, the projectile electrons that interact with the outer-shell electrons do not have enough energy to eject them out of the orbit to ionize them; rather, the interactions that occur are enough to cause excitations of these outer-shell electrons, raising their energy levels. With this excitation and need to level off their raised energy levels, outer-shell electrons emit a large amount of infrared heat or radiation, which is equal to approximately 99% of the kinetic energy of the initial projectile electrons. The remaining less than 1% of kinetic energy is available for the production of x-radiation.

149. **D**

Deep inhalation moves the diaphragm inferiorly and allows for greater lung expansion.

150. **C**

The air-gap technique may be used to minimize the amount of scatter reaching the IR when a grid is not available.

151. **A**

A 14″ × 17″ crosswise IR is the best choice for a hypersthenic patient in order to include the costophrenic angles.

152. **C**

The most radioresistant phase of the cell cycle is dependent on cell division. The most radioresistant phase is during midsynthesis to late synthesis.

153. **B**

Metformin (Glucophage) should be stopped 1 day before the procedure.

154. **B**

The central ray is directed to T6–T7, which is at the level of the inferior scapula.

155. **D**

Bremsstrahlung radiation refers to the interaction of the projectile electron that is influenced by the nuclear field of the target atom.

156. **A**

The most radiosensitive phase of the cell cycle is dependent on cell division. The most radiosensitive phase is during interphase and passage from late G_1 into early S.

157. **D**

Centering 4″ below the jugular notch brings the central ray to the level of T6–T7.

158. **C**

GFR evaluates kidney function and an abnormal GFR means they should not have an intravenous urography exam.

159. **C**

Main-chain scission is represented by a breakage in the backbone of the long-chain macromolecule. This breakage results in reduction of a long, single molecule into many smaller molecules, reducing viscosity.

160. **B**

A 40″ SID would cause the heart to appear magnified, so a 72″ SID is appropriate.

161. **A**

The majority of radiation that results from interactions at the target atom is classified as bremsstrahlung.

162. **C**

Long-scale contrast allows visualization of the thoracic structures by demonstrating shades of white, gray, and black. Short-scale contrast would demonstrate only black and white.

163. **D**

Water-soluble contrast should be used for patients with a suspected perforated bowel.

164. **C**

When a projectile electron interacts with an inner-shell electron and succeeds in totally removing it from its orbital shells, an ion is produced. This process is referred to as *ionization*. In addition, the resulting open space in the shell is replaced by an outer-shell electron dropping into this slot through a process referred to as *transition*. Transition is accompanied by the release of characteristic radiation and energy resulting from the difference between the binding energies of the orbital shells involved in this replacement process.

165. **B**

Long-scale contrast requires higher kVp.

166. **A**

Cross-linking is represented by small, spurlike structures that develop after irradiation of the main chain of a macromolecule, which cause the main chain to become sticky. In addition, these spurs may attach to neighboring macromolecules or another segment of the same molecule, thereby increasing viscosity.

167. **A**

Having the patient stand 12″ in front of the IR and lean back against it pushes the clavicles superior to the apices.

168. **D**

A stoma is a surgically created external opening in the bowel.

169. **C**

Point lesions result in disruption of single chemical bonds through interaction with radiation and are not detectable. In addition, small changes may occur which will result in cell malfunction. Should point lesions that result from low radiation doses occur, the cellular damage that results will present as late effects at the whole-body level.

170. **A**

When a projectile electron interacts with an inner-shell electron, totally removing it, and the resulting open space is filled by an outer-shell electron dropping into this open slot, the process is called *transition*. This transition is accompanied by the release of characteristic radiation and energy resulting from the difference between the binding energies of the orbital shells involved in the replacement process.

171. **B**

A 10-degree to 15-degree oblique will remove superimposed tissue.

172. **D**

Viscosity is the thickness of the contrast agent.

173. **B**

DNA contains the genetic information for each cell. Radiation may result in damage that is not visibly detected but causes abnormal metabolic activity. In addition, observable damage may result from considerable radiation exposure. Point or genetic mutations are common with low LET radiations and may be transferred incorrectly to daughter cells.

174. **A**

The effective energy of characteristic x-rays decreases with target elements of lower Z. The x-ray energies associated with characteristic radiation have precisely fixed energies and form discrete spectrums.

175. **C**

A 60-degree LAO is required for a heart study.

176. **B**

The LAO position will move the spine away from the right ribs.

177. **B**

The hypothalamus regulates body temperature.

178. **D**

When cells are irradiated, observable effects may include cell death, malignant disease, genetic damage, or radiolysis of water. Transition refers to the movement of low energy to high energy in the electron shells when ionization occurs.

179. **A**

An LPO will place the left posterior ribs closest to the IR and the spine away from the area of interest.

180. **C**

Characteristic x-rays may occur in orbital shells other than the k-orbit, but it is only the k-characteristic x-rays of tungsten that are useful in imaging; characteristic x-rays other than k x-rays possess energies that are too low for general diagnostic use.

181. **D**

Inherent filtration aids in reducing the exposure to the patient's skin and superficial tissue by absorbing most of the lower-energy photons, which increases the quality of the beam. Inherent filtration includes the material used in the construction of the tube.

182. **C**

Exhalation will push the diaphragm up, away from the lower ribs.

183. **B**

Barium sulfate can cause impaction in the large intestine.

184. **C**

A 40″ SID is appropriate for rib imaging.

185. **A**

Added filtration provides additional protection and consists of interchangeable aluminum sheets of varying thickness outside the glass window of the tube housing above the collimator shutters.

186. **C**

Electromagnetic radiation in the form of x-rays possesses wavelength and frequency; the relationship between these properties is inverse.

187. **D**

Epinephrine is commonly found in a crash cart.

188. **B**

Inhalation will push the diaphragm down, away from the upper ribs.

189. **A**

Electromagnetic radiation is inversely related to the square of the distance from the source. Should the distance from the source of radiation decrease by one-half, the intensity of the radiation is increased by 25%, or one-fourth.

190. **C**

Bronchial edema occurs with a severe reaction to contrast media.

191. **A**

Inhalation will push the sternum away from the thoracic cavity, allowing better visualization of the sternum.

192. **D**

Total filtration is determined by the kVp of an x-ray unit: for fixed units operating below 50 kVp, 0.5 mm aluminum equivalent; for fixed units operating between 50 and 70 kVp, 1.5 mm aluminum equivalent; for fixed units operating above 70 kVp, 2.5 mm aluminum equivalent. Mobile and fluoroscopic units require total permanent filtration of 2.5 mm aluminum equivalent.

193. **C**

Urticaria is the proper medical term for hives.

194. **A**

A 15-degree to 20-degree RAO will move the sternum away from the spine but into the heart shadow to better demonstrate the sternum.

195. **B**

Pectus excavatum is a condition in which the chest is concave, rather than convex.

196. **B**

A change that occurs to kVp or tube voltage will result in either an increase or decrease in amplitude and energy. There will be no effect to target material or filtration.

197. **A**

Aluminum (Z = 13) is the metal most frequently used because of its ability to effectively remove low-energy x-rays without decreasing the intensity of the beam.

198. **D**

A patient may experience a reaction to contrast material up to 30 minutes after injection.

199. **B**

In mobile C-arm fluoroscopy, there is potential for large radiation doses to patients and operators. Therefore, it is imperative that a minimal source-to-end of collimator assembly distance be set at a distance of 12″ (30 cm).

200. **A**

Pectus carinatum is a condition in which the chest protrudes excessively.

201. **C**

A change that occurs to mA/s or tube current will result in either an increase or decrease in amplitude only.

202. **A**

Control-booth barriers protect the radiographer during an examination, and personnel must remain completely behind the booth for maximal protection. The barrier intercepts only leakage and scatter radiation.

203. **B**

Hypersthenic patients require less obliquity.

204. **D**

Pyrexia is the medical term for fever.

205. **A**

Asthenic patients require more obliquity than hypersthenic patients.

206. **D**

Primary barriers consist of ⅟₁₆″ lead or lead equivalent and extend 7 feet from the floor with the x-ray tube 5 to 7 feet from the primary wall.

207. **C**

Adding filtration to the useful x-ray beam absorbs low-energy x-rays, leaving behind a higher-quality beam. This hardened x-ray beam is more efficient in energy but contains less x-rays in its intensity. Therefore, added filtration increases the energy of the beam, increasing its quality by decreasing the amount of soft or low-energy x-rays.

208. **B**

Autotomography will help blur out vascular markings, allowing better visualization of the sternum.

209. **C**

A partially ambulatory patient can be assisted from a gurney to a wheelchair by helping the patient roll onto his or her side, then sit upright.

210. **B**

By changing target material, there is a change in the peak of the continuous and discrete spectrums. The greater the Z, the greater the efficiency of the radiation that is produced. In addition, the high-energy x-rays increase in number over the low-energy x-rays.

211. **A**

Diaphoretic patients are those experiencing cold sweats.

212. **A**

The joint closest to the IR will be demonstrated when the patient is in an anterior oblique position.

213. **D**

An anterior oblique position brings the S-C joint closest to the IR and decreases magnification/distortion.

214. **C**

Hospice provides palliative care.

215. **B**

Generators such as three-phase or high-frequency types are more efficient than single-phase types. As the efficiency of the generator increases, less voltage ripple will occur, which will increase the intensity and energy of the x-ray beam produced.

216. **B**

Demonstration of the psoas muscles is a good indicator that there is sufficient penetration and that there isn't too much density. Too much density may obscure pathology.

217. **D**

Drugs are metabolized in the liver.

218. **A**

Primary radiation is produced at the x-ray tube and emerges from the x-ray tube target as a result of projectile electrons interacting with the target atoms through bombardment.

219. **A**

Exhalation brings the diaphragm up, away from the abdominal region.

220. **C**

Distortion is defined as the misrepresentation of either the size or the shape of an object on a radiograph.

Answers to Comprehensive Exam 2

1. **A**

   When irradiation occurs in the human body, the resulting effect will either be a direct or indirect action. The human body is composed of approximately 80% water and therefore is more prone to damaging effects caused by radiation. Indirect action indicates that the x-ray photon interacts with a water molecule, which results in the creation of ions and reactive free radicals. These resulting ions and free radicals have the ability to produce toxic substances to cause biologic damage.

2. **D**

   Photoelectric absorption produces ionizing radiation through the interaction of the incoming x-ray photon and an inner-shell electron and energy transfer. Movement of electrons through this interaction results in ionization and therefore useful radiation to produce x-ray images.

3. **C**

   Compton scattering results in scatter of radiation in all directions, which becomes a consideration for the protection of patients and medical personnel during radiologic procedures.

4. **C**

   Through ionization of water molecules, x-ray photons in the human body may cause separation of these molecules into other components. With an HOH+, the resulting smaller molecules will produce H+ and OH*.

5. **B**

   Through ionization of water molecules, x-ray photons in the human body may cause separation of these molecules into other components. With an HOH−, the smaller molecules will produce an OH− and an H*.

6. **A**

   The free radicals OH* and H* are volatile for the short time that they are present and have the ability to break chemical bonds, resulting in further biologic damage.

7. **B**

   Mature cells and tissues with a low metabolic rate are at a lower risk for genetic mutation due to their limited, if not nonexistent, ability to enter into the cell division cycle.

8. **C**

   Mature cells and tissues with a low metabolic rate are at a lower risk for genetic mutation due to their limited, if not nonexistent, ability to enter into the cell division cycle.

9. **D**

   Immature cells and tissues with a high metabolic rate are at a higher risk for genetic mutation due to their increased ability to enter into the cell division cycle.

10. **A**

    Linear energy transfer is the amount of energy that is transferred from ionizing radiation to soft tissue and is another method for expressing the quality of radiation as it relates to radiation protection. As LET increases, so does the ability of the radiation used to cause a damaging biologic response.

11. **B**

    Linear energy transfer is the amount of energy that is transferred from ionizing radiation to soft tissue and is another method for expressing the quality of radiation as it relates to radiation protection. As LET decreases, ability of the radiation used to cause a damaging biologic response reduces as well.

12. **D**

When radiation is administered over a long period of time but at a lower rate, the effect of a large dose is lessened. The continual dosing of radiation through protraction allows for less effect because the body is allowed time for repair of cellular organisms as well as recovery of tissues affected.

13. **A**

When radiation is administered in equal fractions separated by 24 hours, the dose given is said to be fractionated and reduces effect because cells undergo repair and recovery between doses. This type of radiation dosing is most frequently used in radiation oncology.

14. **D**

Tissue is more radiosensitive when placed in an oxygen-rich environment. The response of tissue is a result of a characteristic referred to as the *OER*, which is a numeric value used to enhance radiosensitivity of tumors to make them more responsive to radiation therapy.

15. **C**

Bone marrow contains stem cells which are more immature than the cells within the nervous system. Immature cells are more available to enter into the cell cycle through rapid cell division.

16. **C**

Generally speaking, tissue that is irradiated in a fully oxygenated environment is more radiosensitive than tissues in an anoxic environment.

17. **A**

Deterministic radiation responses result from a high-dose exposure that occurs in an acute exposure and presents as an early response. An example of this would be a radiation-induced skin burn.

18. **B**

Stochastic radiation responses result from a low-dose exposure that occurs in chronic exposure and presents as a late response. An example of this would be cancer, leukemia, or genetic effects.

19. **A**

In a linear, nonthreshold dose-response relationship, a response will be exhibited regardless of size or dose.

20. **C**

The inflection point in a nonlinear, threshold indicates that incremental doses, such as those used in fluoroscopy, become less effective at the uppermost level of the dose curve. Effects to the skin that result from high-dose fluoroscopy follow this S-type or sigmoid type dose-response relationship, which may also be described as nonlinear and threshold.

21. **D**

A lethal dose administered to a population resulting in 50% of that population to die within 30 days is referred to as $LD_{50/30}$. It is expected that if death is to occur postradiation, it will happen within 30 days of exposure. Acute radiation lethality in humans is approximately 350 rad (3.5 Gy [Gy]).

22. **A**

Radiosensitizing agents increase the enhancement of radiation by 2.

23. **B**

Leakage radiation must be minimized within the protective tube housing. Federal regulation mandates that leakage radiation must not exceed 100 mR/hr at a distance of 1 m from the protective tube housing.

24. **B**

Anaphase is the third stage of mitosis, in which centromeres divide and sister chromatids detach and are pulled to an opposite pole. Resulting chromatids are now separate chromosomes and are two complete and distinct sets.

25. **A**

Prophase is the first stage of mitosis, in which the chromosomes condense and spindle fibers that are formed between centrioles move toward opposite poles of the cell. In addition, the nuclear membrane disappears and there is no visible nucleolus.

26. **B**

Metaphase is the second stage of mitosis, in which spindle fibers from each centriole attach to the centromeres of the chromosomes and paired chromosomes line up at the cell's equator. Additionally, there is complete disappearance of the nuclear membrane and centromeres divide.

27. **D**

Telophase is the final stage of mitosis, in which the chromosome sets elongate and become thinner and indistinct as they reach the cell poles. DNA unravels to form chromatin and formation of new nuclear membranes occurs along with the reappearance of the nucleolus. Cell division is almost complete. The final steps include division of the cytoplasm with a new cell membrane and two daughter cells are formed.

28. **C**

Lymphocytes, spermatogonia, erythroblasts, and intestinal crypt cells are considered to be greatly affected by radiation exposure; endothelial cells, osteoblasts, spermatids, and fibroblasts are affected by radiation but on a lesser scale. Finally, muscle cells, nerve cells, and chondrocytes have a low radiosensitivity; however, this sensitivity depends on where the cell may be located within the cell cycle.

29. **D**

The most radioresistant phase of the cell cycle is dependent on cell division. The most radioresistant phase is during midsynthesis to late synthesis.

30. **C**

The most radiosensitive phase of the cell cycle is dependent on cell division. The most radiosensitive phase is during mitosis and passage from late G_1 into early S.

31. **B**

Main-chain scission is represented by a breakage in the backbone of the long-chain macromolecule. This breakage results in reduction of a long, single molecule into many smaller molecules, reducing viscosity.

32. **B**

Cross-linking is represented by small, spur-like structures that develop after irradiation off the main chain of a macromolecule, which causes the main chain to become sticky. In addition, these spurs may attach to neighboring macromolecules or another segment of the same molecule, thereby increasing viscosity.

33. **C**

Point lesions result in disruption of single chemical bonds through interaction with radiation and are not detectable. In addition, small changes may occur, which will cause it to result in cell malfunction. Should point lesions that result from low radiation doses occur, the cellular damage that results will present as late effects at the whole-body level.

34. **A**

DNA contains the genetic information for each cell and may result in damage that is not visibly detected but causes abnormal metabolic activity. In addition, observable damage may result from considerable radiation exposure. Point or genetic mutations are common with low LET radiations and may be transferred incorrectly to daughter cells.

35. **D**

When cells are irradiated, there are effects that may be observed, which may include cell death, malignant disease, genetic damage, or radiolysis of water. Transition refers to the movement of low energy to high energy in the electron shells when ionization occurs.

36. **A**

Inherent filtration aids in reducing the exposure to the patient's skin and superficial tissue by absorbing most of the lower-energy photons, which increases the quality of the beam and includes the material used in the construction of the tube.

37. **B**

Added filtration provides additional protection and consists of interchangeable aluminum sheets of varying thickness outside the glass window of the tube housing above the collimator shutters.

38. **C**

Total filtration is determined by the kVp of an x-ray unit. For fixed units operating below 50 kVp, 0.5 mm aluminum equivalent; for fixed units operating between 50 and 70 kVp, 1.5 mm aluminum equivalent; for fixed unit operating above 70 kVp, 2.5 mm aluminum equivalent; mobile and fluoroscopic units require total permanent filtration of 2.5 mm aluminum equivalent.

39. **A**

Aluminum (Z = 13) is the metal most frequently used due to its ability to effectively remove low-energy x-rays without decreasing the intensity of the beam.

40. **D**

In mobile C-arm fluoroscopy, there is potential for large radiation doses to patients and operators. Therefore, it is imperative that a minimal source-to-end of collimator assembly should be a distance of 12″ (30 cm).

41. **C**

Control-booth barriers protect the radiographer during an examination, and personnel must remain completely behind the booth for maximal protection. The barrier intercepts only leakage and scatter radiation.

42. **D**

Primary barriers consist of ⅟₁₆″ lead or lead equivalent and extend 7 feet from the floor with the x-ray tube and 5 to 7 feet from the primary wall.

43. **A**

While the radiographer should maintain appropriate distance and remain available for assistance during radiographic procedures, he or she should be dressed adequately. Protective aprons of 0.5 mm lead equivalent must be worn with protective lead gloves of 0.25 mm lead equivalent. In addition, thyroid shields of 0.5 mm lead equivalent should also be worn.

44. **B**

The NCRP mandates that the SSD should be no less than 15″ for stationary fluoroscopes and no less than 12″ for mobile fluoroscopes.

45. **D**

A 35-degree angle is appropriate for females due to the lumbosacral curve.

46. **B**

A 30-degree angle is used for imaging the SI joints for male patients.

47. **A**

A cephalic angle is appropriate when the patient is supine on the imaging table to open the SI joints and L5–S1 junction.

48. **A**

Centering 2″ below the iliac crest will place the central ray at the midpoint of the SI joints.

49. **B**

When the head is flexed too much, the lower margin of the front teeth is superimposed over the odontoid.

50. **C**

The Judd view is performed PA and decreases thyroid dose when the dens is of interest.

51. **C**

Positioning the patient PA reduces the thyroid dose.

52. **D**

The head and neck are rotated anteriorly 15 degrees to 20 degrees. Internally rotating the entire leg will place the neck parallel for a true AP image of the hip.

53. **D**

The average angle of the neck to shaft is 125 degrees, with a possible 15-degree variance based on the width of the patient's pelvis.

54. **A**

70-degree oblique or 20 degrees off lateral would best demonstrate the zygapophyseal joints of the thoracic spine.

55. **A**

HNP is when the inner material of the vertebral disk extrudes from the annulus fibrosis.

56. **B**

Spondylolisthesis involves forward slipping of one vertebra onto another, commonly due to a defect in the pars interarticularis.

57. **B**

Posterior oblique positions demonstrate the down side zygapophyseal joints.

58. **A**

Flexion/extension laterals will demonstrate the mobility of the spine.

59. **B**

The measurement of tabletop to ASIS allows the radiographer to angle the tube correctly and brings the tube parallel with the joint space.

60. **C**

A 45-degree medial oblique of the knee will move the fibula away from the tibia.

61. **D**

A medial oblique of the knee will demonstrate the proximal tibiofibular joint space open.

62. **B**

A 20-degree to 30-degree knee flexion opens the femoropatellar joint space.

63. **A**

A cross-table lateral knee with a horizontal central ray will demonstrate an effusion.

64. **A**

The patella and tibial tubercle are seen in profile in a properly positioned lateral knee.

65. **C**

The femoropatellar joint space should be open on a lateral knee.

66. **B**

The adductor tubercle will be demonstrated if the knee is underrotated.

67. **D**

Sinding-Larsen-Johansson is a ligament disorder that pulls on the apex of the patella.

68. **B**

Osgood-Schlatter disease is a patellar ligament disorder that attaches to the tibial tuberosity and is best demonstrated on a lateral knee image.

69. **B**

Intercondylar fossa views will better demonstrate the tibial eminences and possible degenerative joint disease.

70. **C**

The femoral epicondyles are perpendicular to the IR in a lateral knee image.

71. **A**

Dropping the patient's shoulders helps to move the clavicles inferiorly from the apices.

72. **A**

Double inhalation helps to moves the diaphragm more inferior versus single inhalation and allows for greater lung expansion.

73. **D**

A 14″ × 17″ lengthwise is the best choice for a hyposthenic patient in order to include the entire lung field.

74. **B**

The central ray is directed to T6–T7, which is also at the level of the inferior scapula.

75. **A**

Centering 4″ below the jugular notch brings the central ray to the level of T6–T7.

76. **C**

A 40″ SID would cause the heart to appear magnified, so a 72″ SID is used to reduce the magnification of the heart.

77. **C**

Long-scale contrast allows for lung tissue to be visualized by demonstrating white, gray, and black structures.

78. **C**

Long-scale contrast requires higher kVp.

79. **A**

Having the patient stand 12″ in front of the IR and lean against it pushes the clavicles superior to the apices, demonstrating the apical region of the lungs.

80. **D**

A 10-degree to 15-degree oblique image will remove superimposed tissue.

81. **D**

A 60-degree LAO is required for a heart study.

82. **B**

The RPO position will best demonstrate the right posterior ribs.

83. **B**

Lower ribs require exhalation because it will push the diaphragm up to improve visualization of the ribs.

84. **C**

An LPO image of the ribs will demonstrate the left posterior ribs.

85. **D**

An LAO image of the ribs will demonstrate the right anterior ribs.

86. **A**

For lower ribs, exhalation will move the diaphragm up and improve visualization.

87. **C**

Inhalation will push the sternum away from the thoracic cavity, allowing better visualization of the sternum.

88. **A**

A 15-degree to 20-degree RAO will move the sternum away from the spine and into the heart shadow to better demonstrate the sternum.

89. **B**

Pectus excavatum is a condition in which the chest is concave rather than convex and is best demonstrated on a lateral image of the sternum.

90. **D**

Pectus excavatum is a chest that is positioned in a sunken or funnel position.

91. **A**

Hypersthenic patients require less obliquity.

92. **B**

Asthenic patients require more obliquity than hypersthenic patients.

93. **C**

Autotomography will help blur out vascular markings, allowing better visualization of the sternum.

94. **C**

The joint closest to the IR will be demonstrated when the patient is an anterior oblique position.

95. **A**

An anterior oblique position brings the S-C joint closest to the IR and decreases magnification/distortion.

96. **D**

The symphysis pubis is the appropriate landmark to ensure the bladder will appear on an abdominal radiograph (KUB) as the distal part of the bladder terminates at the symphysis pubis.

97. **A**

The diaphragm must be demonstrated on an erect abdominal radiograph to determine if free air is under diaphragm.

98. **C**

When the patient is placed prone, the small intestines are closest to the IR because the kidneys are located in the anterior region of the abdominal cavity.

99. **B**

The erect abdomen image should be performed first because the patient is ambulatory and has been upright for the minimum requirement of 5 minutes. The AP supine image should be performed second.

100. **B**

To best demonstrate free air in the abdomen of a nonambulatory patient, a decubitus projection should be performed because the patient would not be able to stand for an erect abdomen.

101. **A**

The mA would be halved for a soft tissue analog neck radiograph, which would better demonstrate soft tissue rather than bone.

102. **D**

The lateromedial lateral position of the ankle is the best position to demonstrate a displaced ankle fracture.

103. **C**

A fracture ½″ distal to the base of the 5th metatarsal (Jones fracture) is common.

104. **C**

More angle is required for a patient with high arches.

105. **A**

Less angle is required for a patient with flat feet.

106. **B**

The 3rd through 5th metatarsals are free of superimposition, whereas the 1st and 2nd metatarsals are superimposed.

107. **B**

A medial oblique view will superimpose medial anatomy; however, it will demonstrate lateral anatomy.

108. **D**

Dorsoplantar axial projections of the calcaneus will demonstrate medial or lateral displacement of the calcaneus.

109. **A**

When performing a weight-bearing lateral image of the foot, the patient should put his or her full weight onto the affected foot.

110. **B**

When a patient is positioned prone (Lewis method) to demonstrate the sesamoids, the central ray is directed tangential to the sesamoids.

111. **C**

A patient would be supine and instructed to dorsiflex the foot, placing the calcaneus in contact with the IR.

112. **B**

A 7-degree to 10-degree posterior angle is required to open tarsal interspaces.

113. **C**

Lateral weight-bearing radiographs demonstrate the true integrity of a patient's arch.

114. **A**

The base of the 5th metatarsal is a common site of fracture.

115. **D**

A 15-degree to 20-degree internal rotation of the ankle brings the intermalleolar line parallel to the IR and opens the mortise.

116. **C**

A 45-degree internal oblique allows the distal tibio-fibular joint space to open.

117. **A**

A lateral (external) oblique view of the ankle will demonstrate the posterior malleolus.

118. **B**

The 15-degree mortise most accurately demonstrates the ankle joint.

119. **A**

Eversion stress places stress on the medial compartment of the ankle, demonstrating possible medial ligament tears.

120. **D**

Zenker diverticulum is a large outpouching of the proximal esophagus.

121. **C**

The aorta and left primary bronchus cause two indentations in the esophagus.

122. **D**

The timer is used to control the amount of time the x-ray is on (duration).

123. **A**

The anode rotates inside the x-ray tube and is positively charged.

124. **C**

The filaments are two different-sized wires that emit electrons during thermionic emission.

125. **B**

The outer edge of the anode is made of tungsten.

126. **B**

The rotating anode is an induction motor that contains a stator and a rotor.

127. **D**

AEC can be adjusted in exposure settings in small increments that are commonly from −2 up to a +2 density.

128. **B**

AEC units have three different ionization chambers that can be selected by the radiographer prior to patient exposure.

129. **D**

AEC uses ionization chambers (detectors) to determine the appropriate amount of radiation for an imaging study.

130. **C**

An aperture diaphragm is considered a beam restriction device.

131. **D**

A beam restriction device reduces patient exposure, improves image quality, and can be a manual or automatic collimator.

132. **A**

The rectifier changes the current from AC to DC.

133. **A**

Incoming power needs to be converted from AC to DC.

134. **B**

The power in the United States is 60 Hz AC.

135. **C**

Three phase x-ray systems are generally used in general radiography, fluoroscopy, and angiography units.

136. **B**

In a digital fluoroscopic unit, the flat panel detectors replace the image intensifier.

137. **D**

DR uses flat panel detectors.

138. **D**

Dedicated chest units can be either a CR system, a DR system, or a conventional film-type system.

139. **A**

A tomography unit creates a pivot point or fulcrum between the x-ray tube and IR.

140. **C**

Grids increase image quality.

141. **A**

True statements regarding quality assurance testing for light field and radiation field testing would include radiopaque markers on the edge of the light field, a fluorescent plate, and a plastic or aluminum tube for beam alignment.

142. **A**

When x-ray equipment malfunctions, it can endanger the patient and the operator; the procedure should be stopped immediately, and the issue should be reported to maintenance.

143. **B**

Digital imaging receptors are subject to artifacts.

144. **B**

A ghost image can occur with DR when the previous exposure is trapped.

145. **C**

Incomplete system erasures on CR and DR systems can contribute to imaging artifacts.

146. **D**

An SMPTE pattern can be used to check for sharpness, distortion, and luminescence.

147. **A**

The manual exposure setting should be used when checking lead aprons to prevent excessive radiation.

148. **C**

The rotor is made up of soft iron and copper bars.

149. **C**

There are three critical elements that must occur in order for radiation to be emitted from the x-ray tube. These elements include (1) the source of the free electrons, which are located in the focusing cup of the tube as a result of thermionic emissions; (2) the focusing of these electrons to be accelerated from the cathode to the anode through the use of kV; and (3) the target of the anode, which acts as the site of interaction of the projectile electrons, resulting in the projectile electrons either slowing down as they come close to the nuclear field or interacting with the orbital electrons located in the target atom.

150. **B**

Infrared radiation makes up approximately 99% of the kinetic energy of the projectile electrons.

151. **D**

Bremsstrahlung radiation refers to the interaction of the projectile electron that is influenced by the nuclear field of the target atom.

152. **D**

The majority of radiation that results from interactions at the target atom is classified as Bremsstrahlung.

153. **C**

When a projectile electron interacts with an inner-shell electron and succeeds in totally removing it from its orbital shells, an ion is produced. This process is referred to as *ionization*. In addition, the resulting open space in the shell is replaced by an outer-shell electron dropping into this slot through a process referred to as *transition*. Transition is accompanied by the release of characteristic radiation and energy resulting from the difference between the binding energies of the orbital shells involved in this replacement process.

154. **A**

Characteristic radiation produced in other orbital shells than the k-orbit produces radiation that is of lower energy and not useful for imaging.

155. **B**

The effective energy of characteristic x-rays decreases with target elements of lower Z. The x-ray energies associated with characteristic radiation have precisely fixed energies and form discrete spectrums.

156. **B**

Bremsstrahlung radiation is dependent on the electron speed used and the proximity to the nucleus.

157. **C**

Electromagnetic radiation in the form of x-rays possesses wavelength and frequency; the relationship between these properties is inverse.

158. **A**

Electromagnetic radiation is inversely related to the square of the distance from the source. Should the distance from the source of radiation increase by one-half, the intensity of the radiation is reduced by 25%, or one-fourth.

159. **D**

A change that occurs to kVp or tube voltage will result in either an increase or decrease in amplitude and energy. There will be no effect to target material or filtration.

160. **A**

A change that occurs to mA/s or tube current will result in only either an increase or decrease in amplitude.

161. **B**

Added filtration will decrease the intensity of the x-ray produced.

162. **B**

The higher the Z of the target material, the greater the efficiency of brems radiation produced.

163. **D**

Generators such as a three-phase or high-frequency types are more efficient than single-phase types. As the efficiency of the generator increases, less voltage ripple will occur, which will increase the intensity and energy of the x-ray beam produced.

164. **C**

Leakage radiation is any radiation that is not considered a primary radiation.

165. **A**

Primary radiation is produced when the target is bombarded by electrons.

166. **A**

Consent forms are not transferrable to another date even for the same procedure.

167. **C**

Battery is the physical touching of a person without his or her consent.

168. **B**

DNR stands for *do not resuscitate* and no efforts to restart the heart or respiratory function can be done on the patient.

169. **D**

Normal floras are pathogens present on or in a person that do not cause infection for the person.

170. **B**

Pathogenicity is defined as the ability of a microorganism to produce disease.

171. **D**

Restraints cannot be applied without a medical order and are considered false imprisonment because the patient cannot free himself or herself from the restraint.

172. **C**

Structured interviews use simple, one-response questions to gather quick, specific information.

173. **A**

The HIPAA privacy practices notification describes how a physician's office uses a patient's personal health information.

174. **C**

Respondeat superior states that the employer is responsible for the actions of the employee.

175. **B**

Virulence defines how likely a pathogen is to result in active disease; the pathogen's degree of pathogenicity.

176. **A**

Iatrogenic illness is acquired through the treatment prescribed by the physician and does not need to occur in the hospital setting.

177. **D**

Autoclave sterilization uses high, moist heat (steam).

178. **D**

Influenza is transmitted in the air with large droplets that cannot travel greater than 3 feet.

179. **B**

A tort is a civil wrong against a person or property that is not punishable by imprisonment.

180. **A**

A normal BP is a systolic of 120 mm Hg or less and a diastolic of 80 mm Hg or less.

181. **B**

Elderly patients commonly do not have a greater support system than young patients due to major life changes such as illness or death of a spouse, no assistance from adult children, or no family in the local area.

182. **C**

The pathogen must have a means to exit the infected person before there can be a mode of transmission or portal of entry.

183. **A**

The five elements of cultural competency include value diversity, capacity for self-assessment, understand cross-cultural interactions, applying cultural knowledge to medical care, and adapting patient services that reflect cultural understanding.

184. **C**

Anaerobes do not require oxygen to survive.

185. **B**

A normal adult respiratory rate is 10 to 20 breaths per minute.

186. **D**

A Pigg-O-Stat can be used for infants during chest radiography.

187. **B**

The radial pulse is most commonly taken with the hands.

188. **A**

The enema bag should be hung 18″ to 24″ above the table during a barium enema.

189. **C**

A cathartic is commonly administered to cleanse the bowel of any remaining fecal material.

190. **D**

Droplets are spread 3 feet or less, so the patient can be placed with another patient who is more than 3 ft away.

191. **B**

The needle should always be positioned bevel up and an angle of 45 degree when injecting contrast media.

192. **C**

The median cubital vein is located in the arm.

193. **B**

Metformin (Glucophage) should be stopped 1 day before a radiographic contrast procedure.

194. **A**

BUN evaluates kidney function and an abnormal level may prohibit an intravenous urography examination.

195. **C**

The height of the enema bag should be reduced to decrease flow and pressure.

196. **D**

Patients with megacolon are at an increased risk for increased fluid in the blood (hypovolemia).

197. **D**

Hygroscopic as it relates to barium sulfate is defined as a substance that absorbs liquid.

198. **B**

The hypothalamus regulates body temperature.

199. **A**

Diarrhea is not a complication of barium sulfate after a barium enema.

200. **C**

Glucagon is commonly found in a crash cart.

201. **B**

An itchy throat may occur with a mild reaction to contrast media.

202. **D**

Ecchymosis is the proper medical terminology for "black and blue."

203. **D**

A patient may experience a severe reaction to latex-based products.

204. **C**

Hypothermia is the medical term for a body temperature below 95°F.

205. **A**

A patient with a spinal cord trauma injury may exhibit flaccid paralysis.

206. **D**

Patients with pyrexia experience fever and have an increased pulse rate.

207. **B**

Hospice provides palliative care.

208. **D**

Drugs can be secreted through the urine, sweat, and feces.

209. **C**

Contrast is defined as the visible difference between two densities on an image.

210. **A**

mA/s affects radiographic density.

211. **A**

As mA/s decreases, density decreases as a result of decreased thermionic emission.

212. **B**

kVp is the main controlling factor of contrast.

213. **C**

The law of reciprocity states that different combinations of mA and time that produce the same mA/s produce the same density.

214. **B**

The law of reproducibility states that every time the same combination of mA and time is set on the same x-ray unit, the resulting image will demonstrate the same density.

215. **C**

mA affects radiation quantity.

216. **D**

Film-screen speed and density are directly proportional. As film-screen speed increases, density increases.

217. **A**

The inverse square law states that the intensity of radiation is inversely proportional to the square of the distance from the x-ray source.

218. **C**

A minimum air gap of 6″ will have an effect on density.

219. **B**

The air-gap technique may be used to minimize the amount of scatter reaching the IR when a grid is not available.

ARRT Content Specifications for the Examination in Radiography

CONTENT SPECIFICATIONS FOR THE EXAMINATION IN RADIOGRAPHY

Publication Date: August 2010
Implementation Date: January 2012

The purpose of the ARRT Examination in Radiography is to assess the knowledge and cognitive skills underlying the intelligent performance of the tasks typically required of the staff technologist at entry into the profession. To identify the knowledge and skills covered by the examination, the ARRT periodically conducts practice analysis studies involving a nationwide sample of staff technologists[1]. The results of the most recent practice analysis are reflected in this document. The complete task inventory, which serves as the basis for these content specifications, is available from our website *www.arrt.org.*

The table below presents the five major content categories, along with the number and percentage of test questions appearing in each category. The remaining pages provide a detailed listing of topics addressed within each major content category.

This document is not intended to serve as a curriculum guide. Although certification programs and educational programs may have related purposes, their functions are clearly different. Educational programs are generally broader in scope and address subject matter not included in these content specifications.

	CONTENT CATEGORY	PERCENT OF TEST	NUMBER OF QUESTIONS [2]
A.	Radiation Protection	22.5%	45
B.	Equipment Operation and Quality Control	11.0%	22
C.	Image Acquisition and Evaluation	22.5%	45
D.	Imaging Procedures	29.0%	58
E.	Patient Care and Education	15.0%	30
		100%	200

1. A special debt of gratitude is due to the hundreds of professionals participating in this project as committee members, survey respondents, and reviewers.

2. Each exam includes up to an additional 20 unscored (pilot) questions. On the pages that follow, the approximate number of test questions allocated to each content category appears in parentheses.

A. RADIATION PROTECTION (45)

1. Biological Aspects of Radiation (10)

A. Radiosensitivity

1. dose-response relationships
2. relative tissue radiosensitivities (e.g., LET, RBE)
3. cell survival and recovery (LD_{50})
4. oxygen effect

B. Somatic Effects

1. short-term versus long-term effects
2. acute versus chronic effects
3. carcinogenesis
4. organ and tissue response (e.g., eye, thyroid, breast, bone marrow, skin, gonadal)

C. Acute Radiation Syndromes

1. CNS
2. hemopoietic
3. GI

D. Embryonic and Fetal Risks

E. Genetic Impact

1. genetic significant dose
2. goals of gonadal shielding

F. Photon Interactions with Matter

1. Compton effect
2. photoelectric absorption
3. coherent (classical) scatter
4. attenuation by various tissues
   a. thickness of body part (density)
   b. type of tissue (atomic number)

2. Minimizing Patient Exposure (15)

A. Exposure Factors

1. kVp
2. mAs

B. Shielding

1. rationale for use
2. types
3. placement

C. Beam Restriction

1. purpose of primary beam restriction
2. types (e.g., collimators)

D. Filtration

1. effect on skin and organ exposure
2. effect on average beam energy
3. NCRP recommendations (NCRP #102, minimum filtration in useful beam)

E. Exposure Reduction

1. patient positioning
2. automatic exposure control (AEC)
3. patient communication
4. digital imaging
5. pediatric dose reduction
6. ALARA

F. Image Receptors (e.g., types, relative speed, digital versus film)

G. Grids

H. Fluoroscopy

1. pulsed
2. exposure factors
3. grids
4. positioning
5. fluoroscopy time

(Section A continues on the following page)

A. RADIATION PROTECTION (cont.)

3. Personnel Protection (11)

A. Sources of Radiation Exposure

   1. primary x-ray beam

   2. secondary radiation

      a. scatter

      b. leakage

   3. patient as source

B. Basic Methods of Protection

   1. time

   2. distance

   3. shielding

C. Protective Devices

   1. types

   2. attenuation properties

   3. minimum lead equivalent (NCRP #102)

D. Special Considerations

   1. portable (mobile) units

   2. fluoroscopy

      a. protective drapes

      b. protective Bucky slot cover

      c. cumulative timer

   3. guidelines for fluoroscopy and portable units (NCRP #102, CFR-21)

      a. fluoroscopy exposure rates

      b. exposure switch guidelines

4. Radiation Exposure and Monitoring (9)

A. Units of Measurement*

   1. absorbed dose

   2. dose equivalent

   3. exposure

B. Dosimeters

   1. types

   2. proper use

C. NCRP Recommendations for Personnel Monitoring (NCRP #116)

   1. occupational exposure

   2. public exposure

   3. embryo/fetus exposure

   4. ALARA and dose equivalent limits

   5. evaluation and maintenance of personnel dosimetry records

D. Medical Exposure of Patients (NCRP #160)

   1. typical effective dose per exam

   2. comparison of typical doses by modality

---

*Conventional units are generally used. However, questions referenced to specific reports (e.g., NCRP) will use SI units to be consistent with such reports.

B. EQUIPMENT OPERATION AND QUALITY CONTROL (22)

1. **Principles of Radiation Physics (9)**

    A. X-Ray Production

       1. source of free electrons (e.g., thermionic emission)
       2. acceleration of electrons
       3. focusing of electrons
       4. deceleration of electrons

    B. Target Interactions

       1. bremsstrahlung
       2. characteristic

    C. X-Ray Beam

       1. frequency and wavelength
       2. beam characteristics
          a. quality
          b. quantity
          c. primary versus remnant (exit)
       3. inverse square law
       4. fundamental properties (e.g., travel in straight lines, ionize matter)

2. **Imaging Equipment (9)**

    A. Components of Radiographic Unit (fixed or mobile)

       1. operating console
       2. x-ray tube construction
          a. electron sources
          b. target materials
          c. induction motor
       3. automatic exposure control (AEC)
          a. radiation detectors
          b. back-up timer
          c. density adjustment (e.g., +1 or −1)
       4. manual exposure controls
       5. beam restriction devices

    B. X-Ray Generator, Transformers, and Rectification System

       1. basic principles
       2. phase, pulse, and frequency

    C. Components of Fluoroscopic Unit (fixed or mobile)

       1. image intensifier
       2. viewing systems
       3. recording systems
       4. automatic brightness control (ABC)

    D. Components of Digital Imaging (CR and DR)

       1. PSP - photo-stimulable phosphor
       2. flat panel detectors - direct and indirect
       3. start up and shut down
       4. CR plate erasure
       5. equipment cleanliness (imaging plates, CR plates)

    E. Types of Units

       1. dedicated chest unit
       2. tomography unit

    F. Accessories

       1. stationary grids
       2. Bucky assembly
       3. image receptors

3. **Quality Control of Imaging Equipment and Accessories (4)**

    A. Beam Restriction

       1. light field to radiation field alignment
       2. central ray alignment

    B. Recognition and Reporting of Malfunctions

    C. Digital Imaging Receptor Systems

       1. artifacts (e.g., non-uniformity, erasure)
       2. maintenance (e.g., detector fog)
       3. display monitor quality assurance

    D. Shielding Accessories (e.g., lead apron and glove testing)

C. IMAGE ACQUISITION AND EVALUATION (45)

1. **Selection of Technical Factors (20)**

    A. Factors Affecting Radiographic Quality. Refer to Attachment C to clarify terms that may occur on the exam. (X indicates topics covered on the examination)

	1. Density/Brightness	2. Contrast/Gray Scale	3. Recorded Detail/Spatial Resolution	4. Distortion
a. mAs	X			
b. kVp	X	X		
c. OID		X (air gap)	X	X
d. SID	X		X	X
e. focal spot size			X	
f. grids*	X	X		
g. filtration	X	X		
h. film-screen	X		X	
i. beam restriction	X	X		
j. motion			X	
k. anode heel effect	X			
l. patient factors (size, pathology)	X	X	X	X
m. angle (tube, part, or receptor)			X	X

  * Includes conversion factors for grids

B. Technique Charts

  1. pre-programmed techniques – anatomically programmed radiography (APR)
  2. caliper measurement
  3. fixed versus variable kVp
  4. special considerations
      a. casts
      b. anatomic and pathologic factors
      c. pediatrics
      d. contrast media

C. Automatic Exposure Control (AEC)

  1. effects of changing exposure factors on radiographic quality
  2. detector selection
  3. anatomic alignment
  4. density control (+1 or −1)

D. Digital Imaging Characteristics

  1. spatial resolution
      a. sampling frequency
      b. DEL (detector element size)
      c. receptor size and matrix size
  2. image signal (exposure related)
      a. quantum mottle (noise)
      b. SNR (signal to noise ratio) or CNR (contrast to noise ratio)

(Section C continues on the following page)

C. IMAGE ACQUISITION AND EVALUATION (cont.)

2. Image Processing and Quality Assurance (12)

A. Image Identification

1. methods (e.g., photographic, radiographic, electronic)
2. legal considerations (e.g., patient data, examination data)

B. Film Screen Processing

1. film storage
2. components*
   a. developer
   b. fixer
3. maintenance/malfunction
   a. start up and shut down procedure
   b. possible causes of malfunction (e.g., improper temperature, contamination, replenishment, water flow)

C. Digital Imaging Processing

1. electronic collimation (masking)
2. grayscale rendition (look-up table (LUT), histogram)
3. edge enhancement/noise suppression
4. contrast enhancement
5. system malfunctions (e.g., ghost image, banding, erasure, dead pixels, readout problems)
6. CR reader components

D. Image Display

1. viewing conditions (i.e., luminance, ambient lighting
2. spatial resolution
3. contrast resolution/dynamic range
4. DICOM gray scale function
5. window level and width function

E. Digital Image Display Informatics

1. PACS
2. HIS
3. RIS (modality work list)
4. Networking (e.g., HL7, DICOM)
5. Workflow (inappropriate documentation, lost images, mismatched images, corrupt data)

* Specific chemicals in the processing solutions will not be covered (e.g., glutaraldehyde).

3. Criteria for Image Evaluation (13)

A. Brightness/Density (e.g., mAs, distance)

B. Contrast/Gray Scale (e.g., kVp, filtration, grids)

C. Recorded Detail (e.g., motion, poor film-screen contact)

D. Distortion (e.g., magnification, OID, SID)

E. Demonstration of Anatomical Structures (e.g., positioning, tube-part-image receptor alignment)

F. Identification Markers (e.g., anatomical, patient, date)

G. Patient Considerations (e.g., pathologic conditions)

H. Image artifacts (e.g., film handling, static, pressure, grid lines, Moiré effect or aliasing)

I. Fog (e.g., age, chemical, radiation, temperature, safelight)

J. Noise

K. Acceptable Range of Exposure

L. Exposure Indicator Determination

M. Gross Exposure Error (e.g., mottle, light or dark, low contrast)

D. IMAGING PROCEDURES (58)

This section addresses imaging procedures for the anatomic regions listed below (1 through 7). Questions will cover the following topics:

1. Positioning (e.g., topographic landmarks, body positions, path of central ray, immobilization devices).

2. Anatomy (e.g., including physiology, basic pathology, and related medical terminology).

3. Technical factors (e.g., including adjustments for circumstances such as body habitus, trauma, pathology, breathing techniques).

The specific radiographic positions and projections within each anatomic region that may be covered on the examination are listed in Attachment A. A guide to positioning terminology appears in Attachment B.

---

1. **Thorax (10)**
   A. Chest
   B. Ribs
   C. Sternum
   D. Soft Tissue Neck

2. **Abdomen and GI Studies (8)**
   A. Abdomen
   B. Esophagus
   C. Swallowing Dysfunction Study
   D. Upper GI Series, Single or Double Contrast
   E. Small Bowel Series
   F. Barium Enema, Single or Double Contrast
   G. Surgical Cholangiography
   H. ERCP

3. **Urological Studies (3)**
   A. Cystography
   B. Cystourethrography
   C. Intravenous Urography
   D. Retrograde Pyelography

4. **Spine and Pelvis (10)**
   A. Cervical Spine
   B. Thoracic Spine
   C. Scoliosis Series
   D. Lumbar Spine
   E. Sacrum and Coccyx
   F. Sacroiliac Joints
   G. Pelvis and Hip

5. **Head (5)**
   A. Skull
   B. Facial Bones
   C. Mandible
   D. Zygomatic Arch
   E. Temporomandibular Joints
   F. Nasal Bones
   G. Orbits
   H. Paranasal Sinuses

6. **Extremities (20)**
   A. Toes
   B. Foot
   C. Calcaneus (Os Calcis)
   D. Ankle
   E. Tibia, Fibula
   F. Knee
   G. Patella
   H. Femur
   I. Fingers
   J. Hand
   K. Wrist
   L. Forearm
   M. Elbow
   N. Humerus
   O. Shoulder
   P. Scapula
   Q. Clavicle
   R. Acromioclavicular Joints

6. **Extremities (cont.)**
   S. Bone Survey
   T. Long Bone Measurement
   U. Bone Age
   V. Soft Tissue/Foreign Bodies

7. **Other (2)**
   A. Arthrography
   B. Myelography

E. PATIENT CARE AND EDUCATION (30)

1. Ethical and Legal Aspects (4)

A. Patient's Rights

1. informed consent (e.g., written, oral, implied)
2. confidentiality (HIPAA)
3. additional rights (e.g., Patient's Bill of Rights)
   a. privacy
   b. extent of care (e.g., DNR)
   c. access to information
   d. living will; health care proxy
   e. research participation

B. Legal Issues

1. examination documentation (e.g., patient history, clinical diagnosis)
2. common terminology (e.g., battery, negligence, malpractice)
3. legal doctrines (e.g., *respondeat superior*, *res ipsa loquitur*)
4. restraints versus immobilization

C. ARRT Standards of Ethics

2. Interpersonal Communication (5)

A. Modes of Communication

1. verbal/written
2. nonverbal (e.g., eye contact, touching)

B. Challenges in Communication

1. patient characteristics
2. explanation of medical terms
3. strategies to improve understanding
4. cultural diversity

C. Patient Education

1. explanation of current procedure
2. respond to inquiries about other imaging modalities (e.g., CT, MRI, mammography, sonography, nuclear medicine, bone densitometry regarding dose differences, types of radiation, and patient preps)

3. Infection Control (5)

A. Terminology and Basic Concepts

1. asepsis
   a. medical
   b. surgical
   c. sterile technique
2. pathogens
   a. fomites, vehicles, vectors
   b. nosocomial infections

B. Cycle of Infection

1. pathogen
2. source or reservoir of infection
3. susceptible host
4. method of transmission
   a. contact (direct, indirect)
   b. droplet
   c. airborne/suspended
   d. common vehicle
   e. vector borne

C. Standard Precautions

1. handwashing
2. gloves, gowns
3. masks
4. medical asepsis (e.g., equipment disinfection)

D. Additional or Transmission-Based Precautions

1. airborne (e.g., respiratory protection, negative ventilation)
2. droplet (e.g., particulate mask, restricted patient placement)
3. contact (e.g., gloves, gown, restricted patient placement)

E. Disposal of Contaminated Materials

1. linens
2. needles
3. patient supplies (e.g., tubes, emesis basin)

(Section E continues on the following page)

E. PATIENT CARE AND EDUCATION (cont.)

4. Physical Assistance and Transfer (4)

  A. Patient Transfer and Movement

    1. body mechanics (balance, alignment, movement)

    2. patient transfer

  B. Assisting Patients with Medical Equipment

    1. infusion catheters and pumps

    2. oxygen delivery systems

    3. other (e.g., nasogastric tubes, urinary catheters, tracheostomy tubes)

  C. Routine Monitoring

    1. equipment (e.g., stethoscope, sphygmomanometer)

    2. vital signs (e.g., blood pressure, pulse, respiration)

    3. physical signs and symptoms (e.g., motor control, severity of injury)

    4. documentation

5. Medical Emergencies (5)

  A. Allergic Reactions (e.g., contrast media, latex)

  B. Cardiac or Respiratory Arrest (e.g., CPR)

  C. Physical Injury or Trauma

  D. Other Medical Disorders (e.g., seizures, diabetic reactions)

6. Pharmacology (3)

  A. Patient History

    1. medication reconciliation (current medications)

    2. premedications

    3. contraindications

    4. scheduling and sequencing examinations

  B. Complications/Reactions

    1. local effects (e.g., extravasation/ infiltration, phlebitis)

    2. systemic effects

      a. mild

      b. moderate

      c. severe

    3. emergency medications

    4. radiographer's response and documentation

7. Contrast Media (4)

  A. Types and Properties (e.g., iodinated, water soluble, barium, ionic versus non-ionic)

  B. Appropriateness of Contrast Media to Exam

    1. patient condition (e.g., perforated bowel)

    2. patient age and weight

    3. laboratory values (e.g., BUN creatinine, GFR)

  C. Patient Education

    1. verify informed consent

    2. instructions regarding preparation, diet, and medications

    3. pre- and post-examination instructions (e.g., discharge instructions)

  D. Venipuncture

    1. venous anatomy

    2. supplies

    3. procedural technique

  E. Administration

    1. routes (e.g., IV, oral)

    2. supplies (e.g., enema kits, needles)

Attachment A
Radiographic Positions and Projections

1. Thorax
- A. Chest
  1. PA upright
  2. lateral upright
  3. AP Lordotic
  4. AP supine
  5. lateral decubitus
  6. anterior and posterior obliques
- B. Ribs
  1. AP and PA, above and below diaphragm
  2. anterior and posterior oblique
- C. Sternum
  1. lateral
  2. RAO breathing technique
  3. RAO expiration
  4. LAO
  5. PA sternoclavicular joints
  6. anterior oblique sternoclavicular joints
- D. Soft Tissue Neck
  1. AP upper airway
  2. lateral upper airway

2. Abdomen and GI studies
- A. Abdomen
  1. AP supine
  2. AP upright
  3. lateral decubitus
  4. dorsal decubitus
- B. Esophagus
  1. RAO
  2. left lateral
  3. AP
  4. PA
  5. LAO
- C. Swallowing Dysfunction Study
- D. Upper GI series*
  1. AP scout
  2. RAO
  3. PA
  4. right lateral
  5. LPO
  6. AP
- E. Small Bowel Series
  1. PA scout
  2. PA (follow through)
  3. ileocecal spots
  4. enteroclysis procedure
- F. Barium Enema*
  1. left lateral rectum
  2. left lateral decubitus
  3. right lateral decubitus
  4. LPO and RPO
  5. PA
  6. RAO and LAO
  7. AP axial (butterfly)
  8. PA axial (butterfly)
  9. PA post-evacuation
- G. Surgical Cholangiography
  1. AP
- H. ERCP
  1. AP

* single or double contrast

3. Urological Studies
- A. Cystography
  1. AP
  2. LPO and RPO 60º
  3. lateral
  4. AP 10-15º caudad
- B. Cystourethrography
  1. AP voiding cystourethrogram female
  2. RPO 30º, voiding cystogram male
- C. Intravenous Urography
  1. AP, scout, and series
  2. RPO and LPO 30º
  3. PA post-void
  4. AP post-void, upright
  5. nephrotomography
  6. AP ureteric compression
- D. Retrograde Pyelography
  1. AP scout
  2. AP pyelogram
  3. AP ureterogram

4. Spine and Pelvis
- A. Cervical Spine
  1. AP angle cephalad
  2. AP open mouth
  3. lateral
  4. cross table lateral
  5. anterior oblique
  6. posterior oblique
  7. lateral swimmers
  8. lateral flexion and extension
  9. AP dens (Fuchs)
  10. PA dens (Judd)
- B. Thoracic Spine
  1. AP
  2. lateral, breathing
  3. lateral, expiration
- C. Scoliosis Series
  1. AP/PA scoliosis series (Ferguson)
- D. Lumbar Spine
  1. AP
  2. PA
  3. lateral
  4. L5-S1 lateral spot
  5. posterior oblique 45º
  6. anterior oblique 45º
  7. AP L5-S1, 30-35º cephalad
  8. AP right and left bending
  9. lateral flexion and extension
- E. Sacrum and Coccyx
  1. AP sacrum, 15-25º cephalad
  2. AP coccyx, 10-20º caudad
  3. lateral sacrum and coccyx, combined
  4. lateral sacrum or coccyx, separate

- F. Sacroiliac Joints
  1. AP
  2. posterior oblique
  3. anterior oblique
- G. Pelvis and Hip
  1. AP hip only
  2. cross-table lateral hip
  3. unilateral frog-leg, non-trauma
  4. axiolateral inferosuperior, trauma (Clements-Nakayama)
  5. AP pelvis
  6. AP pelvis, bilateral frog-leg
  7. AP pelvis, axial anterior pelvic bones (inlet, outlet)
  8. anterior oblique pelvis, acetabulum (Judet)

5. Head
- A. Skull
  1. AP axial (Towne)
  2. lateral
  3. PA (Caldwell)
  4. PA no angle
  5. submentovertical (full basal)
  6. PA 25-30º angle (Haas)
  7. trauma cross table lateral
  8. trauma AP, 15º cephalad
  9. trauma AP, no angle
  10. trauma AP, axial (Towne)
- B. Facial Bones
  1. lateral
  2. parietoacanthial (Waters)
  3. PA (Caldwell)
  4. PA (modified Waters)
- C. Mandible
  1. axiolateral oblique
  2. PA no angle
  3. AP axial (Towne)
  4. PA semi-axial, 20-25º cephalad
  5. PA (modified Waters)
  6. submentovertical (full basal)
- D. Zygomatic Arch
  1. submentovertical (full basal)
  2. parietoacanthial (Waters)
  3. AP axial (Towne)
  4. axial oblique
  5. lateral
- E. Temporomandibular Joints
  1. lateral (Law)
  2. lateral (Schuller)
  3. AP axial (Towne)
- F. Nasal Bones
  1. parietoacanthial (Waters)
  2. lateral
  3. PA (Caldwell)
- G. Orbits
  1. parietoacanthial (Waters)
  2. lateral
  3. PA (Caldwell)
- H. Paranasal Sinuses
  1. lateral
  2. PA (Caldwell)
  3. parietoacanthial (Waters)
  4. submentovertical (full basal)
  5. open mouth parietoacanthial (Waters)

6. Extremities
   A. Toes
      1. AP, entire foot
      2. oblique toe
      3. lateral toe
   B. Foot
      1. AP angle toward heel
      2. medial oblique
      3. lateral oblique
      4. mediolateral
      5. lateromedial
      6. sesamoids, tangential
      7. AP weight bearing
      8. lateral weight bearing
   C. Calcaneus (Os Calcis)
      1. lateral
      2. plantodorsal, axial
      3. dorsoplantar, axial
   D. Ankle
      1. AP
      2. AP mortise
      3. mediolateral
      4. oblique, 45° internal
      5. lateromedial
      6. AP stress views
   E. Tibia, Fibula
      1. AP
      2. lateral
      3. oblique
   F. Knee
      1. AP
      2. lateral
      3. AP weight bearing
      4. lateral oblique 45°
      5. medial oblique 45°
      6. PA
      7. PA axial – intercondylar
         fossa (tunnel)

   G. Patella
      1. lateral
      2. supine flexion 45° (Merchant)
      3. PA
      4. prone flexion 90° (Settegast)
      5. prone flexion 55° (Hughston)
   H. Femur
      1. AP
      2. mediolateral
   I. Fingers
      1. PA entire hand
      2. PA finger only
      3. lateral
      4. oblique
      5. AP thumb
      6. oblique thumb
      7. lateral thumb
   J. Hand
      1. PA
      2. lateral
      3. oblique
   K. Wrist
      1. PA
      2. oblique 45°
      3. lateral
      4. PA for scaphoid
      5. scaphoid (Stecher)
      6. carpal canal
   L. Forearm
      1. AP
      2. lateral
   M. Elbow
      1. AP
      2. lateral
      3. external oblique
      4. internal oblique
      5. AP partial flexion
      6. axial trauma (Coyle)

   N. Humerus
      1. AP non-trauma
      2. lateral non-trauma
      3. AP neutral trauma
      4. scapular Y trauma
      5. transthoracic lateral trauma
      6. lateral, mid and distal, trauma
   O. Shoulder
      1. AP internal and external
         rotation
      2. inferosuperior axial, non-
         trauma
      3. posterior oblique (Grashey)
      4. tangential non-trauma
      5. AP neutral trauma
      6. transthoracic lateral trauma
      7. scapular Y trauma
   P. Scapula
      1. AP
      2. lateral, anterior oblique
      3. lateral, posterior oblique
   Q. Clavicle
      1. AP
      2. AP angle, 15-30° cephalad
      3. PA angle, 15-30° caudad
   R. Acromioclavicular Joints – AP
      Bilateral With and Without
      Weights
   S. Bone Survey
   T. Long Bone Measurement
   U. Bone Age
   V. Soft Tissue/Foreign Body

7. Other Procedures
   A. Arthrography
   B. Myelography

Attachment B

Standard Terminology
for Positioning and Projection

Radiographic View: Describes the body part as seen by the image receptor or other recording medium, such as a fluoroscopic screen. Restricted to the discussion of a *radiograph* or *image*.

Radiographic Position: Refers to a specific body position, such as supine, prone, recumbent, erect, or Trendelenburg. Restricted to the discussion of the *patient's physical position*.

Radiographic Projection: Restricted to the discussion of the *path of the central ray*.

POSITIONING TERMINOLOGY

A.   Lying Down

    1.   *supine*   –   lying on the back
    2.   *prone*   –   lying face downward
    3.   *decubitus*   –   lying down with a horizontal x-ray beam
    4.   *recumbent*   –   lying down in any position

B.   Erect or Upright

    1.   *anterior position*   –   facing the image receptor
    2.   *posterior position* –   facing the radiographic tube
    3.   *oblique position*   –   erect or lying down

        a.   anterior (facing the image receptor)

            i.   *left anterior oblique*   body rotated with the left anterior portion closest to the image receptor
            ii.   *right anterior oblique*   body rotated with the right anterior portion closest to the image receptor

        b.   posterior (facing the radiographic tube)

            i.   *left posterior oblique*   body rotated with the left posterior portion closest to the image receptor

            ii.   *right posterior oblique*   body rotated with the right posterior portion closest to the image receptor

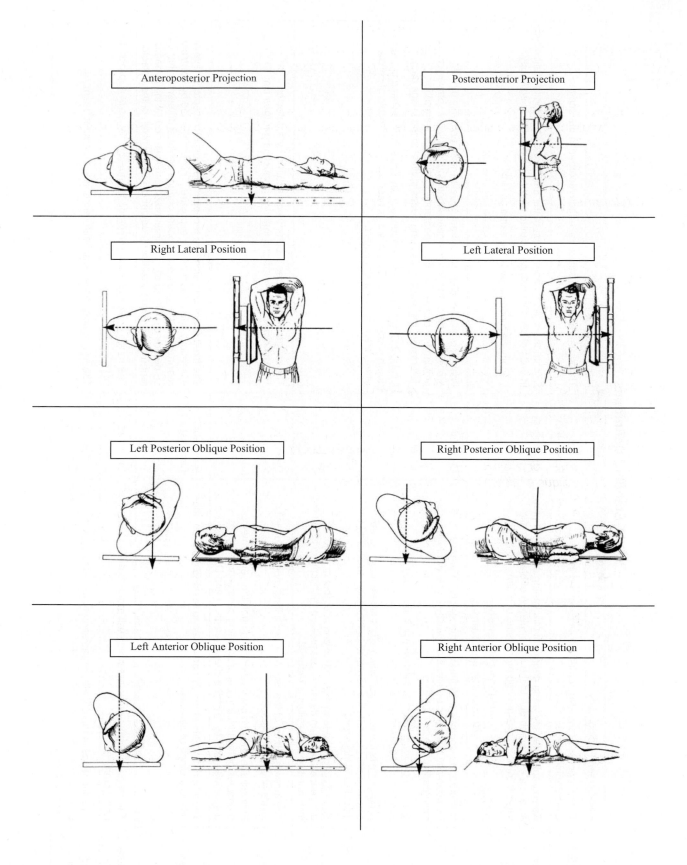

Attachment C
ARRT Standard Definitions

Term	Film-Screen Radiography	Term	Digital Radiography
Recorded Detail	The sharpness of the structural lines as recorded in the radiographic image.	Spatial Resolution	The sharpness of the structural edges recorded in the image.
Density	Radiographic density is the degree of blackening or opacity of an area in a radiograph due to the accumulation of black metallic silver following exposure and processing of a film. $$Density = Log \frac{incident\ light\ intensity}{transmitted\ light\ intensity}$$	Brightness	Brightness is the measurement of the luminance of a monitor calibrated in units of candela (cd) per square meter on a monitor or soft copy. Density on a hard copy is the same as film.
Contrast	Radiographic contrast is defined as the visible differences between any two selected areas of density levels within the radiographic image. _Scale of Contrast_ refers to the number of densities visible (or the number of shades of gray). _Long Scale_ is the term used when slight differences between densities are present (low contrast) but the total number of densities is increased. _Short Scale_ is the term used when considerable or major differences between densities are present (high contrast) but the total number of densities is reduced.	Contrast	Image contrast of display contrast is determined primarily by the processing algorithm (mathematical codes used by the software to provide the desired image appearance). The default algorithm determines the initial processing codes applied to the image data. _Scale of Contrast_ is synonymous to "gray scale" and is linked to the bit depth of the system. 'Gray scale' is used instead of "scale of contrast" when referring to digital images.
Film Latitude	The inherent ability of the film to record a long range of density levels on the radiograph. Film latitude and film contrast depend upon the sensitometric properties of the film and the processing conditions, and are determined directly from the characteristic H and D curve.	Dynamic Range	The range of exposures that may be captured by a detector. The dynamic range for digital imaging is much larger than film.
Film Contrast	The inherent ability of the film emulsion to react to radiation and record a range of densities.	Receptor Contrast	The fixed characteristic of the receptor. Most digital receptors have an essentially linear response to exposure. This is impacted by **contrast resolution** (the smallest exposure change or signal difference that can be detected). Ultimately, contrast resolution is limited by the dynamic range and the **quantization** (number of bits per pixel) of the detector.
Exposure Latitude	The range of exposure factors which will produce a diagnostic radiograph.	Exposure Latitude	The range of exposures which produces quality images at appropriate patient dose.
Subject Contrast	The difference in the quantity of radiation transmitted by a particular part as a result of the different absorption characteristics of the tissues and structures making up that part.	Subject Contrast	The magnitude of the signal difference in the remnant beam.

GLOSSARY

15% rule—in order to double the density of an image, a 15% increase in kVp is required

Absolute risk—predicts that a set number or excess cancers will occur from exposure to radiation

Absorbed dose—energy transferred from ionizing radiation per unit mass of irradiated material; expressed in rad or gray

Absorption—transfer of energy from an electromagnetic field to matter; removal of x-rays from a beam via the photoelectric effect

Actual focal spot—the size of the area on the anode which is struck by electrons

Acute radiation syndromes—relationship of the signs and symptoms to an organism's exposure to whole body radiation

Added filtration—thin sheet of aluminum provided by the manufacturer located between the tube and collimator

Additive pathologies—require an increase in technique

Adjustable collimator—rectangular shutters located below the x-ray tube that open and close based on the desired field of view

Aggravating or alleviating factors—things that either intensify, relive, or modify symptoms

Airborne transmission—mode of transmitting infection by dust containing spores or droplet nuclei, which are particles measuring 5 μm or smaller that contain microorganisms and remain in the air for long periods of time

Aliasing (moiré)—electronic artifacts that appear as wavy lines due to improper sampling of pixels

Alternating current (AC)—converted to direct current in order for radiation to be produced

Anabolism—production of large molecules from small parts

Anaphase—third stage of mitosis, in which centromeres divide and chromatids detach and are pulled to opposite poles

Anaphylactic shock—an exaggerated, life-threatening hypersensitivy reaction to a previously encountered antigen

Anatomically preprogrammed radiography (APR)—allows the radiographer to select an anatomical area from a menu on the control panel that contains preprogrammed exposure factors for that particular anatomy

Anode—positively charged component of the x-ray tube

Anode heel effect—states that radiation intensity exiting the x-ray tube is higher on the side of the cathode and lower on the side of the anode

Antibodies—provide a defensive front to infection and disease that may attack a person

Antihistamine—any substance capable of reducing the physiological and pharmacological effects of histamine; used to treat allergies

Aperture diaphragm—flat piece of lead with a hole cut out of the center and used as a collimation device

Assault—the threat of touching in an injurious way

Associated manifestations—additional symptoms that occur at time of primary complaint

Auditory learner—learns best through verbal explanations

Automatic exposure control (AEC)—device incorporated into the x-ray system that measures the correct amount of radiation reaching the image detectors

Autotransformer—allows the operator to select the voltage needed to make an x-ray exposure

Bacteria—small, unicellular microorganisms

Banding—artifact that occurs during processing where densities in the form of stripes of wide lines are displayed across an image

Barium sulfate—radiopaque medium used as a diagnostic aid in gastrointestinal radiography

Battery—the unlawful use of force against a person

Blood pressure—pressure exerted by the blood against the walls of the blood vessels, especially the arteries

Blood urea nitrogen (BUN) or serum urea nitrogen—clinical laboratory test of kidney function

Borrowed servant—physician liable for those acting under his or her orders

Bradycardia—heart condition in which the ventricles contract at a rate of fewer than 60 bpm

Bremsstrahlung radiation (breaking radiation)—type of radiation found in the primary beam that results from interaction of the projectile electron with a target nucleus

Calipers—measuring devices that are used to accurately determine the thickness of an anatomical area

Capsules—drug dosage form consisting of either a hard or soft gelatin shell that encloses the active ingredient

Carbohydrates—provide main source of energy within the body for cell metabolism

Carcinogenesis—creation of cancer

Cardiac arrest—sudden cessation of cardiac output and effective circulation. Usually precipitated by ventricular fibrillation or ventricular asystole

Catabolism—breaking down of macromolecules into smaller parts

Cathode—negatively charged component of the x-ray tube that emits electrons

Characteristic radiation—type of radiation found in the primary beam that is released as a result of photoelectric effect; discrete energies as determined by the respective electron binding energy

Chronic obstructive pulmonary disease (COPD)—a progressive and irreversible condition characterized by diminished inspiratory and expiratory capacity of the lungs

Chronology—onset, duration, frequency, and progression of symptoms

Cinefluorography—recording of fluoroscopic images on movie film

Civil offense—violation of the rights or duties of an individual or society but is not punishable by imprisonment

Coherent scattering—results in no loss of energy as x-ray scatter

Colonization—multiplication of a microorganism that does not result in cellular injury

Components of a radiographic unit—operating console, power switch, kVp control, mA control, and timer

Compton scattering—most of the scattered radiation produced during imaging

Cones and cylinders—collimation device with an opening cut out but an extended flange that attaches below the x-ray tube

Congestive heart failure (CHF)—abnormal condition that reflects impaired cardiac pumping caused by myocardial infarction, ischemic heart disease, or cardiomyopathy

Contact transmission—direct or indirect way that infection is spread

Contraindications—the presence of a disease or physical condition that makes it impossible or undesirable to treat a particular patient in the usual manner or to prescribe medicines that might otherwise be suitable

Contrast—the visible difference between any two selected areas of density levels within the radiographic image (gray scale)

Contrast enhancement—converts the digital signal to an image with either increased or decreased contrast

Contrast-to-noise ratio—overall grayscale quality of an image and how an image is perceived by the viewer

Contributory malpractice—malpractice in which the behavior of the injured party contributed to the injury

Corporate malpractice—facility is responsible as a whole

Creatine—found in the blood, urine, and muscle tissue and is tested as an indicator of kidney function

Criminal offense—crime that violates a state or federal law and is punishable by fine or imprisonment

Cultural diversity—difference in gender, race, generation, geography, or sexual preference

Cyanosis—bluish discoloration of the skin and mucous membranes caused by an excess of deoxygenated hemoglobin in the blood or a structural defect in the hemoglobin molecule

Cycle of infection—outlines the process by which microorganisms infect an individual and cause disease

Cytoplasm—major structure that contains all molecular components except DNA

Dead pixels—occurs when DR panel fails to produce a charge in an area and does not produce an image in that particular pixel

Density—degree of blackening or opacity of an area in a radiograph due to the accumulation of black metallic silver following exposure and processing of a film

Dermis—middle layer of connective tissue

Destructive pathologies—require a decrease in technique

Detector element size (DEL)—determines the size of the electronic charge detector

Deterministic—radiation responses that usually follow a high-dose exposure and result in an early response such as a radiation-induced skin burn

Developer—used during film processing and turns the silver halide crystals to black metallic silver

Diabetic hyperosmolar syndrome—when a patient's blood sugar is in excess of 600 milligrams per deciliter

Diabetic hypoglycemia—there is an excess amount of insulin and blood glucose levels are low

Diabetic ketoacidosis—when the body produces high levels of ketones when there is an insufficient amount of insulin in the body

Diaphoresis—secretion of sweat, especially the profuse secretion associated with an elevated body temperature, physical exertion, exposure to heat, and mental or emotional stress

Diastolic pressure—the blood pressure at the instant of maximum cardiac relaxation

DICOM Grayscale Standard Display Function—standard within DICOM to derive a common grayscale standard or consistency that can be used between different manufacturers when viewing images

Digital imaging receptor systems—refers to either computed radiography imaging plate and indirect or direct digital systems

Direct current (DC)—needed to generate x-rays because the anode and cathode both need corresponding positive and negative charges to operate

Direct square law—law that allows for a change in density/intensity to compensate for a change in distance

Distortion—misrepresentation of either the size or the shape of an object

Droplet transmission—when droplet nuclei that are greater than 5 μm can travel through the air for up to 3 ft

Dual-focus tube—having two filaments

Duty of care—individuals must adhere to reasonable standard of care

Dynamic range—the number of densities or shades of gray of different levels compared in an image

Dyspnea—difficult or painful breathing that may be caused by certain heart conditions, lung conditions, asthma, strenuous exercise, or anxiety

Edge enhancement—algorithm and function of postprocessing to increase spatial resolution by refining or sharpening a digital image along the edges of the pixels

Effective focal spot—the size of the focal spot area beneath the anode and is influenced by the anode target angle

Electromagnetic (EM) radiation—oscillating electric and magnetic fields that travel in a vacuum with the velocity of light. Includes x-rays, gamma rays, and some nonionizing radiation

Endoplasmic reticulum—acts as a channel or series of channels that allows for communication between the nucleus and the cytoplasm

Enzymes—molecules that allow biochemical reactions to progress within the body

Epidermis—outer layer of skin

Epilepsy—a group of neurological disorders characterized by recurrent episodes of convulsive seizures, sensory disturbances, abnormal behavior, loss of consciousness, or all of these

Excretion—how the drug exits the body once it has been metabolized

Exposure—measure of the ionization produced in air by x-rays or gamma rays. Quantity of radiation intensity expressed in roentgen (R), coulomb per kilogram (C/kg), or air kerma (Gy)

Extravasation—passage or escape from a blood or lymph vessel into the tissues, usually of blood, serum, or lymph

False imprisonment—the intentional unjustified, nonconsensual detention or confinement of a person for any length of time

Felony—crime declared by statute to be more serious than a misdemeanor and deserving a more severe punishment

Fetus exposure—exposure value delivered to the fetus

Film fog—artifact on an image from radiation, expired films, high processor temperatures, chemical contamination, or poor safelights

Film-screen speed—relative speed index

Fixer—used during film processing and dissolves and removes the unexposed silver halide crystals on the film and stops any further developing

Flaccid paralysis—occurs to the skeletal muscles—loss of sensation, respiratory distress, unstable blood pressure, bradycardia, and incontinence

Focal spot size—affects the amount of geometric unsharpness and recorded detail that exist on the image

Follicles—accessory hair structures that originate out of the dermis and are actively growing

Fomites—nonliving material such as bed linen that may transmit microorganisms

Force—that which changes the motion of an object; a push or a pull. Expressed in newton (N)

Fractionation—indicates a dose of radiation that is delivered at the same dose rate but in equal fractions of dose over a 24-hour period

Fraud—willful attempt to misrepresent information that may cause harm or loss to another person

Frequency—number of cycles or wavelengths of a simple harmonic motion per unit time. Expressed in hertz (Hz) (1 Hz = 1 cycle/s)

Fungi—type of organism that requires an external carbon source, including molds and yeasts

Genetic or germ—sexually reproducing cells

Genetically significant dose (GSD)—assesses the impact of gonadal dose and is based on the genetic influence of low doses of radiation to the entire population

Ghosting—occurs when an imaging plate is not completely erased and a faint image of the previous exam is shown along with the new image

Global learner—can look at entire picture at once to learn information

Glomerular filtration rate (GFR)—flow rate of filtered fluid through the kidney

Grayscale rendition (LUT)—records all intensity values in a radiographic image into a lookup table and are applied by an exposure algorithm of a digital system

Grid conversion factor—relates to each grid ratio and is applied to a formula to determine the mA/s needed when that grid ratio is used

Grid frequency—the number of lead lines per inch or centimeter with the usual ranges between 25 and 45 lines/cm

Grid ratio—rate between the height of the lead lines and the distance between them

Grids—device used to reduce the intensity of scatter radiation in the remnant x-ray beam

Gross malpractice—reckless disregard for a person

Halo sign—visible cerebrospinal fluid due to injury to the base of the skull

Health Insurance Portability and Accountability Act (HIPAA)—protects the release of protected health information without the patient's written consent and standardizes how electronic data is shared

Health Level Seven International (HL7) DICOM—standard universal language that is networked for the exchange and sharing of electronic health information

Hemoptysis—coughing up blood

Hertz (Hz)—the number of wavelengths that pass the point of observation per second

Histogram—determines different intensity values on an XY scale on a digital system

Hormesis—the idea that small amounts of radiation are beneficial due to their ability to stimulate hormones and immune responses to other toxic environmental agents

Hormones—molecules that provide regulatory control over body functions and are secreted by glands within the human body

Hospital information system (HIS)—a system to manage all aspects of patient care that allows access to clinical information to administration and all departments of a hospital

Hygroscopic—tending to absorb moisture

Hyperosmolar—increases in the number of particles when it dissociates

Hyperpyrexia—temperature between 105.8° and 111.2°F

Hypertensive crisis—patients with a blood pressure greater than 180 mm Hg systolic or 110 mm Hg diastolic

Hypervolemia—abnormal increase in the amount of intravascular fluid, particularly in the volume of circulating blood or its components

Hypothermia—temperature 95°F or lower

Image intensifier—electronic vacuum tube that amplifies a fluoroscopic image to reduce patient dose

Imaging equipment—refer to the components of an x-ray unit

Immobilization—used to keep patients from moving during radiographic procedures and do not require a physician order to be applied

Induction motor—made of high heat resistance material that is made up of the stator and rotor

Infection—invasion and multiplication of a microorganism that does result in cellular injury

Infiltration—the process whereby a fluid passes into the tissues, such as when a local anesthetic is administered or an intravenous infusion leaks form a vein

Informed consent—permission obtained from a patient to perform a specific test or procedure

Inherent filtration—filtration of useful x-ray beams provided by the permanently installed components of an x-ray tube housing assembly and the glass window of an x-ray tube

Interphase—first phase of the cell cycle; separated into G1, S, and G2

Inverse square law—the intensity of radiation is inversely proportional to the square of the distance from the source

Iodinated—refers to substances to which iodine has been added, especially types of contrast media prepared with iodine compounds, which absorb radiation to a greater degree than blood or soft tissues and therefore produce a more clearly visible white or light shadow on the radiographic image

Ionic—pertaining to a compound that separates into charged particles in solution

Ionization—removal of an orbital electron from an atom

Ionization chambers—instrument that detects and measures the radiation intensity in areas outside of protective barriers

Kilovoltage peak—determines the energy level of the photons in the x-ray beam

Kinesthetic learner—learns through demonstration and return demonstration

kVp—kilovolts peak-controlling factor for quality of radiation

Latent stage—response to radiation exposure that does not present symptoms in affected individuals

Law of linearity—states that doubling the mA/s doubles the amount of density of the resulting imaging, while halving the mA/s halves the density

Law of reciprocity—states that the different combination of mA and time that produce the same mA/s will produce the same density

LD$_{50/30}$—refers to the lethal dose required to kill 50% of a population in a 30-day time period and requires no medical intervention

Libel—false accusation written printed, or typewritten, or presented in a picture or a sign that is made with malicious intent to defame the reputation of a person who is living or the memory of a person who is dead, resulting in public embarrassment, contempt, ridicule, or hatred

Linear energy transfer (LET)—measure of the rate at which energy is transferred from ionizing radiation to soft tissue

Linear learner—needs to learn information in sequential steps/order

Lipids—provide structure to cell membranes, insulate the body, and provide energy to the body

Localization—precise area involved

Lysosomes—small pealike sacs that contain enzymes which help control contamination within the cell by digesting cellular fragments and itself

Macromolecules—molecule containing a large number of atoms linked together

Main-chain scission—breakage of the backbone of the long-chain macromolecule

Manifest illness stage—response to radiation exposure where there is noticeable illness in specific organ systems that are damaged

Masking—electronic collimation

Matrix—rows and columns or an array

Medical asepsis—reduces the probability of pathogens being present and able to cause infection

Medication reconciliation—comprehensive list of all medication being taken by the patient

Meiosis—cell cycle in which genetic cells reproduce

Metabolism—anabolism and catabolism; the aggregate of all chemical processes that take plan in living organisms, resulting in growth, generation of energy, elimination of waste, and other body functions as they relate to the distribution of nutrient in the blood after digestion

Metaphase—second phase of mitosis where spindle fibers attach to the centromeres of the chromosomes

Milliamperes per second—product of the electron tube current and the amount of time in seconds that the x-ray tube is activated

Misdemeanor—criminal offense that is considered less serious than a felony and carries a lesser penalty, usually a fine or imprisonment for less than a year

Mitochondria—large bean-shaped structure that digest macromolecules in order to produce energy for the cell

Mitosis—cell cycle in which somatic cells replicate

Modes of transmission—bridge in the cycle of infection connecting the reservoir and the susceptible host

Myocardial infarction (MI)—a heart attack; necrosis of heart muscle tissue caused by coronary artery thrombosis or occlusion

Negative contrast agent—appear black on x-ray images

Negligence—the commission of an act that a prudent person would not have done or the omission of a duty that a prudent person would have fulfilled, resulting in injury or harm to another person

Noise (quantum mottle)—grainy pattern on an image due to low radiation exposure

Noise suppression—low-pass filtering or smoothing that reduces image contrast and noise on a digital image

Noniodinated—contrast material that does not contain iodine

Nonionic—pertaining to compounds that do not dissociate into charged particles within a solution

Nonverbal—a way of communication with a patient that does not require spoken words (eye contact, touch, appearance, body language)

Nosocomial infections—hospital-acquired infections

Nucleolus—rounded structure attached to the nuclear membrane that contains most of the RNA

Nucleus—major structure that contains the target molecule, DNA, some RNA, protein, and water

Object-to-image distance (OID)—distance from the object being imaged to the image receptor

Occupational exposure—radiation exposure received by radiation workers

Onset—explanation by the patient of what the patient was doing when the condition began

Osmolality—the concentration of particles in a solution

Ostomies—when a portion of the intestine is removed

Oxygen enhancement ratio (OER)—ratio of radiation dose required to cause a particular biological response in cells or organisms in an environment deprived of oxygen to radiation dose required to cause the exact response in an environment with natural oxygenation

Pair production—interaction between the x-ray and the nuclear electric field that causes the x-ray to disappear and that causes two electrons—one positive and one negative—to take its place

Pathogenicity—ability of an organism to produce disease

Pathogens—any microorganism capable of producing disease

Patient's Bill of Rights—12 rights for all of patients

Periorbital ecchymoses—facial nerve injury

Pharmacokinetics—the study of how drugs enter the body, are absorbed, reach their site of action, are metabolized, and exit the body

Phlebitis—inflammation of a vein

Photodisintegration—interaction that occurs about 10 MeV in high-energy radiation therapy treatment machines

Photoelectric absorption—interaction between x-ray photons and atoms of the patient's body

Photostimulable phosphor (PSP)—component of an imaging system; phosphor crystal that will either emit light when exposed to radiation or store radiation energies

Picture Archiving and Communication System (PACS)—a system in which digital images and patient information can be stored and delivered to various sites through a digital network

Pixel size—size in microns or millimeters of the picture element found in digital systems

Point lesions—not detectable lesions that may cause small changes that will cause it to result in cell malfunction

Prehypertensive—patients with a blood pressure ranging between 120 and 139 over 80 and 89 mm Hg

Priapism—presence of a painful and persistent erection of the penis unrelated to sexual stimulation

Primary beam—radiation that passes through the tube window and interacts with the patient's body

Prions—infectious protein that causes irreversible neurologic damage

Prodromal stage—response to radiation exposure that can occur with a dose as low as 50 rad

Prophase—first phase of mitosis where chromosomes condense and spindle fibers are formed

Protozoans—single-celled microorganism of the subkingdom protozoa

Protraction—indicates a dose of radiation that is delivered continuously but at a lower dose rate

Public exposure—exposure value acceptable to the general public

Pulmonary edema—the accumulation of extravascular fluid in lung tissues and alveoli caused most commonly by congestive heart failure

Pulmonary embolism (PE)—occurs when one or more pulmonary arteries are occluded by a thrombus

Pulse—pressure wave in an artery when blood is expelled from the left ventricle

Pyrexia—abnormal elevation of body temperature above 37°C (98.6°F)

Quality—description of the character of the symptoms

Quality control (QC)—all actions necessary to control and verify the performance of equipment; part of quality assurance

Quantum mottle—Noisy or grainy appearance on an image

Radiation protection—minimizing and reducing radiation exposure

Radiology information system—system to help manage images and other information in a radiology department including patient information, reports, schedules, billing, and so forth

Recorded detail (spatial resolution)—sharpness of the structural edges that are demonstrated in the radiographic image

Rectified—to change from AC to DC

Relative biologic effectiveness (RBE)—effect of ionizing radiation influenced by the dose, dose rate and the quality of the radiation

Relative risk—predicts that the number of excess cancers will increase as the natural incidence of cancer increases within an aging population

Relative speed index (RSI)—image receptor speed

Remnant radiation—the primary beam that exits the patient and is responsible for forming the image

Res ipsa loquitur—legal doctrine applied when negligence and loss are so apparent they would be obvious to anyone. Literally, "the thing speaks for itself"

Respiration—breathing; the process of the molecular exchange of oxygen and carbon dioxide within the body's tissues from the lungs to cellular oxidation

Respiratory arrest—the cessation of breathing caused by obstruction of the airway by a foreign object or by tracheal or bronchial edema

Respondeat superior—legal doctrine that holds employers responsible for negligent acts of their employees that occurs in the course of their work. Literally, "let the master respond"

Restraints—used to prevent people from harming themselves or others and require a physician order to be applied

Ribosomes—small speck-like structures located throughout the cytoplasm or the endoplasmic reticulum and is the site where protein synthesis occurs

Roentgen Equivalent Man (rem)—dosage of radiation that will cause the same biological injury as one rad of x-rays

Rotor—rotating part of an electromagnetic induction motor that is located inside the glass envelope

Rule of personal liability—each person responsible is liable for himself or herself

Sebaceous glands—secrete oil

Seizure—hyperexcitation of neurons in the brain leading to a sudden, violent involuntary series of contractions of a group of muscles

Sensory receptors—allows for touch

Severity—intensity of the condition

Shielding accessories—lead apron, lead glove, and thyroid shield

Signal-to-noise ratio—comparing signal (resultant exposure displayed on a computer workstation) and noise (quantum mottle). The higher the ratio, the better the image

Single phase—system that uses one source of power, operates at 60 cycles per second, and consists of positive and a negative pulse

Slander—any words spoken with malice that are untrue and prejudicial to the reputation, professional practice, commercial trade, office, or business of another person

Somatic—all cells in the body that are not sexually reproducing

Source—origin of radiation

Source-to-image distance (SID)—refers to the distance from the x-ray source to the image receptor

Spatial resolution (digital systems)—amount of detail in a digital image which is measured in pixels

Sphygmomanometer—instrument of indirect measurement of blood pressure

Stage I hypertensive—patients with a blood pressure ranging between 140 and 159 over 90 and 99 mm Hg

Stage II hypertensive—patients with a blood pressure ranging between 160 and 169 over 100 and 109 mm Hg

Standard precautions—reduce the risk of transmission of infectious microorganisms and apply to all blood, body fluids, secretions, and excretions from any patient

Stator—stationary coil windings that is part of the electromagnetic induction motor located in the protective housing but outside the x-rays tube glass envelope

Step-down transformer—incoming voltage is stepped down to supply voltage to the filament of the x-ray tube

Sterile fields—specified area, such as within a tray or on a sterile towel, that is considered free of microorganisms

Stochastic—radiation responses that usually follow a low-dose exposure and result in a late radiation response such as cancer

Stoma—pore, orifice, or opening on a surface; the external opening of a colostomy or ileostomy

Subconjunctival hemorrhage—hearing loss

Subcutaneous—layer of fat and connective tissue

Suppositories—solid dosage forms generally designed for vaginal or rectal delivery

Surgical asepsis—complete destruction of pathogens and spores from equipment

Sweat glands—secrete water

Syncope—brief lapse in consciousness caused by transient cerebral hypoxia. Same as fainting

Systemic effects—involving the whole body rather than a localized area or regional part of the body

Systolic pressure—blood pressure measured at the peak of ventricular contraction

Tablets—drug dosage form consisting of an active ingredient, various fillers and disintegrators, dyes, flavoring agents, and an outside coating

Tachycardia—abnormally rapid pulse; a condition in which the heart beats at a rate greater than 100 bpm

Target—region of an x-ray tube anode that is struck by electrons emitted by the filament

Telophase—final stage of mitosis where CAN unravels to form chromatic and form new nuclear membranes

Temperature—value that indicated the body's heat loss and production within its tissues

Thermionic emission—emission of electrons from a heated surface

Three phase—generation of three simultaneous voltage waveforms out of step with one another; thus, voltage never drops to zero during exposure

Tomography—imaging modality that brings into focus only the anatomic structure lying in a plane of interest, while structures on either side of that plan are blurred

Tort—civil wrong, such as negligence, false imprisonment, assault, and battery

Troches—drugs in solid form designed to dissolve in the mouth

Type 1 diabetes—juvenile/insulin dependent—patient do not produce enough insulin in the pancreas, prohibiting cells from using glucose

Type 2 diabetes—adult onset/non–insulin dependent—patients do not produce enough insulin or their cells do not use the insulin produced

Vector—an animal in whose body a pathogen multiplies or develops before becoming infective to a new host

Vehicles—any substance, such as food or water, that can serve as a mode of transmission for infectious agents

Velocity—rate of change of an object's position over time; speed

Verbal—how a radiographer speaks to the patient prior to, during, and after an examination

Vicarious liability—responsibility of a superior for the acts of his or her subordinate

Virulence—degree of pathogenicity

Virus—minute parasitic microorganism much smaller than a bacterium that, having no independent metabolic activity, may replicate only within a cell of a living plant or animal host

Viscosity—the ability or inability of a fluid solution to flow easily

Visual learner—material is best presented in picture or graphic format

Wavelength—the distance from one crest or point on a sine wave to another or the next

Width function—allows the operator to change contrast levels to conform to his or her visual perception

Window level—allows the operator to lighten or darken an image to conform to his or her visual perception

Written—form of communication with patients in which words are made visible for the patient to read

INDEX

Page numbers followed by *f* indicate figures and those followed by *t* indicate tables.